The
Breastfeeding
Bible

DR. PENNY STANWAY

AUTHOR OF *THE NATURAL GUIDE TO WOMEN'S HEALTH*
PROFESSIONAL ADVISER TO LA LECHE LEAGUE INTERNATIONAL

The
Breastfeeding
Bible

EVERYTHING YOU NEED TO KNOW
FROM FIRST LATCH TO FINAL FEEDING

PLAIN SIGHT PUBLISHING
AN IMPRINT OF CEDAR FORT, INC.
SPRINGVILLE, UTAH

ISBN 13: 978-1-4621-1283-8

Published in the USA by Plain Sight Publishing, an Imprint of Cedar Fort, Inc.
2373 W. 700 S., Springville, UT 84663
Distributed by Cedar Fort, Inc., www.cedarfort.com

Cover design by Angela D. Olsen
Cover design © 2013 by Lyle Mortimer
Edited and typeset by Whitney Lindsley and Eileen Leavitt

Printed in the United States of America

10 9 8 7 6 5 4 3 2 1

To Susannah, Amy, and Ben

By the same author

Contents

one

two

three

four

five

six

Contents

Chapter Contents

three

eight

nine

ten

thirteen

fourteen

fifteen

sixteen

seventeen

Acknowledgments

I would like to thank all the mothers who, over many decades, have helped me to so many insights. Thanks also to my husband, Andrew Stanway, who has contributed so much to this sixth edition.

Notes

If you would like to know more about any study mentioned in the text, enter a few keywords into an Internet search engine, plus the journal's name and year.

Advice on medical matters given in the book should not take the place of professional help. If you feel you need to, consult your doctor, midwife, or health visitor. For additional information or advice on more practical matters, talk with a certified lactation consultant, National Childbirth Trust breastfeeding counselor, or La Leche League leader.

Throughout the text, and after some soul searching, I have used "he" to refer to a baby, since saying "he or she" each time seemed so cumbersome. The alternative was to use "he" and "she" in alternate chapters, but "she" referring to the baby could sometimes be confused with "she" referring to the mother.

Introduction

Does it really matter in the twenty-first century whether babies are breast-fed? After all, millions of women feed their children cows'-milk formula and they seem to do perfectly well.

The answer is that although babies can be adequately fed with the milk of another animal, breastfeeding is, provably, the best and safest way of nourishing your baby, wherever in the world you live. Experts agree that breastfeeding confers unique benefits on both mother and baby. Where things have become muddled is that first-world peoples have confused feeding a baby with nutrients, with giving the "nourishment" that arises from the special mother-baby relationship that's an integral part of breastfeeding. When you choose to breastfeed, you're signing up for far more than just giving milk.

The Breastfeeding Bible was written 35 years ago and has been updated many times since. It is based on the collective wisdom of countless women's feedback; on my personal experience as a mother with many years of breastfeeding behind me; on the input I've had over decades from those I've helped, worked with, and taught; and on research reported in peer-reviewed medical journals.

But why, as breastfeeding is the natural way of feeding a baby, might a woman need a book to help her do it successfully? The truth is that although breastfeeding is what Nature intended, the "art" of doing it is unfamiliar to many women, and to many midwives, nurses, and doctors. And it is indeed an art. While techniques can be learned—and this book is full of them—the magic, delight, creativity, and sense of connection that many breastfeeding women experience are part of the intuitive art of mothering a baby. This art, like any other, can be learned, perfected, and honed.

I hope *The Breastfeeding Bible* will help new generations of mothers to breastfeed successfully for as long as they want, because the pleasures and advantages of feeding a baby naturally are as worthwhile and rewarding today as they ever were.

Penny Stanway
London, 2012

one

Breastfeeding Today

Breastfeeding isn't just a way of *feeding* a baby; it's a unique way of *mothering* him too.

Breastfeeding is endorsed by many official bodies, including the World Health Organization (WHO), the American Academy of Pediatrics, and the UK Department of Health. Indeed, in 2001, WHO recommended exclusive breastfeeding (giving no other milk, food, or drink) for six months, then continued breastfeeding along with other food and drink for up to two years or beyond.

Once, there was no choice. A woman either breastfed, or her baby died unless someone else—paid or unpaid—breastfed for her. The advent of cows'-milk formula feeds in the first half of the twentieth century offered an alternative that was easier and cheaper than hiring a wet nurse. But this apparent advance has had two worrying results. One is that formula-fed babies today have a higher risk of immediate, short-term, and long-term health problems. The other is that fewer people are now familiar with the womanly art of breastfeeding, so women often don't breastfeed for as long as they want to.

Several major changes in lifestyle over the last few decades have had an important influence on breastfeeding. In developed countries, for example, the number of babies born each year has been shrinking, the number born to women over age 30 has been growing, more babies are being born to single mothers, and more mothers are working. Choosing how to feed her baby can have particular implications for an older woman, for one who will probably have only one or two babies, and for one who is unpartnered or returns to work when her baby is very young.

When choosing how to feed your baby, you'll probably consider the benefits of breastfeeding to his health, development, and contentment, and to your health, well-being, convenience, and relationship with him. You may start to think how your choice will impact on your partner and other children. You'll also factor in any previous experiences of feeding, your observations of how other women feed, and your perception of other people's attitudes to breastfeeding. Finally, you'll have your own ideas, preconceptions, and prejudices about how breastfeeding could affect your love life, weight, figure, sleep, self-confidence, and freedom, and what it will mean at a deeper level in terms of loving, giving, and receiving.

With good information and support, nearly every woman can breast-feed successfully for as long as she or her baby wants.

How popular is breastfeeding?

The breastfeeding rates in these developed countries are

	% Breastfed when newborn	% Breastfed at six months
Norway	99	56
Australia	92	48
Portugal	92	No Data
Canada	90	54
Italy	85	19
UK	81	29
Spain	80	24
Netherlands	78	37
US	74	43
Brazil	93	29
France	63	No Data
Ireland	56	11

Breastfeeding rates have improved in many developed countries over the past 30 years or so.

Large surveys commissioned by the UK Department of Health give an interesting comparison of the numbers of women in England and Wales breastfeeding (at all, not just exclusively) at different stages from 1975 to 2005 (at the time of writing, there's only one preliminary figure for 2010).

	1975	1980	1985	1990	1995	2000	2005	2010
Birth	51	67	65	62	66	69	76	81

1 week	42	58	56	54	58	57	63	-
2 weeks	35	54	53	51	54	54	60	-
6 weeks	24	42	40	39	44	43	48	-
4 months	13	27	26	25	28	29	34	-
6 months	9	23	21	21	22	22	25	-
9 months	0	12	11	12	14	14	18	-

In developing countries the rates are by and large high. In Ghana, for example, 97 percent of mothers start off breastfeeding. The worry is that the potential for financial gain for formula companies is much greater in these countries, thus encouraging them to put pressure on mothers to discontinue breastfeeding and start using their products.

Exclusive breastfeeding

Globally, less than 40 percent of babies are exclusively breastfed for the World Health Organization's goal of six months, according to UNICEF.

And the UK is nowhere near achieving this goal. In 2005, the figure was astonishingly low, at only 1 percent, mostly because of the introduction of formula.

Australia comes a little closer to the goal, with 15 percent of babies exclusively breastfed at six months (2011). And so does the US, with 14 percent of babies exclusively breastfed until 6 months (2008).

But in many developing countries the rates are much higher. For example, in Rwanda in central Africa, 94 percent of babies are still being exclusively breastfed at four months.

Why not bottle-feed?

Humans have reared milk-producing animals for the last ten thousand years or so. During the early nineteenth-century, feeding babies a formula based on cows' or other animals' milk became more popular in westernized countries. But only in the last 80 years has the use of cows'-milk formula become widespread as an infant food. Giving babies formula deprives them of the unique milk nature intended. And giving cows' milk formula to babies at so crucial a time in their life is an intervention without parallel in history. It's a massive change that's been called the "greatest uncontrolled trial ever done on humans." But the stark fact is that huge numbers of studies suggest it can be hazardous to both short- and long-term health.

The first doubts arose when scientists pointed out that compared with breast milk, cows' milk lacked vitamins B6 and E and linoleic acid (a fatty acid), and had too much protein, phosphorus, and sodium. As the years passed, they found that breast milk contained high levels of antibodies against disease. They then discovered that formula doesn't contain the live cells, enzymes, and hormones found in breast milk. They also found that the protein in formula could encourage allergy by leaking from a baby's gut into his blood. Last, it became clear that each mother's milk is designed to meet her own baby's needs at each developmental stage.

Formula manufacturers have repeatedly changed their products to try to keep pace with these ongoing discoveries. There's even been talk of vaccinating cows to give them immunity against human diseases, so formula could protect human babies. But the facts are that breast milk is impossible to replicate.

Given the provable benefits of breastfeeding but the comparatively low rates of doing it, what can be done to help?

School education

Nowadays, most modern westernized families are small. So a girl can reach motherhood without ever seeing a baby at the breast. Yet studies show that a girl who sees a baby being breastfed is much more likely to become a breastfeeder later.

So teachers are doing something very valuable if they ask a woman to talk to a biology or parenting class about breastfeeding, and, baby permitting, breastfeed in front of them. It's even better if the father can come too. The children also benefit from the opportunity to discuss breastfeeding. The subject can be introduced at any age, and teachers can be creative in the way their class learns. If it's left until the teen years, many girls and boys in mixed classes are too embarrassed to learn anything much.

As for education in general, it is well recognized that the higher a woman's level of education, the more likely she is to breastfeed.

Mother's age

In the UK, the older the mother, the more likely she is to breastfeed. In 2010, 58 percent of women under age 20 breastfed, 67 percent of 20- to 24-year-olds, 76 percent of 25- to 29-year-olds, and 87 percent of those aged 30 and older.

Friends, relatives, and neighbors

Women have helped each other with feeding in all cultures throughout history.

However, some people are more familiar with bottle-feeding than breastfeeding and may try to persuade a pregnant or newly delivered woman that bottle-fed babies are as contented and healthy as breastfed. If you've decided to breastfeed, it might help to arm yourself and, ideally, your partner, with information and a positive attitude in case you come into contact with anyone unsupportive of your decision. I look at this more on page 195.

Any country that wants to improve its breastfeeding rates must remember to educate everyone about breastfeeding, not just mothers-to-be and their professional helpers.

Professional backup

Professional helpers can have an enormously influential role. For example, studies show that a pediatrician who is enthusiastic about breastfeeding can make all the difference to the numbers of women who breastfeed their newborn babies. He or she can also encourage other health professionals (and perhaps also the cleaners, store clerks, and others who come into contact with mothers) to work together to make sure their hospital is "baby friendly" (page 90). Health professionals can also encourage breastfeeding by ensuring that women have good prenatal education, continuous care during childbirth, and early close contact with their newborns. They can also make sure that mothers in the hospital are allowed to have their baby by them all the time (known as "rooming in") and are offered expert help in positioning him at the breast and helping him latch on (take the nipple and areola into his mouth). They can encourage unrestricted feeding. And they can promote women's confidence in themselves as breastfeeders and help them overcome any problems.

Thankfully, breastfeeding education for doctors, midwives, and other professional helpers has improved, but it's vital for all helpers to maintain their standards and enthusiasm through ongoing in-service training.

Work

Today's young woman is brought up to think of herself as a wage-earner and a career woman. When she leaves her parents' home, she'll

7

almost certainly need an income to buy or rent a place of her own, and it may be difficult for her and her partner to surrender this income when they have a baby.

Pregnant women tend to think of themselves more in relation to their career and partner than to their unborn baby—the birth is often as far ahead as they see. Few give much thought to breastfeeding.

But when her baby arrives, a woman comes face-to-face with the reality of the choice between caring for him full-time or working. And if she decides to work, should she do so full or part time, and away from home or at home?

It is often claimed that many mothers don't breastfeed because they return to work so soon. But in developed countries only a small percentage of women return to work while their children are very young.

It would be good to have a more realistic and informed debate about the lifestyle choices women face once they have a baby. This is probably best done before pregnancy.

Governments and nongovernmental organizations

Companies selling infant formula and other drinks and foods for babies have a lot to gain by promoting their products. It's a highly lucrative industry. And it's growing. In 2005, worldwide sales of infant formula market reached $7.9 billion a year. But in 2010, the figure was $20.2 billion.

The International Code of Marketing of Breast Milk Substitutes, adopted by the World Health Assembly in 1981, aims to protect breastfeeding by controlling how companies market their products. It says they should not promote formula. Nor should they promote feeding bottles and teats; bottled water, juice, tea, glucose solution, or cereal for babies under six months; or, for babies over six months, promote these products or follow-on milks as a replacement for that part of the diet best met by breast milk. They should also not market any infant food in a way that undermines breastfeeding.

In practice, this means they shouldn't advertise to mothers or health workers, imply their products are equal to breast milk, claim health benefits for formula, or provide free samples or supplies to hospitals or to mothers at any time. Company representatives should make no contact with pregnant women or mothers of young children. There should be no promotion of products through health care facilities—no posters, leaflets, videos, lectures, or sponsorship of events, for example. There should be no advertising in stores and no discount coupons, premiums, special sales, loss leaders, and tie-in sales. And companies shouldn't give gifts to mothers or health workers. The reason is that all these can provably undermine a mother's knowledge about and confidence in breastfeeding.

The Code has been very helpful in certain countries. In Brazil, for example, it has been associated with a change from breastfeeding lasting for less than three months in the 1970s, to it lasting for ten months in 2008.

By 2012, as many as 84 countries had put in place legislation implementing all or many of the provisions of the Code. But even in certain countries with the Code fully in place, some formula companies blatantly violate its guidelines, to the detriment of women who want to breastfeed.

The US government, following strong lobbying by the formula industry, has not adopted the Code. Not only is formula heavily marketed in the US, but it is also subsidized by the state. In 2004, more than half the formula sold went via the Special Supplemental Nutrition Program for Women, Infants, and Children (WIC) to women of low socioeconomic status. Although this at first sounds noble, the pity is that free formula discourages breastfeeding. Yet breastfeeding is particularly valuable because babies born into relative poverty are at greater risk of ill health. The stark fact is that writing a check for formula is cheap and easy for the state. But it would be better to give mothers sound information about the benefits of breastfeeding, and then provide good support from nurses trained in lactation assistance, or from trained lactation consultants.

The money spent on marketing formula is colossal. In the UK, for example, in 2001, the government spent £1.60 (approx. $2.30) per baby on promoting breastfeeding, while formula companies spent £18 (approx. $26) per baby on promoting formula.

What we need is for all governments to protect, promote, and support breastfeeding meaningfully and wholeheartedly.

We should also applaud nongovernmental organizations such as the International Baby Food Action Network for their vitally important work of helping to monitor companies' promotional tactics and holding them to account.

The status of mothers

Fewer babies are being born in developed countries nowadays, and our society doesn't seem to value mothers as it once did, so mothering is less often seen as a rewarding career in itself. Also, it is widely accepted that grandmothers, child care providers, nursery nurses, au pairs, mother's helpers, and nannies are interchangeable with mothers. Not only do many millions of people now believe that breast milk isn't essential, but large numbers also seem to think mothers aren't all that important either.

What we need is encouragement for women to think well of themselves not only for for breastfeeding but also for mothering in general. They are doing a unique job that is an invaluable contribution to society.

The media

Newspapers, magazines, TV, radio, and the Internet have an important role to play in the promotion of breastfeeding.

They can do this by featuring the stories and views of breastfeeding women, and by giving space to groups campaigning for the public acceptance of breastfeeding, and facilities to make it easier.

However, some people who work in the media—just like some who don't—are not "breastfeeding-friendly." If they broadcast their opinions about baby feeding in print, online, on social networks, or on TV or radio, they may influence large numbers of women. Often this is not for the better. There's no answer to this other than to remember that they're expressing only their personal, often uninformed, views.

Peer support

Breastfeeding counselors or leaders in organizations such as La Leche League, the Australian Breastfeeding Association and, in the UK, the National Childbirth Trust, have breastfed for long periods themselves. They have also learned from their experience with many women, as well as from books and courses. They are committed to positive attitudes and practices in a way health professionals find hard to equal. They have time to focus on breastfeeding. And they can offer a degree of one-to-one support that few professionals—because of other commitments and a lack of experience—can match.

two

Best for Baby

Breast milk has the perfect composition for a baby's development and well-being. And both breast milk and breastfeeding have many advantages to his health.

Less illness

Breastfed babies—especially those exclusively breastfed—are less likely to be ill in their first year and less likely to be hospitalized. This is because breast milk has considerable anti-infective power, whereas formula has little or none. Most important, breastfeeding saves lives:

- The World Health Organization estimates that breastfeeding could save the lives of 1.5 million children under age five a year worldwide. The main reason formula-feeding can be life-threatening in developing countries is because it encourages pneumonia and diarrhea

- Researchers at Harvard Medical School, Massachusetts, say that if 9 in 10 US mothers breastfed exclusively for 6 months, 911 lives would be saved each year, and there would be $13 billion savings in healthcare (*Pediatrics*, 2010).

Fewer infections

Breast milk helps protect against infections with bacteria, viruses, yeasts, and protozoa such as giardia and cryptosporidium. In particular, breastfeeding helps protect against diarrhea caused by infective gastroenteritis, pneumonia, and bronchiolitis; ear, urine, and eye infections; meningitis; and septicemia ("blood poisoning").

Many of the anti-infective factors in cows' milk are destroyed when it's processed to produce formula, or aren't appropriate for human babies anyway.

You might think formula is sterile. But it isn't:

- Of 82 samples of powdered formula in one UK study, 8 contained gastrointestinal bacteria (*Food Microbiology*, 2004).

The bacteria count of prepared formula doubles every half-hour at room temperature. Even in the refrigerator, the count doubles every 10 hours. However, these bacteria almost never cause infection in full-term babies (those born from 37 to 42 weeks) provided that adequate hygiene precautions are taken when making up powdered formula, and safe storage is observed if made-up formula is stored for any amount of time.

Diarrhea

A newborn's gut is bacteria-free, and the very first feed initiates its colonization by billions of bacteria and other microorganisms. The balance of types varies according to the individual baby, the length of pregnancy, the type of delivery, whether he has had antibiotics, and, most important, his feeding. Breast milk encourages a more beneficial proportion of "good" (protective or "probiotic") and "bad" (potentially harmful) bacteria than does formula.

The proportions of bacteria help account for the the sweetish smell of a breastfed baby's motions. In contrast, those of a formula-fed baby smell relatively unpleasant.

Lactobacilli are the predominant probiotics in a breastfed baby's bowel. They aid digestion and produce acetic and lactic acids which discourage the growth of certain disease-producing organisms, including *Escherichia coli*, dysentery bacilli, and candida.

Although dairy products containing probiotic bacteria are widely available to consumers, manufacturers haven't yet added them to infant formula.

Among their many benefits, the high proportion of probiotic bacteria in a breastfed baby's bowel helps prevent diarrhea caused by infective gastroenteritis.

In developed countries—

- Of 15,890 UK babies, those exclusively breastfed were less likely to be hospitalized for diarrhea The researchers think exclusive breastfeeding could have prevented 53 percent of the hospitalizations, and partial breastfeeding 31 percent. The protection wore off when breastfeeding stopped (*Pediatrics*, 2007).

- Formula-fed babies had nearly four times as much diarrhea as exclusively breastfed ones in this study in England (*Archives of Disease in Childhood*, 2006).

- Babies born in the US to relatively affluent families and breast-fed for the first year had only half the diarrhea of formula-feds (*Journal of Pediatrics*, 1995). This is an important study as many people wrongly believe that breastfeeding is advantageous only to babies born into poverty in developing countries.

In developing countries—The risk of diarrhea from infective gastro-enteritis in formula-fed babies is very high if there's

- Dirty water, as this makes a baby up to 25 times more likely to die from diarrhea.

- Insufficient fuel, as this is needed to boil water to add to dried formula, and to sterilize bottle-feeding equipment.

- Poor sanitation, as this encourages the spread of diarrhea germs.

- Poverty, as this often means a mother can't afford as much for-mula as her baby needs. She's then likely to give over-dilute for-mula, which encourages malnutrition.

The combination of diarrhea, dehydration, and malnutrition is called "bottle-baby disease" and is a frequent killer in developing countries.

Respiratory infection

In developing countries breastfeeding helps protect babies from bron-chiolitis (infection in the lungs' small airways) and pneumonia. The evi-dence from developed countries is mixed.

- Of 4, 164 babies in the Netherlands, those exclusively breastfed for 4 months, then partially breastfed for longer, had less upper and lower respiratory infection (and gastrointestinal infection) in the first 6 months, compared with those who were formula-fed or only partially breastfed. They also had less lower respiratory infection in the second 6 months (*Pediatrics*, 2010).

- Babies in the US exclusively breastfed for 6 months or more had a lower risk of pneumonia than those exclusively breastfed for 4–6 months (*Pediatrics*, 2006).

- Analysis of 33 studies found that formula-fed babies had more than 3 times the risk of needing hospital treatment for respiratory infections (and asthma) compared with breastfeds (*Archives of Pediatric and Adolescent Medicine*, 2003).

Middle-ear infection

There's good evidence that breastfed babies are less prone to middle-ear infection (*otitis media*). This is important because this condition is painful and, without proper treatment, can lead to deafness. Also, bacteria readily travel from the middle ear along the Eustachian tube to the throat, then to the stomach and gut, where they can cause diarrhea.

Breastfed babies have a lower risk because a breastfeeding mother tends to hold her baby more upright, so milk is less likely to go from the throat along the Eustachian tube to the middle ear. Also, breast milk's anti-infective and anti-inflammatory factors discourage infection in any milk that does enter the middle ear. And the way a breastfed baby sucks and milks the breast tends to widen the Eustachian tubes. This encourages any fluid to drain from the middle ears, making infection less likely.

- Babies exclusively breastfed for six months or more had a lower risk of recurrent midde-ear infection than those exclusively breastfed for four to six months, according to a study in the US (*Pediatrics*, 2006).

- Among babies in the US born to relatively affluent families and breastfed for the first year, middle-ear infections lasting more than 10 days were 80 percent less likely (*Journal of Pediatrics*, 1995). This study clearly shows that breastfeeding is advantageous to all babies, not only to those born into poverty in developing countries.

Urine infection

This is less likely in breastfed babies. One reason is that breast-milk sugars called oligosaccharides make *Escherichia coli* bacteria less able to stick to the urinary-tract lining. Another is that a breastfed baby's urine contains more IgA, lactoferrin, and lysozme than that of a formula-fed baby. These can't have come from breast milk as they aren't absorbed by his gut, so must have been made in the baby's urinary system. This means breastfeeding must encourage a better immune response in the urinary system.

- A Swedish study compared 200 children up to six years old who had a first-time urine infection, with 336 controls. Exclusive breastfeeding was associated with a lower risk, particularly soon after birth. Longer breastfeeding was associated with a lower risk after weaning, indicating a long-term mechanism (*Acta Paediatrica*, 2007).

Sticky eye

Bacterial infection of the surface of the eye (conjunctivitis) is common in newborns. Women in India, Jamaica, Brazil, the Middle East, and North Africa often help prevent it by putting a few drops of colostrum (the earliest breast milk) into their baby's eyes. And an eighteenth-century London Pharmacopoeia says, "Breast milk . . . cureth Red Eye immediately."

- Researchers in New Delhi reported that only 6 percent of babies who had colostrum put into their eyes developed an eye infection, compared with 35 percent of those who didn't (*Journal of Tropical Pediatrics*, 1982).

Meningitis

Limited evidence suggests this is less common in breastfed babies.

- Researchers investigating a 2.5-fold increase in the incidence of *Haemophilus influenzae* meningitis in Orebro County, Sweden, noted that breastfeeding was a strong protective factor (*International Journal of Epidemiology*, 1999).

Septicemia

Breastfed babies might be less likely to get septicemia (blood poisoning):

- Even partial breastfeeding was a great help in protecting against septicemia, according to a study in Pakistan (*Archives of Disease in Childhood*, 1991).

Better response to immunization

Breastfed babies make more antibodies when immunized, possibly because breastfeeding helps to mature their immune system.

- When given *Haemophilus influenzae* type b (Hib) vaccine at two, four, and six months, breastfed babies had significantly higher levels of Hib antibodies at seven, and twelve months than formula-feds (*Lancet*, 1990).

Protection from infections or immunizations a mother has had?

Many mothers wonder if antibodies in their milk resulting from their own immunity to illnesses they've had or have been immunized against will protect their baby. The answer is that they might, but only a little. This is because the antibodies that give long-term resistance to infections we've encountered are the immunoglobulin G (IgG) type, but breast milk's main antibodies are largely immunoglobulin A. The small amounts of IgG in breast milk may offer a little protection, but not enough to "immunize" a baby. Most of any protection from the mother's IgG comes via her placenta before birth and is lost by six to eight months after.

Less obesity

Formula-fed babies drink more milk and gain weight more rapidly than do breastfeds. Their increased weight gain is predominantly from increased fat stores. In contrast, breastfed babies gain proportionately more lean body mass. Research shows that rapid weight gain in babyhood is associated with a greater likelihood of childhood obesity. The concern is that formula feeding and nonexclusive breastfeeding may be contributing to the obesity epidemic among children in the US and the UK, for example. Astonishingly, researchers estimate that 15–20 percent of obese children in the US are obese because they were formula-fed!

- Formula-fed babies are 11–28 percent more likely to be overweight or obese in later life, according to an overview of five research reviews by Australian researchers (*Public Health Nutrition*, 2010).

The US Breastfeeding Committee recommends breastfeeding as as a way of discouraging overweight and obesity and promoting a healthy weight throughout life. It's also one of the most cost-effective strategies available. Research suggests that exclusive breastfeeding is more effective than nonexclusive breastfeeding, or formula-feeding. One possible reason is that it programs a baby's metabolism in a different way. Another is that breastfed babies may grow up in families in which they learn to make healthier food choices.

- A study of 14,297 children aged 9–14 in the US found that overweight and obesity was 10 percent less likely if they'd been only or mostly breastfed for at least seven months. The researchers ruled out the effects of other factors associated with weight gain, including sexual maturity, calorie intake, time spent watching television, physical activity, mother's body mass index, and other variables reflecting social, economic and lifestyle factors (*JAMA*, 2001).

A formula-fed baby also has more chance of being overweight or obese 20–30 years later. In the US, for example, one in three adults is now obese. The concern is that obese adults are more prone to high blood pressure, diabetes (page 31), heart disease, varicose veins, and gallstones.

Lower blood pressure

A breastfed baby can expect lower blood pressure as an adult:

- Adults who'd been breastfed had lower blood pressure than those who were formula-fed, according to 30 studies reviewed by experts at the World Health Organization (WHO) and researchers at the University of Pelotas, Brazil. This held even in large studies and after accounting for socioeconomic and demographic variables (WHO, 2007).

Less allergy and food sensitivity

Many studies suggest that breastfeeding for at least four to six months discourages allergic disease, particularly atopic eczema and wheezing, in the early years. But any effect is small. And we don't yet know if exclusive breastfeeding helps prevent allergy in later life, particularly in babies with an "atopic" family history (having eczema, asthma or hay fever in the family). This is partly because we lack large, well conducted studies that account for other risk factors, distinguish between partial and exclusive breastfeeding, and note the duration of breastfeeding.

However, experts agree that as far as we currently know, it's particularly wise to breastfeed for at least four to six months if there's allergy in a baby's family.

Breastfeeding may also help prevent the sort of food sensitivity that results from a nonallergic slow-onset immune response. This is more common than food allergy.

Food allergy and nonallergic food sensitivity

In a susceptible baby, a food allergen can inflame the gut lining, stimulating an abnormal immune response with the production of IgE antibodies that trigger symptoms such as diarrhea within hours. In contrast, a nonallergic immune reaction involves the production of IgG antibodies that trigger symptoms two or three days and sometimes a week or more later.

Three factors encourage food allergy. First is an inherited risk. A baby has a higher risk of eczema, asthma, hay fever, and food allergy if there's allergy in the family—especially on both sides.

Second is diarrhea. Babies with a food allergy have often had many more attacks of diarrhea than other babies. Whether diarrhea encourages food allergy (by inflaming the gut, which makes it easier for food allergens to pass through its lining into the bloodstream), or whether it's just an early sign of food allergy is unclear. But we know that breastfeeding discourages diarrhea.

Third is exposure to a potential allergy trigger. A young baby's immune system is immature. Exposure to a potential trigger readily sensitizes a susceptible baby, making him prone to food allergy and other allergies. Besides certain food proteins, possible triggers include house-dust-mite droppings, viral infections, smoky or otherwise polluted air, and certain pollens and molds.

The trigger that first sensitizes a baby is called the primary allergy trigger. Allergists believe that once a baby is sensitized, he subsequently reacts more readily to other allergy triggers.

Cows' milk—the most common primary allergy trigger

This isn't surprising, as it contains the first foreign food protein many babies encounter. And formula-fed babies get it in extraordinarily large amounts.

- Allergy to cows' milk affects 2–3 percent of babies in developed countries and is the most common food allergy in early childhood, according to researchers in Denmark (*Annals of Allergy, Asthma and Immunology*, 2002).

This said, it can be difficult to know whether cows'-milk formula is the primary allergy trigger, since it occasionally sensitizes a baby without immediately provoking allergic symptoms. Also, cows'-milk-antibody levels fall after the initial sensitization, so aren't a reliable gauge of cows'-milk allergy unless measured before and immediately after the first formula feed. What's more, breastfeeding women who drink a lot of cows' milk may have traces of its proteins in their breast milk, so cows' milk could be the primary allergy trigger even in an exclusively breastfed baby, though this is extremely unlikely.

How is breast milk protective?

Breast milk might help protect against allergy in three ways:

By preventing a "leaky gut"—The leaky-gut hypothesis suggests that in a susceptible baby, foreign proteins can leak from his gut into his blood, travel elsewhere in his body, then either trigger an immediate food-allergic response, or sensitize him so he reacts to allergy triggers in future, or trigger a nonallergic sensitivity from a slow-onset immune reaction.

Breast milk may help prevent all this. For a start, the most common potential sensitizer in cows'-milk formula, beta-lactoglobulin, isn't present in breast milk.

What's more, several breast-milk constituents (including cortisone, an epidermal growth factor) encourage a baby's gut lining to mature and become impervious to foreign proteins. They also encourage his immune system to mature. And breast milk's immunoglobulin A (IgA) antibodies coat the gut lining, which is thought to help prevent foreign food proteins leaking into the blood. It takes several months for a baby to make useful amounts of IgA himself. The IgA coating is thought to disappear fairly rapidly after a breastfeed, as the turnover of gut-lining cells is so rapid. So if breastfeeds are widely spaced, and interspersed with feeds of formula or solids, traces of cows' milk protein or other foreign food protein could enter the blood.

Formula-fed babies lack IgA, because even if formula's IgA were useful to them, it's spoiled by heat treatment during formula manufacture.

So the leaky-gut hypothesis favors exclusive breastfeeding with frequent feeds for the first few months, especially if a baby has a family history of allergy.

By protecting against diarrhea—as it influences the population of microorganisms in a baby's gut. Repeated diarrhea can be associated with damage to the gut lining, which encourages foreign food proteins to leak into the blood. So breast milk may help protect against both allergic reactions, and nonallergic slow-onset immune reactions.

By protecting against respiratory infections—this is important because such infections encourage respiratory allergy.

Eczema

Most but not all studies suggest breastfeeding can help prevent eczema, particularly the atopic sort, which runs in families.

Asthma and wheezing

Most but not all studies suggest breastfeeding discourages asthma and wheezing. The lack of agreement may be because many researchers call all wheezing "asthma," rather than distinguish between allergic asthma, wheezing associated with viral infection, and "transient infantile wheezing." It's possible that breastfeeding helps protect against the wheezing associated with viral infections, but not against allergic asthma.

- Among 3,963 children, those who'd been breastfed for more than 16 weeks had a reduced risk of asthma at 3–8 years old, regardless of any family history of allergy, according to a study in the Netherlands (*Thorax*, 2009).

- A research review concluded that breastfeeding for 4 months discouraged asthma (*Allergy*, 2003).

- Analysis of 12 studies involving 8, 183 babies found that in those exclusively breastfed for at least 3 months, the risk of asthma in childhood was reduced by a quarter in all children, and halved if there was asthma, eczema, or hay fever in the family (*Journal of Pediatrics*, 2001).

Hay fever (allergic rhinitis)

Breastfeeding might help prevent hay fever:

- Exclusive breastfeeding for at least three months gave substantial protection against hay fever in children with or without an allergic family history, according to a review of six studies (*Acta Paediatrica*, 2002).

Breastfeeding and solids

Some experts suggest that if a breastfeeding mother introduces "solids" to her baby, her breast milk helps protect against them triggering allergy.

And some experts believe that introducing solids sooner rather than later might help protect against allergy if a mother is still breastfeeding. Indeed, researchers are currently investigating whether the risk of allergy might be reduced if very small amounts of potential triggers were introduced when a breastfed baby is three months old. A study in London is comparing breastfed babies given solids including peanuts and eggs from three months, with babies exclusively breastfed for six months.

Food exclusion and challenge for a baby

The best way to discover whether a baby's allergic symptoms are being caused by cows'-milk formula is to give only breast milk for three weeks. Then, if the symptoms disappear, to reintroduce a small amount of formula to see if they recur. Repeat this "challenge" twice.

If you want to do this, discuss it with your doctor first and increase your milk supply if necessary. *Expert supervision by a doctor or state-registered dietitian will ensure your baby has adequate nourishment.*

Note that between one-in-five and one-in-two cows'-milk-allergic babies can't tolerate hydrolyzed-soy formula either. As for goats' milk, this doesn't contain the right proportions of nutrients for babies even when diluted. It is deficient in folate. Most isn't pasteurized. And up to 60 percent of cows'-milk-allergic babies are also sensitive to goats' milk.

Breast milk is best for a cows'-milk-allergic baby. With time and patience, even if you've never breastfed, you can build up your milk supply to provide some or all of your baby's needs.

Should a breastfeeding mother avoid potential food-allergens?

Several good studies suggest that doing this reduces a baby's risk of allergy. But several others don't. They're difficult to compare because of variations in size and in how they were done.

- The Australasian Society of Clinical Immunology and Asthma summarized the evidence by saying that dietary restrictions by a breastfeeding mother couldn't be recommended for preventing allergy in her baby. This is because there was no convincing evidence that they had a protective effect (*Medical Journal of Australia*, 2005).

• A research review concluded that avoidance of potential food allergens by a breastfeeding mother might discourage eczema in a baby with a family history of allergy. And for babies who already had atopic eczema (the sort that runs in families) it might reduce its severity. But larger trials were needed to be sure (*Cochrane Database*, 2003).

But what about "Nature's immunization"?—Some immunologists claim that traces of undigested food proteins in breast milk prepare a baby's digestive and immune systems for contact with these foods later, thereby reducing the risk of allergy.

Until we know whether this is correct, breastfeeding women may want to avoid consuming large amounts of cows' milk, egg, nuts, fish, citrus fruits, and wheat, as there's an unproven risk that traces of these in breast milk might trigger allergy in susceptible babies. And breastfeeding mothers of a baby with allergy in his family might think it wise to avoid cows' milk, eggs, nuts, and fish completely.

Food exclusion and challenge for a breastfeeding mother

If you want to know whether your baby's symptoms could result from something you've eaten, you could do a food-exclusion trial followed by a challenge in which you take the food again. But do this under the guidance of a doctor or registered dietitian to ensure your diet remains sound and neither your baby's health nor yours is put at risk.

When choosing what to avoid first, record in your diary whether the baby's symptoms relate to what you eat. Cows' milk is often high on the list because many women drink it so frequently and in such large amounts. The fact is there's no need to drink any cows' milk at all when you are breastfeeding.

Avoid one food at a time, or you'll be none the wiser, and avoid it for about a week. If your baby's symptoms improve, try adding the food back into your diet to see if his symptoms return. If so, repeat this "challenge" twice to be sure.

Less dental decay

Most studies agree that children who were breastfed have less dental decay. Any decay that does occur also tends to be less severe. It has been suggested that this is because breastfeeding is more popular with women from higher socioeconomic groups, as they are less likely to give their babies sugary snacks. But this can't be the whole answer, because exclusively breastfed babies are pretty much immune from decay. And partially breastfed babies get less decay than do formula-feds. So something about breastfeeding or breast milk must be protective.

- Researchers found that most of the 26 formulas tested in an adult's mouth made the mouth more acidic. This would encourage decay (*Pediatric Dentistry*, 1998).

Breastfeeding

When a baby bottle-feeds, milk tends to pool around any teeth before being swallowed. The more reclined he is, the more likely this is. Formula can encourage decay, especially if it lingers around the teeth.

In contrast, when a baby breastfeeds, the milk emerges from the nipple way back in the mouth and is swallowed very quickly.

Researchers say that decay generally occurs in breastfed babies only if they are also given sweet drinks, or foods, containing refined carbohydrates such as sugar and white flour. So if you are partially breastfeeding, take care to clean your baby's teeth after giving him foods containing refined flour (such as white or brown bread, rusks, or cookies) or any sugar-containing foods.

Anti-infective factors

Breast milk's lactoferrin and immunoglobulins help prevent decay, whereas these are lacking in cows'-milk formula.

Fluoride

In childhood, fluoride helps prevent dental decay. Much of it comes from drinking water and a level of 0.7–1.2 mg/L (or parts per million) is considered the most protective.

In infancy, things are different. Fluoride is very poorly transferred from a mother's blood into her milk, so her breastfed baby gets almost none. The risk of decay in children who were breastfed is lower than in those who were formula-fed (regardless of sugar intake). This shows it's breastfeeding, not fluoride, that in infancy helps protect against future decay.

Too much fluoride can cause white mottling of teeth and, at worst, brown marks, pitting, and roughness. This "dental fluorosis" accounts for another possible disadvantage of formula-feeding. This arises because most mothers make up formula by adding sterilized drinking water to powdered formula or concentrated liquid formula. The worry is, firstly, that the made-up feed's fluoride level can be up to 200 times higher than that of the breast milk of a mother who drinks the water (because of the poor transfer of fluoride into her milk). Second, a baby's body retains about 86 percent of his intake, which is about half as much again as an adult's body retains.

The more fluoride in the water, the greater the risk of tooth mottling from formula made up with that water.

A baby whose formula is made up with drinking water not only consumes much more fluoride than does a breastfed baby, but *he also consumes more fluoride per 2.2 pounds (1 kg) body weight than people in any other age group in the population supplied by that water, while a breastfed baby consumes the least.*

Fluoride in drinking water can be naturally present calcium fluoride, or added sodium fluoride or silicofluorides (sodium fluorosilicate or fluorosilicic acid). Its concentration ranges from very low, at up to 0.2 mg/L, to very high, at 2 mg/L or more. The World Health Organization's guideline is 1.5 mg/L. In the US, at the time of writing, the amount recommended by the Environmental Protection Agency (EPA) is 0.7–1.2 mg/L; and the maximum allowed is 4 mg/L. But the US government is proposing making the recommended amount a flat 0.7 mg/L. It's also considering reducing the maximum allowed. In the UK, the target level in natural or artificially fluoridated water is 1 mg/L. A higher natural level is diluted to achieve this result. In continental Europe, fluoride is added not to water but to table salt. Ask your local water company about your water supply's fluoride level.

A mother whose tap water is high in fluoride can reduce her formula-fed baby's risk of consuming too much by making up formula with low-fluoride bottled water some or all of the time. This means buying deionized, purified, demineralized, or distilled water.

There are also unproven—and sometimes vigorously contested—suspicions that too much fluoride can reduce intelligence and encourage an underactive thyroid, stiff and painful joints, and hip fractures in later life.

Better jaw and mouth development

Many specialists report fewer problems of jaw and mouth development in children who were breastfed. In one survey only 2 of nearly 500 children with such problems had been breastfed!

Breastfeeding exercises the mouth, jaw, and face muscles much better than bottle-feeding. Indeed, it uses 60 times more energy! And different movements are involved in sucking from and milking the breast compared with sucking from a bottle. As a baby's face and jaw grow, their shape is influenced by the strength and balance of the pull of their muscles.

Some but not all researchers report that the longer breastfeeding continues, the more likely are the jaw and palate to grow into an optimal shape. In contrast, formula-fed babies and those breastfed for four months or less seem more likely to develop a narrow dental arch. The teeth are therefore less well spaced, which encourages malocclusion (the top and bottom teeth not meeting as they should).

- The longer a baby is breastfed, the lower his risk of a posterior crossbite, says a study in Brazil of 1377 children aged 3–6. This "malocclusion" results from the upper and lower jaws not meeting properly, usually because the upper jaw is too narrow. Children breastfed for more than a year had a 20-fold lower risk compared with those never breastfed, and a 4-fold lower risk compared with those breastfed for 6–12 months (*American Journal of Orthodontics and Dentofacial Orthopedics*, 2010).

Less colic

Babies are often said to have colic if they frequently have unexplained bouts of crying for several hours a day. This usually happens in the evening, is distressing for all, and tends to stop by three months. It's often due to gas, though investigations don't back this up. Intolerance to cows'-milk protein in formula is another possibility. It seems much less likely in babies that are breastfed on demand and held or carried a lot.

- Colic is only about half as likely in breastfed babies as in formula-feds, according to a study of 1,100 babies by researchers at the University of Pelotas, Brazil (*Journal de Pediatria*, 2003).

Less celiac disease

Some children develop celiac disease when they begin to eat foods such as bread, rusk, and breakfast cereal that contain cereal grain. It results from sensitivity to a protein called gliadin in gluten, a "compound" protein found in wheat, barley, rye and, perhaps, oats. It represents a slow-onset immune response, leads to the production of antibodies to gliadin, and can cause abdominal pain, diarrhea, and poor absorption of nutrients.

In a baby who has been sensitized to gluten, eating a gluten-containing food (especially in large amounts) triggers the production of gliadin antibodies that can damage his gut lining. Possible symptoms include abdominal pain, diarrhea, gas, abdominal swelling, foul-smelling bowel motions, and weight loss. Other possibilities are fatigue, headaches, joint pains, seizures (convulsions or fits), and mouth ulcers.

The World Health Organization recommends exclusive breastfeeding for babies of less than six months. One reason is to avoid sensitizing them to gluten while their digestive and immune systems are immature. But experts aren't yet sure whether this is the best course of action.

- One US study found that celiac disease was more likely if babies had a gluten-containing food for the first time either before three months or after six months (*Journal of the American Medical Association*, 2005).

Research shows that sensitization to gluten is less likely if a baby is still being breastfed.

- Analysis of six studies involving 900 children with celiac disease and almost 3,500 controls, at Central Manchester Children's University Hospital in the UK, found that in all but one small study, babies still breastfed when introduced to gluten-containing foods had only half the risk of celiac disease (*Archives of Disease in Childhood*, 2006).

Less pyloric stenosis

This narrowing of the opening of the stomach into the gut can make a baby vomit and is reported to be less common in breastfed babies.

Less likelihood of meconium plugs and meconium ileus

These conditions can cause a blockage in the gut requiring surgery. Both are less common and, if they do occur, less severe, in breastfed babies. This is because colostrum encourages the easy passage of meconium—a baby's very sticky and tar-like first bowel motions.

Less appendicitis

Breastfeeding may make appendicitis less likely in later life:

- Italian research found that being breastfed for at least seven months halved the risk of appendicitis later (*British Medical Journal*, 1995).

Less colitis

Of these three types of colitis (inflammation of the colon), the first is definitely less common in breastfed babies, and the others may prove to be too.

Necrotizing enterocolitis

This is a serious and potentially fatal type of bowel inflammation. The lower a newborn's birthweight and post-conception age, the more likely it is. It affects 1 in 10 babies who have a birthweight of less than 1,500g and just under 4 in 1000 of those whose birthweight was 1,500–2,500g.

It is 10 times more likely in formula-fed infants, and kills 15–25 percent of affected babies.

- Researchers in Cambridge, England, studied 926 pre-term babies, 51 of whom developed necrotizing enterocolitis. This was six to ten times more common in those exclusively formula-fed than in those fed breastmilk alone. And it was three times more common in those exclusively formula-fed as in those who had formula and breast milk. Among babies born at more than 30 weeks, it was rare in those who received some breast-milk, but 20 times more common in those fed formula only. Pasteurized donor milk seemed as protective as a mother's own raw milk (*Lancet*, 1990).

Researchers suspect that freshly expressed or pumped milk is more protective than frozen breast milk.

Less ulcerative colitis and Crohn's disease?

These inflammatory bowel diseases may be associated with the feeding method:

- An Italian study found that not being breastfed increased the risk of ulcerative colitis and Crohn's disease (*International Journal of Epidemiology*, 1998).

- A Canadian study found that both formula-feeding and early diarrhea encouraged Crohn's disease in childhood. Having been breastfed had no protective effect against ulcerative colitis in childhood (*British Medical Journal*, 1989).

The latter study contrasts with another study which found that adults with ulcerative colitis were twice as likely as other people not to have been breastfed.

Less colitis in general

Breast-milk fats are mainly unsaturated. But cows'-milk fats—as in formula—are mainly saturated, which could encourage colitis.

- Researchers at the University of Chicago reported that a diet high in cows'-milk fats boosted the proportion of *Bilophilia wadsworthia* bacteria in the gut from virtually nothing to 6 percent. Within 6 months 60 percent of these mice developed colitis (*Nature*, 2012).

Note that breast milk can also cause colitis, though rarely (page 43).

Fewer complications in very-low-birthweight babies

Breast milk discourages necrotizing enterocolitis (above), retinopathy of prematurity (a potentially blinding eye disorder), late-onset sepsis (potentially overwhelming infection), intolerance to tube feeds, chronic lung disease, and cognitive and behavioral problems associated with nerve damage.

Less acrodermatitis enteropathica

This rare disease is thought to result from an inherited defect of zinc metabolism. It is almost never seen in breastfed children. Breast milk—ideally colostrum—provides the only treatment, possibly because it's rich in zinc, and this zinc is particularly well absorbed.

Fewer SIDS deaths

It seems likely that breastfeeding offers considerable protection against sudden infant death syndrome (SIDS).

- A review of 18 studies concluded that the risk for babies who received any breast milk at all was only two-fifths that of babies who had none. The risk in babies breastfed exclusively, for however short a time, was less than one-third of that in formula-fed babies (*Pediatrics*, 2011).

Because of the nature of these studies, this review doesn't prove that breastfeeding directly helps to prevent SIDS. But there are good reasons (see below) why this could be so.

Interestingly, three boy babies succumb to every two girls. Researchers don't know why. But one possible reason may be that fewer boys are breastfed than girls, and those who are breastfed tend to be breastfed for fewer months than are girls.

Why breastfeeding is probably protective
Breastfed babies

Are more easily aroused. Two- to three-month-old babies are usually more easily aroused from sleep if they are breastfed than if they are formula-fed. And two to four months old is the peak age for SIDS to occur.

Receive anti-infective factors from breast milk. This could be important because it's thought that some babes die from SIDS because they get a viral infection (perhaps even just a mild one) that their immune system can't fight. Breast milk helps protect against certain viral infections.

Aren't exposed to cows' milk protein. It has been suggested that in some babies, SIDS results from a sudden overwhelming response to a foreign protein. Cows'-milk protein is by far the most common foreign protein that formula-fed babies get, and formula-feds consume huge amounts of it.

Tend to feed more often than do formula-feds. Babies who die from SIDS tend to have had a gap of more than six hours between their last feed and their death. If this is indeed important, it's noteworthy that successfully breastfed babies have more frequent feeds than do formula-feds, especially early on in life and at night. The resulting more frequent nourishment and physical contact may be protective.

Frequently fed babies have more sucking and milking time and more "comfort-sucking" time than those who are less frequently fed. A longer time at the breast may be important as it keeps the mouth and throat muscles active for longer, thus keeping these muscles fit and "well toned." They might then be better able to keep the baby's airway open.

- Using a pacifier, especially when going off to sleep during the day or at night, discourages SIDS, according to US researchers who reviewed seven studies. They recommend offering babies a pacifier up to a year old. But breastfeeding should be well established before offering one to a breastfed baby (*Pediatrics*, 2005).

- New Zealand research suggested that a pacifier helped protect against SIDS, possibly because by keeping the mouth and throat muscles more active and "toned," they can keep the airway well open (*Archives of Diseases in Childhood*, 1993).

Note that having your baby in the same room as you at night encourages more frequent breastfeeds and also discourages SIDS:

- A study in 20 areas of Europe, of 745 SIDS babies and 2,411 controls, attributed more than one in three deaths to the baby sleeping in a separate room (*Lancet*, 2004).

- Bed-sharing mothers breastfed three times more often than those whose baby slept separately (*Early Human Development*, 1994). *This frequent contact and feeding might help explain why sleeping in the same room as your breastfed baby discourages SIDS.*

Risk factors

It looks likely, as we've seen, that formula-feeding is a risk factor for SIDS and breastfeeding is protective. But it's sensible to avoid other risk factors too. These include

- Not putting your baby on his back to sleep.
- Having a very soft mattress or mattress pad, or a water mattress.
- You or your partner being a smoker.
- Overheating—though this is so only if babies sleep on their front, which isn't advisable anyway.
- Parental alcohol consumption.
- Parental exhaustion.
- Sleeping with your baby on a sofa or chair.

- Your baby being pre-term.

- Your family being in a low socioeconomic group (probably because of associated risk factors).

- Your baby having an inherited factor (an identical twin of a SIDS baby has a higher risk).

- You having postpartum depression.

- Possibly—sleeping with your baby in bed. But if you exclude the above risk factors, any risk is small, and its existence is anyway contested by many experts. One study (*British Medical Journal*, 1999). found that if neither parent was a smoker, there was an increased risk only in babies less than 14 weeks old. Another study (*Pediatrics*, 2001) of 130 babies in Alaska who died from SIDS found that of the 40 who were sleeping with a parent, all but one had one of the following recognized risk factors—sleeping on their tummy, sleeping with a drug-using parent, or sleeping on a water mattress.

See page 141 for tips on how to minimize the risk of smothering.

Less autoimmune disease

Autoimmune diseases include type 1 diabetes (the sort that comes on suddenly in young people), juvenile rheumatoid arthritis, multiple sclerosis, and Crohn's disease (page 27). They result from a trigger such as a viral infection or stress, making the body produce rogue antibodies that attack certain cells instead of being protective. Breastfeeding seems to reduce a baby's lifetime risk.

Diabetes

Studies strongly suggest that formula-feeding encourages type 1 diabetes:

- A study of 7,208 2½-year-olds in Sweden associated stopping breastfeeding before 2 months with a raised risk of having antibodies to the insulin-producing cells of the pancreas (*British Journal of Nutrition*, 2006).

- Among 350 overweight or obese 8-year-olds and 33 normal-weight controls, those who'd been formula-fed were less sensitive to insulin and produced less of it than those exclusively breastfed for 4 months (*Journal of the American College of Nutrition*, 2011).

- A research review found that people with type 1 diabetes were more likely to have been breastfed for less than 3 months, and to have been exposed to cows' milk before 4 months. The reviewers estimated that early exposure to cows' milk may increase the risk by 1.5 times (*Diabetes Care*, 1994).

It also seems to encourage type 2 diabetes (the type that usually has a late onset):

- People breastfed as babies have a 37 percent lower risk of type 2 diabetes, according to a review of five studies, by experts at the World Health Organization (WHO) and the University of Pelotas, Brazil, This reduction is similar to that when someone with pre-diabetes exercises more and eats more healthily (WHO, 2007).

- A US study of Pima Indians aged 10–39 showed that being exclusively breastfed in their first 2 months was associated with a lower rate of type 2 diabetes. The odds of having type 2 diabetes were 59 percent lower in those who'd been exclusively breastfed than in those exclusively bottle-fed (*Lancet*, 1997).

Juvenile rheumatoid arthritis

Breastfeeding may be protective.

- Children with juvenile rheumatoid arthritis are less likely to have been breastfed (*Journal of Rheumatology*, 1995).

Multiple sclerosis

Several studies suggest a link between formula-feeding and the later development of multiple sclerosis (MS). Two studies showed no link, though they didn't consider the duration of breastfeeding.

- Italian researchers found that adults with MS were less likely than healthy controls to have been breastfed. If they were breast-fed, this was on average for 8.4 months, compared with 12.5 months for controls.

- This "dose" finding is important. Suggested reasons for any pro-tection from prolonged breastfeeding include differences in the amounts and proportions of polyunsaturated fatty acids in breast milk and formula (*British Medical Journal*, 1994).

- Researchers reported that the brains of formula-fed babies had different proportions of fatty acids compared with those of breastfed ones (*Lancet*, 1992).

It's possible, though unproven, that the fatty-acid composition of a formula-fed baby's brain could allow easier viral damage, or make the myelin coating of certain nerves age faster. Breastfeeding also influences a baby's developing immunity, so might affect the immune response to certain triggers in later life.

Less lymph-system cancer

Some but not all studies suggest that children with this sort of cancer are more likely to have been formula-fed. The most recent one is negative:

- The risk of acute lymphoblastic leukemia was investigated as part of the Northern California Childhood Leukemia Study. Whether or not a child had been breastfed had no effect up to age 14 (*British Journal of Cancer*, 2005).

However, several have been positive:

- Analysis of 14 studies by US researchers found that children who'd been breastfed had a lower risk of acute lymphoblastic leukemia and acute myeloblastic leukemia (*Public Health Reports*, 2004).

- Children aged 2–14 with a lymphoma or lymphocytic leukemia had been breastfed for fewer months than had healthy controls, according to research in the United Arab Emirates (*European Journal of Cancer*, 2001).

- Babies breastfed for more than six months had a lower risk of lymphoma—especially Hodgkin's lymphoma—before six years, according to research in China (*International Journal of Epidemiology*, 1995).

More successful kidney transplants

Children with kidney failure who receive a kidney transplant from their mother, brother, or sister (but not their father) have a dramatically better chance of the kidney working successful if they were breastfed as babies.

Better brain and nerve development

Good evidence suggests that breastfeeding encourages better brain and nerve development.

Earlier walking

Two studies have shown that breastfed babies walk earlier than formula-feds. This finding holds even after allowing for differences in weight, and after excluding babies whose mothers went out to work—because their babies might have had less encouragement to walk.

Fewer minor nerve problems

Breastfeeding might be protective:

- Dutch researchers reported that by 9 years, children who'd been exclusively breastfed had half the number of minor neurological (nerve) problems as those who'd received any formula. The researchers thought the concentrations of certain polyunsaturated fats in breast milk (particularly arachidonic and docosahexaenoic acids) might account for this difference (*Lancet*, 1994).

Better intelligence and development tests

Overall, evidence suggests an association between breastfeeding and intelligence, even allowing for other significant factors. It's likely that human milk provides optimal nourishment for the development of the brain, which grows extraordinarily fast in the first year and fastest of all in pre-term babies.

- The longer breastfeeding continues, the greater the brain growth, suggest researchers in England and Northern Ireland. They compared the brain and body size of various mammals with the time they fed their young with their milk and carried them (*Proceedings of the National Academy of Science*, 2011).

- A study of more than 1,000 children from before birth until age ten found that boys who were predominantly breastfed for at least six months did 10 percent better in maths and writing, 8 percent better in spelling and 6 percent better in reading. The researchers say these findings held even after accounting for factors such as the family's income and the mother's educational level. They suggest that the estrogens in breast milk—which are

thought to help protect brain cells—may be particularly beneficial to boy babies. They also point out that the amount a parent
reads to a child aged three to five is, statistically speaking, a much
more important factor (*Pediatrics*, 2010).

- Data from 2,232 children in England and Wales found that
breastfeeding increased IQ by seven points in the nine in ten who
had a particular version of a gene that produces an enzyme which
helps produce docosahexaenoic and arachidonic acids from other
polyunsaturated fatty acids (PUFAs). These long-chain PUFAs
accumulate in the brain and are vital for nerve-message trans-
mission and brain growth. Factors that could skew the findings,
including a baby's growth during pregnancy, mother's intelligence, and socioeconomic class, were ruled out (*Proceedings of the
National Academy of Science*, 2007).

- Being breastfed causes a difference of three to seven points in
IQ, says a review of eight studies by experts at the World Health
Organization (WHO) and the University of Pelotas, Brazil
(WHO, 2007).

Pre-term babies

Breast milk is particularly important for nerve and brain development in pre-term babies:

- An English study found that small-for-dates babies had a higher
developmental score at 9 and 18 months if breastfed than if fed
with standard or enriched formula (*Pediatrics*, 2004).

- Researchers in Cambridge, England, reported that pre-terms given
breast milk had a higher IQ at eight years, even allowing for their
mothers' education, smoking, and socioeconomic status. This suggests that something in breast milk promotes brain growth and
maturation. This may be its arachidonic and docosahexanoic acids,
hormones, and growth factors. But there may also, or instead, be
some other as yet unidentified factor about those mothers who provide breast milk that benefits their babies (*Lancet*, 1992).

Better visual development and eyesight

Breast milk is good for eyesight:

- A US study found that very low-birthweight babies who received breast milk were less likely to develop eye problems due to a retinal disorder called retinopathy of prematurity (*Journal of Perinatology*, 2001).

- Australian researchers found that formula-fed babies had similar visual development to breastfeds only if the formula was enriched with the omega-3 long-chain fatty acids docosahexaenoic and arachidonic acids (*Lancet*, 1995).

Further work suggests these outcomes may result from the different fatty-acid profiles of breast milk and formula. Many pre-term and some full-term babies may be unable to manufacture particular omega-3 fatty acids (including docosahexaenoic and arachidonic acids). Following European recommendations, formula manufacturers now add certain fatty acids to some of their products.

Less vitamin A deficiency

In some developing countries, including Bangladesh, long-term breastfeeding protects children from vitamin A deficiency. This condition can cause dangerously dry eyes (xerophthalmia) and blinds a million children worldwide each year.

- Children with xerophthalmia in Malawi, Africa, were more than three times as likely as others to have stopped breastfeeding before two years old (*American Journal of Clinical Nutrition*, 1986).

Enables spacing between children

The contraceptive effect of long-term unrestricted breastfeeding means that women using no other family planning method have longer gaps between their children. In a developing country, this means a baby has a better chance of surviving and being healthy.

- Chinese research in the largely rural province of Shaanxi found the child-spacing effect of breastfeeding had a marked effect on survival in infancy and early childhood (*Social Science and Medicine*, 1989).

Different activation of gut genes

Breast milk activates certain protective genes in gut-lining cells that formula doesn't:

- Differences in the activation of hundreds of genes in the gut were found between twelve breastfed and ten formula-fed babies, according to research in the US. For example, certain genes expressed only in breastfed babies enhance the gut's immune response to infection (*American Journal of Physiology, Gastrointestinal and Liver Physiology*, 2010).

Less prone to inflammation?

People who are prone to inflammatory disorders, including heart disease, have a higher level of an inflammation-marker called C-reactive protein. People who were breastfed may have a relatively low level, suggesting a reduced risk of such disorders:

- Researchers found a strong relationship in women between how long they'd been breastfed and their level of C-reactive protein. The longer the breastfeeding, the lower their C-reactive protein (*Journal of Epidemiology and Community Health*, 2006).

Healthier cholesterol?

Having been breastfed might reduce the risk of unhealthy cholesterol levels in later life:

- People breastfed as babies are 22 percent less likely to have high cholesterol, says a research review by the World Health Organization (WHO) and the University of Pelotas, Brazil. The effect was bigger than from making dietary changes as an adult (WHO, 2007).

Less heart disease?

Being formula-fed as a baby is associated with a raised risk in later life of certain risk factors for heart disease, including obesity, diabetes and high cholesterol, blood pressure and C-reactive protein. This may be because babies have different hormonal responses to breast milk and infant formula.

- Of 624 babies born in Amsterdam from 1943–1946, at the time of the Dutch famine, 83 percent were exclusively breastfed for at least 10 days. The rest were completely or partially bottle-fed with cows' milk or buttermilk. As adults aged 48–53, those who'd been bottle-fed also had less healthy cholesterol levels (higher low-density-lipoprotein cholesterol, and lower high-density-lipoprotein cholesterol). Those who'd been bottle-fed had impaired insulin function, which is known to encourage diabetes and other ailments. Neither blood pressure nor body mass index were affected by the type of infant feeding (*Archives of Disease in Childhood*, 2000).

Less breast cancer?

One study associated having been breastfed with a lower risk of breast cancer in later life:

- A study of 1,130 women from New York found that if they had been breastfed, regardless of how long, their risk of both pre-menopausal and postmenopausal breast cancer was about 25 percent lower than if they'd been only formula-fed (*Epidemiology*, 1994).

No "acidosis"

This condition is relatively unknown yet potentially very important. Our body fluid's balance of acidity and alkalinity is indicated by its pH (potential of Hydrogen: a pH of 0–7 is acidic, 7 neutral and 7–14 alkaline). Blood, for example, has an alkaline pH that's kept within a very narrow range. Only with certain illnesses does its pH stray outside this range by becoming more alkaline ("alkalosis") or less alkaline (confusingly called "acidosis"). Either can cause symptoms.

Various foods make our body fluids more or less alkaline while still staying within the normal pH range. Being less alkaline creates "low-grade metabolic acidosis." Certain researchers claim that almost everyone eating a typical Western diet has low-grade acidosis. And we now know this can cause symptoms (For an excellent review, read "Diet-Induced Acidosis: Is It Real and Clinically Relevant?" (*British Journal of Nutrition*, 2010). But can formula cause it in a baby? It seems probable.

Foods that make the pH relatively more alkaline are called

alkali-producing foods; those that make it relatively less alkaline are called acid-producing foods. Now the crunch. *Breast milk is an alkali-producing food* and so too is fresh, unprocessed cows' milk. In contrast, cows'-milk formula is an acid-producing food because the processing it undergoes during manufacture (which, depending on the make, can include homogenization and pasteurization) changes its nature.

So it's possible, though unproven, that formula-feeding can cause chronic low-grade metabolic acidosis. If so, this could encourage a wide variety of health conditions, including anxiety, asthma, cancer, convulsions, dental decay, diabetes, drowsiness, eczema, fatigue, food allergy, indigestion, inflammation, hyperactivity, obesity, pain, and urine infection.

Less diaper rash?

One survey showed that formula-fed babies were twice as likely as breastfeds to get diaper rash.

Fewer inguinal hernias?

Breastfeeding might offer some protection:

- Babies with an inguinal hernia (a "rupture" or weakness in the groin) were much more likely than other babies never to have been breastfed, according to Italian researchers. They suggest that certain hormones (such as gonadotropin-releasing hormone) in breast milk may help prevent inguinal hernias (*Journal of Pediatrics*, 1995).

Different emotional and behavioral development?

The influences of breastfeeding on emotional and behavioral development are impossible to pinpoint with certainty. However, studies suggest that breastfed babies spend less time in their cribs and more with their mothers than do formula-feds.

In communities that encourage unrestricted breastfeeding, babies hardly ever cry, whereas in many developed countries babies are often left to cry because "it isn't time for a feed" or "they might be spoiled if they're picked up." It is reasonable to assert that a baby offered the breast for food or comfort whenever he wants it will grow up feeling more confident that his needs will be met.

The researcher Jean Liedloff studied two neighboring tropical islands whose inhabitants reared children very differently. On one island, babies were carried or held almost all the time. They slept with their mother. When with her, they could breastfeed frequently and more or less as much as they wanted. As they grew up, they scarcely ever cried and appeared much happier and less aggressive than those on the other island. These others were reared in a way more akin to how many people in developed countries bring up their babies—neither carried nor held much, nor breastfed in an unrestricted way. Research shows that a breastfeeder is more likely to kiss, rock, touch, and talk to her baby, while a bottle-feeder is more likely to rub, pat, and jiggle her baby and is much more concerned about "gas."

- More than nine in ten long-term American and Canadian breast-feeders considered the benefits to their babies of being breastfed to be emotional security, happiness, and the earlier development of independence (*Journal of Tropical Pediatrics*, 1987).

Better attachment to mother?

A closer relationship between a mother and her breastfed baby seems likely, if only because he depends on her for food, and greater physical intimacy is involved. But proof is lacking.

Better mental-health development?

Breastfeeding even for a few weeks might, though we most certainly don't yet have enough proof, discourage alcoholism and schizophrenia:

- Adults who hadn't been breastfed as babies, or who'd been breast-fed for less than a month, were more likely to have been hospitalized for alcoholism, according to a large study in Copenhagen, Denmark. This held even after ruling out other factors known to encourage alcoholism (*American Journal of Psychiatry*, 2006).

- When teachers rated anxiety in ten-year-olds, those who'd been breastfed had a much lower risk of anxiety after their parents' separation or divorce than did those who'd been formula-fed (*Archives of Disease in Childhood*, 2006).

- Adults who'd been breastfed for less than two weeks, or who'd never been breastfed, were twice as likely to have been diagnosed with schizophrenia (*Acta Psychiatrica Scandinavia*, 2005).

Possible disadvantages to your baby

The possible disadvantages to a baby of being breastfed are very few.

Lack of vitamin B12 in the babies of some vegetarians or vegans

Some strict vegetarians, or vegans (who eat no foods from animal sources at all), have too little vitamin B12 in their breast milk, and their babies develop deficiency symptoms. This is sometimes because such a woman hasn't grown up in a family that knows how to choose and prepare nutritious vegetarian or vegan foods. Good advice about what to eat, plus extra vitamin B12 for vegan mothers, puts this right.

Lack of vitamin B1 in babies of mothers with beriberi

In certain developing countries, some women risk getting beriberi, a disease caused by a deficiency of vitamin B1 (thiamine). This is because they eat large amounts of polished rice. Breastfed babies of women with beriberi can become acutely ill with infantile beriberi. Polishing brown rice to produce white rice removes the outer layers of each grain, but vitamin B1 is lost at the same time. The solution is to eat unpolished brown rice.

Insufficient milk

Babies that don't get enough breast milk can become dangerously dehydrated and can starve.

Tell your midwife, doctor, or, in the UK, health visitor, if your baby isn't feeding well, or doesn't have six to eight really wet cloth diapers or five to six really wet disposables a day after your milk has come in. Using the steps on page 204 should increase your milk production within two to three days. If the health professional doesn't think your baby can wait that long, meet your baby's needs for fluid and nourishment during those few days by giving donated breast milk or infant formula by cup after a breastfeed, or via a supplementer (page 170) during a breastfeed.

Malnourishment

If a breastfeeding woman's diet is grossly deficient in protein and fat, her baby is liable to go short too. The World Health Organization now concentrates famine-relief monies on food for breastfeeding mothers instead of only on formula for babies. This is because in famine circumstances formula-fed babies are much more likely to die because of the enormous risk of gastroenteritis from unsterilized bottles and water. Mothers in such circumstances are also likely to give bottle-fed babies diluted feeds so as to save milk powder in case they can't get any or afford it the next day.

Learning to cope with stress by eating?

Frequent feeds are important for young babies. As they grow, they may not always want the breast every time they fidget or cry. But one of the only times it's ever sensible to cut down on breastfeeds is if you're giving very frequent feeds, your baby latches on properly and you let your milk down well, but you've got into the habit of misinterpreting restlessness or cries as signs that he wants the breast when what he really needs is attention of some other kind (for example, to be talked to, listened to, played with, or simply accompanied when feeling grumpy). A crying or fidgeting baby will probably feed even if not hungry. However, if milk isn't what he needs, this could be an early lesson in how to use food as a tranquilizer at times of stress.

Many distressed and/or overweight adults turn to food for comfort in the face of stress or emotional pain that has little or nothing to do with being hungry for food. A baby's experiences affect behavior in adult life, and it's possible, though unproven, that early experiences at the breast could encourage eating disorders and other attempts to find solutions to emotional distress in later life.

So how best can we help babies grow up believing the world is a good place, and they can get their needs met?

Offering your baby the breast whenever he seems to need it is an excellent way of making him feel cared for. If he's hungry or thirsty or needs the nonspecific comfort of sucking and being intimately close to you, continuing to breastfeed is a good idea. If he doesn't seem very interested, and you think he might need something else, try to identify what this might be. In this way you'll teach a variety of methods of dealing with emotional situations such as boredom, loneliness, anger, frustration and so on. The sort of mothering that fits a baby's needs this precisely calls for more thought and effort than simply pacifying him with indiscriminate breastfeeding. But it may pay dividends later in life.

Breast-milk colitis

A baby with blood-stained bowel motions and, perhaps, colic, may have a rare condition known as breast-milk colitis. The cause is unclear, though it may be associated with sensitivity to a breast-milk protein, or to traces of protein in foods the mother has eaten and that have "leaked" through her gut wall into her blood, then entered her milk. The usual medical recommendation is to stop breastfeeding. If breast milk is the cause, the symptoms then resolve within about seven to 10 days, but recur if the baby again has breast milk.

Although some of these possible disadvantages of breastfeeding to your baby might sound alarming, there's absolutely no doubt that its potential advantages greatly outweigh them.

It's a good idea to identify and air any concerns you have about breast-feeding, whether you're pregnant, breastfeeding or neither. This is because bottling up such questions, doubts or worries could make them more powerful in your conscious or unconscious mind. That way, if you're pregnant, they might prevent you deciding to breastfeed. If you're breastfeeding, they might stop you breastfeeding sooner than you might otherwise have done. And if you're neither pregnant nor breastfeeding, they could lead you to instil doubt in women who are pregnant, to criticize those who are breastfeeding, or just generally to "diss" breastfeeding.

Breastfeeding is now fully accepted at scientific and international levels as the normal way of feeding babies. And breastfeeding is the most common way of feeding young babies in virtually every country.

Some years ago, prenatal clinic staff used to ask pregnant women whether they were going to breastfeed or formula-feed—which they euphemistically called "bottle-feed." This very question implied that breastfeeding and formula-feeding were choices of equal value. But we now know from a literally vast amount of medical research that they are not. Breastfeeding is best not only for babies but also for their mothers. It's also better for society as a whole.

So the expectation should be that a baby will be breastfed unless a woman asserts her intention to formula-feed. There is no ill-will in this expectation. And there should be absolutely no bullying, criticism or judgment from other people, health professionals or others, of a woman who says she is going to, or does, formula-feed. It is in her gift alone to make the decision and everyone should respect her right to make it and support her however she feeds her baby (page 334).

Hopefully, this chapter will have clarified the fact that breastfeeding is without any shadow of a doubt best for babies. Women's concerns about breastfeeding mostly relate to the possibility that it might be disadvantageous to them (page 59). For example, they might imagine that breastfeeding will make their breasts sag or that the whole undertaking will be too tying. These concerns are particularly important as they are they ones most likely to prevent or stop them breastfeeding. Hopefully, reading what's been said here and in the next chapter and, perhaps, airing your concerns with other women will either make them evaporate or will at least minimize them.

three

Best for You

Breastfeeding has a surprising number of advantages to a mother. Before exploring them, it'll help to consider the biological perspective.

The biological perspective

Human females develop breasts several years before they are physically ready to bear children, whereas most other mammals develop mammary glands only when needed to feed their offspring. This difference is because human breasts serve purposes other than feeding babies, the chief being sexual attraction and arousal.

Humans have probably been on earth for about five million years, though the earliest evidence of the "modern" human, *Homo sapiens*, comes from fossils dating back only 195,000 years. These predecessors lived as hunter-gatherers and ate a mainly vegetarian diet until around 10,000 years ago, when they started living in agricultural settlements.

Studies of the few hunter-gatherer tribes remaining today suggest that their reproductive life is very different from that of most westernized people.

The best studied present-day hunter-gatherers are the !Kung of Botswana and Namibia. !Kung women start menstruating at 17 to 18, which is late by Western standards. And their menopause is earlier, at about 38. So their reproductive span is about 20 years, whereas ours— between the average ages of 13 and 51—is about 38. The average !Kung woman has six or seven children. Because she breastfeeds each one on an unrestricted basis for many years, she has comparatively few menstrual cycles. Such women become fertile, menstruate a few times, have their first child and breastfeed for several years. Then, as they breastfeed less often and therefore start to ovulate again, they become pregnant again and repeat the cycle.

So hunter-gatherer women are either pregnant or breastfeeding for most of their reproductive life and only ever have 20 to 30 menstrual cycles. This was the picture for all women until a mere 10,000 years ago, which is very recent in evolutionary terms.

While we're biologically akin to these hunter-gatherers, we've dramatically changed our way of life over the past 200 years of industrialization. The average modern girl eats more and therefore weighs more, so she starts menstruating much earlier. She has very few pregnancies and breastfeeds each child for only a few months, if at all. So until her menopause she has perhaps 400–450 menstrual cycles. Researchers think the accompanying surges of hormones encourage certain health problems.

Obviously breastfeeding one or two children for a few months or even a year or so each won't transform a modern woman into a hunter-gatherer but it certainly has provable advantages to her health.

Less bleeding after childbirth

Breastfeeding stimulates the production of oxytocin. This hormone encourages the womb to shrink back to normal after childbirth, so bleeding stops sooner than in a formula-feeding woman.

Less breast cancer

Breast cancer is common in developed countries and has become more so over the last 200 years. Yet it's rare in countries where women spend many years breastfeeding.

According to an expert panel convened in 2010 by the World Cancer Research Fund and the American Institute for Cancer Research, there's now convincing evidence that breastfeeding discourages breast cancer.

But it's important to know that it's a long lifetime duration of breastfeeding (the total time a woman spends breastfeeding in her life) that's considered protective. The theory is that this is because it can suppress ovulation and therefore the monthly hormone cycles that can disrupt cells (page 48), for longer. See page 53 for the sort of breastfeeding most likely to do this.

- Of a group of 60,000 mothers in the US Nurses Health Study, those whose mother or sister had had breast cancer were 59 percent less likely to develop premenopausal breast cancer if they breastfed. The reduction in risk was similar to that from taking tamoxifen (an antiestrogen drug) for five years (*Archives of Internal Medicine*, 2009).

- Research at the University of Southern California, involving 1,457 women with breast cancer and 1,455 controls, aged 55 or older, found that breastfeeding discouraged breast cancer. This held even for cancers sensitive to estrogen and progesterone. However, in women who had breastfed and whose first full-term pregnancy had been after 25, invasive breast cancer was more likely (*Cancer Epidemiology, Biomarkers and Prevention*, 2007).

- A Korean study of 110,604 women found a reduced risk of breast cancer in those whose lifetime total of breastfeeding was more than 24 months. The greater the total, the lower the risk (*International Journal of Cancer*, 2003).

- Analysis of 47 studies from 30 countries, involving 50,302 women with invasive breast cancer and 96,973 controls, indicated strong links between breastfeeding and a reduced rate of breast cancer. The risk decreased by over 4 percent for every year of breastfeeding (*Lancet*, 2002).

How might breastfeeding be protective?

There are three theories which, if correct, may act together or separately.

First, exclusive breastfeeding can prevent ovulation, thereby preventing the monthly rises in estrogen, progesterone, and prolactin that can cause new-cell growth and stimulate genetic material in the breast, which might encourage cancer.

Second, if a woman lets her milk dry up, stagnant milk might speed breast-cell multiplication and increase the number of atypical cells, causing a state similar to that known to encourage cancer. This is because stagnant milk is slightly less acidic than freshly produced milk. And cells are more likely to multiply rapidly and become abnormal in such an environment. Interestingly, the Tanka boat-women of Hong Kong, who feed only from their right breast, are very unlikely to get cancer in this breast. But their cancer-risk in the left breast is relatively high and similar of that of women in the US.

Third, breastfeeding might flush out potentially carcinogenic (cancer-encouraging) chemicals that have entered milk glands from food.

So what should you do?

In the light of current knowledge, choose to breastfeed on an unrestricted basis, don't give your baby solids for six months, and breastfeed each child for at least a year. This usually prevents ovulation for many months, which delays the return of the monthly disruption of breast cells. Evidence suggests this reduces the risk of breast cancer.

However "breast-aware" you are, if you develop breast cancer while breastfeeding, you might notice it later than if you weren't breastfeeding. This is because lactating breasts are often naturally lumpy because of their enlarged milk glands, ducts, and reservoirs.

There's some concern that even though breast cancer in general seems to be less likely in women who have ever breastfed, aggressive breast cancer may be more common. See the University of Southern California trial on page 47 and

- A study in Sweden of 17,035 women, 622 of whom developed breast cancer, found that women who'd breastfed for 6 months or more had an increased risk of any breast cancer being more aggressive. This suggests that a woman who's breastfed for a long time should have more frequent screening (Presented at the European Breast Cancer Conference, 2010).

Until these findings are replicated and we have more information about these particular women, the message to take from this is to be breast-aware and, if you have even a tiny suspicion that something is wrong, to get it checked without delay.

Less ovarian cancer

This cancer is more common in industrialized countries and kills more women than any other cancer. Years of monthly ovulation make it more likely. So it's sensible to predict that the more children a woman has, and the longer she breastfeeds each one, the lower her risk is likely to be.

- Of 149,693 women studied in the US, those who'd breastfed for 18 months or more had a smaller risk of ovarian cancer. Each extra month of breastfeeding was associated with an extra 2 percent decrease in risk (*Cancer Causes and Control*, 2007).

Less uterine cancer

Breastfeeding seems to offer some protection against uterine cancer in later life:

- Women who'd breastfed had a smaller risk of womb [uterine] cancer than those who'd given birth but never breastfed, according to researchers in Japan (*Journal of Experimental Medicine*, 2006).

Less cyclical breast pain

Anecdotal evidence suggests that women who have ever breastfed are less likely to get this each month.

Helps you get your figure back

Breastfeeding uses up some of the fat stored in pregnancy and can help you get back to your prepregnancy shape and weight, provided you eat a healthy diet and exercise regularly. An increased amount of stored fat is mobilized after the first three months of breastfeeding.

Breasts tend to return to their previous shape and size about six months after stopping breastfeeding. Experts agree that any permanent change in body shape is likely to result from factors other than breastfeeding.

- In a US study of 93 women awaiting cosmetic breast surgery, all of whom had been pregnant at least once, 55 percent reported an adverse change in breast shape after pregnancy. Having breastfed was not associated with increased sagging, nor were the number of children breastfed, the duration of breastfeeding or the amount of weight gained in pregnancy. But body mass index, the number of pregnancies, a larger prepregnancy bra size, smoking, and age, all were (Presented at a conference in Baltimore of the American Society of Plastic Surgeons, 2007).

More convenient

A big practical bonus of breastfeeding is that it's more convenient, even at home, with no bottles and nipples to wash and sterilize and no feeds to prepare. Breast milk is always at hand. Going out is easier, as you have no equipment to prepare and take. Holidays and travel become much more practical. Not for you the cooling of a bottle of hot milk by holding it out of the car window! And there's no milk powder to spill in a car, train, or plane.

A breastfeeder needs only her baby and a clean diaper to go anywhere, and it takes only a little ingenuity and forethought to breastfeed without embarrassment to you or anyone else.

Also, it's nearly always possible to comfort an infant with the breast easily and quickly, anywhere and any time, and without overfeeding. But a formula-fed baby often isn't comforted by sucking a bottle or a pacifier and may get too much milk if allowed to feed freely.

Cheaper

In the UK the cost of formula, bottles, nipples, and either sterilizing tablets, or fuel to boil the equipment was estimated to be around £650 (about $1280) a year in 2006 and is probably more today.

A breastfeeder needs to pay for more food so she can get an extra 300–500 calories a day. The actual cost will depend on her preferences— extra calories from best steak and asparagus are more expensive than those from cheese-and-tomato sandwiches. If she simply eats a little more of everything she normally eats, the cost will probably be less than that of formula-feeding. This could be vitally important for certain women in developing countries who can't afford enough formula, but can afford a little extra food for themselves.

Can provide birth control

The contraceptive effect of particular types of breastfeeding can be as efficient as better-known contraceptive methods such as the pill. It's the only contraception available to many of the world's women. And in developing countries there are two reasons why it can be vitally important.

First, it spaces children more widely. In most of the world a child born less than two years after an older sibling is twice as likely to die young as one born after a longer gap.

Second, it does more than any other contraceptive method to contain the population explosion.

Using data gathered from more than 4,000 women in more than 15 countries, an international group of experts stated in 1995 that the contraceptive effect of breastfeeding as part of the lactational amenorrhea method (LAM—see below) is more than 98 percent effective. In other words, it's very safe, though not failsafe.

No popular contraceptive method is 100 percent reliable but the contraceptive effect of LAM equals that of the pill and the condom and is very useful for temporary contraception after childbirth.

The lactational-amenorrhea method (LAM)

This gives a better than 98 percent chance of avoiding pregnancy. But to get this protection

- **Your baby** must be under six months old.

- **Your periods** should not yet have returned.

And you should

- Breastfeed exclusively (give your baby no other drinks or food) or very nearly so.

- Give at least eight (and preferably more) feeds every 24 hours (Fewer than six will let your prolactin fall to a level that might allow ovulation).

- Have a gap from the beginning of one feed to the beginning of the next of no longer than 4 hours by day and 6 hours at night. One study (1992) found that once periods had returned, nine feeds in 24 hours prevented ovulation in 7 in 10 women, whereas six in 24 hours did so in only 3 in 10 women. The more frequent feeders had higher prolactin levels.

Scientists aren't clear why conception is less likely with this sort of breastfeeding. But they know prolactin is involved, as are vigorous sucking and milking by the baby, and frequent breastfeeds with no long gaps day or night.

Prolactin—LAM helps prevent prolactin dipping low enough to allow ovulation. High prolactin seems to prevent ovulation by discouraging the ovaries from responding to follicle-stimulating hormone, a hormone which in non-pregnant, non-breastfeeding women allows an egg to ripen each month.

As time passes, a breastfeeding woman's prolactin falls until it's no longer high enough to prevent ovulation. In exclusively breastfeeding women ovulation doesn't happen until the tenth week after childbirth at the earliest, and only 1 in 20 ovulates before the eighteenth week.

Reliability—Breastfeeding's contraceptive effect differs from woman to woman, even if they breastfeed in similar ways. But the type of breast-feeding makes a very big difference to the return of fertility. The average time before their first period in women who breastfeed exclusively and on an unrestricted basis for six to eight months, then introduce solids but continue to breastfeed frequently for drinks and comfort, is over 14 months! A woman breastfeeding this way can expect an average gap of two to three years between babies, which means ovulation returns, on average, after 15–27 months, the exact timing depending on personal factors.

By contrast, **formula-feeders** ovulate on average eight to ten weeks after giving birth, which means one in two risks becoming pregnant before her baby is eight to ten weeks old if she resumes sexual activity without contraception.

Partially breastfeeding women ovulate on average later than bottle-feeding women but before exclusively breastfeeding ones.

If a breastfeeding woman menstruates in the first six months after delivery, her cycles are likely to be anovulatory (without ovulation), which is why most women can rely on LAM until their first period (Though remember LAM is only for women with babies up to six months). This doesn't mean you can't become pregnant while using LAM—just that you have only a 2 percent chance of doing so.

As the months pass, ovulation before the first period becomes increas-ingly likely. One woman in twenty ovulates before her first period, which is one reason LAM isn't 100 percent effective. But there are several ways of discovering when you're about to ovulate (see "other contraception," on page 54).

Many studies suggest that breastfeeding's contraceptive effect is more powerful and lasts longer in developing countries than in westernized ones. There are several possible reasons, including poor nourishment and taboos against sex with lactating women. But the main reason is undoubt-edly that many women here breastfeed in an unrestricted way, with fre-quent feeds day and night, whereas in developed countries many women breastfeed only five or six times in any 24-hour period, with very few, or no, feeds at night.

Women in developing countries also tend to allow more nonnutri-tive suckling, putting their babies to the breast for comfort and pleasure as well as "proper" feeds. This means that even if their babies have solids or bottle-feeds, they still spend a lot of time at the breast, which helps prevent ovulation.

The first eight weeks—If using LAM, you need no other contraception. It's exceedingly unlikely even for formula-fed women to ovulate now.

After 8 weeks, ask yourself

1. Are you content with 98 percent reliable contraception from LAM (which is better than most women settle for most of the time)?

2. Are you breastfeeding exclusively or very nearly exclusively?

3. Are you still without periods (defined as a recognizable menstrual period or two consecutive days of bleeding or spotting)?

If you answer "no" to any of these questions, breastfeeding alone will give you nowhere near 98 percent reliability, so you'll need to use another contraceptive method.

If you answer "yes" to all three, LAM can be your only contraceptive method until your baby is six months or until such time as your answers change.

If you feel strongly that you don't want to get pregnant again quickly, then—in case you're among the one in 20 exclusively breastfeeding women who ovulate before their first period—you might like to use "extra-safe LAM" and/or additional contraception compatible with breastfeeding and recent childbirth.

Extra-safe LAM—You can delay ovulation and help detect the unlikely event of ovulation before your first period by stimulating your milk supply more. Do this by

- Breastfeeding more often than eight times in 24 hours.

- Checking your baby is well positioned at the breast.

- Allowing nonnutritive ("comfort") sucking.

- Not giving foods or drinks other than your milk until your baby is four to six months old. Once a baby starts solids or other drinks, LAM's reliability falls to 96 percent.

If you or your baby don't want to or can't breastfeed frequently (for example, if he is unwell or disinterested, or you're not with each other) you can mimic the anti-ovulatory effect of breastfeeding to some extent by hand-expressing (or pumping) every two to three hours by day and every four hours or so at night.

Other contraceptive methods compatible with breastfeeding and recent childbirth

When you resume having sex, you could use a condom with spermicidal jelly, or a **diaphragm**. If you've used a diaphragm before, you'll need to be refitted after having a baby because you'll be a different size inside. Another idea is to have an IUD (intrauterine contraceptive device) fitted.

The combined pill is not advisable because it decreases breast milk production. Having a progesterone-containing intrauterine device inserted at six to eight weeks after childbirth dramatically lowers the breastfeeding rate at six months, according to one study. Having a progesterone injection or implant from four to eight weeks is likely to do the same.

According to the World Health Organization, the advantages of monthly progesterone injections or a progesterone implant for breastfeeding women in the first six weeks after delivery outweigh the disadvantages. And the US Centers for Disease Control advised in 2010 that by a month after childbirth, the benefits of progesterone injections or implants outweigh the risk of reducing breastfeeding rates. But doctors in India report that women who have contraceptive injections lose minerals from their bones, leading to lower bone density. So they suggest these injections are unsafe for breastfeeding women.

However, the progestogen-only pill neither interferes with breastfeeding nor affects a breastfed baby.

The sympto-thermal method—is a natural form of birth control. Analysis of five studies shows that when used carefully it is 96.8 percent effective (Used imperfectly, it is only 86.4 percent effective). It involves

- Being aware of the bodily changes that herald impending ovulation and the fertile time of your cycle. These include changes in the amount and nature of vaginal mucus, and in body temperature. The average woman ovulates on day 12 of her cycle, counting the first day of her period as day one. However, ovulation may occur any time between days 10 and 14. In a few women, it occurs at other times. Most women are especially fertile for the six days before and for a few days after ovulation.

- Avoiding sex (or using a condom or diaphragm) if you recognize you're entering a fertile time.

This method can help you identify the unlikely event of ovulation before your first period after childbirth. It can also help you identify whether newly returned periods are associated with ovulation. This becomes even easier as the months pass and you settle back into ovulatory menstrual cycles.

It's wise for a breastfeeding woman to get expert help if she wants reliable contraception from this method. This is because breastfeeding may make the signs indicating your fertile time less obvious.

A small saliva microscope (page 340) can help you identify the fern-like pattern in your saliva that precedes your fertile time. Ovulation-prediction kits (page 340) that test hormone levels in a few drops of urine are another useful aid.

Better for bones

Breastfeeding may reduce the risk of osteoporosis in later life:

- Of 311 women aged 65 or more, those who'd had a baby but never breastfed had twice as many hip fractures as those who had breastfed, according to Australian researchers. The longer a woman breastfed each baby, the lower her risk. Breastfeeding each one for more than nine months reduced the risk to a quarter of that of women who'd never breastfed (*International Journal of Epidemiology*, 1993).

- A South African study showed that breastfeeders had higher bone-mineral density in later life than formula-feeders. Women who developed osteoporosis were four times less likely to have breastfed (*South African Medical Journal*, 1992).

But if breastfeeding protects against osteoporosis, as these studies suggest, this may be so only if done for a cumulatively large number of months or years. Long-term breastfeeding delays the onset of ovulation after a baby. This makes a woman's egg supply last longer, so she continues to ovulate further into middle age. The longer she has menstrual cycles, with their accompanying high estrogen and progesterone, the later is her menopause and the further away the time when low hormone levels encourage osteoporosis.

Less rheumatoid arthritis

Breastfeeding seems to discourage the long-term risk. A suggested mechanism is that women who've breastfed for 12 months or more have higher levels of the anti-inflammatory hormone cortisol that persist past the menopause.

- Women who had breastfed for a longer duration had a lower risk of rheumatoid arthritis than those who had breastfed for less time or never breastfed, according to a study of 18,236 women in Sweden (*Annals of Rheumatic Diseases*, 2008).

- Of 121,700 women in the US Nurses Health Study, 674 developed rheumatoid arthritis (RA). Breastfeeding for more than 12 months reduced the risk; breastfeeding for more than two years halved it (*Arthritis and Rheumatism*, 2004).

- A Norwegian study of 63,090 women, 355 of whom died from RA, found an association between a woman's lifetime duration of breastfeeding and her risk of dying from RA. Those who'd breastfed for 20 months or more had a particularly low risk (*Endocrine Research*, 1994).

Sometimes RA flares up after childbirth, just as it can at other times of great changes in sex hormones. One study found an increased risk of this happening among breastfeeders, but two similar studies found none.

Lower risk of high blood pressure

Breastfeeding is associated with a lower risk of high blood pressure in later life. One theory is that this results from breastfeeding hormones.

- A US study of 139,681 postmenopausal women associated having breastfed for more than a year with a 12 percent reduction in the risk of high blood pressure. Even doing so for at least a month was associated with a lower risk (*Obstetrics and Gynecology*, 2009).

Lower cholesterol

Breastfeeding is associated with a lower risk of high cholesterol in later life. The reasons are unclear but could result from hormones produced while breastfeeding.

- The same study (above) associated having breastfed for more than a year with a 20 percent reduction in the risk of high cholesterol. Even doing so for at least a month was associated with a lower risk (*Obstetrics and Gynecology*, 2009).

Less diabetes

Breastfeeding is associated with a lower risk of diabetes in later life. The reasons for this are unclear but could result from hormones produced while breastfeeding.

- The same study (above) associated having breastfed for more than a year with a 20 percent reduction in the risk of diabetes. Even doing so for at least a month was associated with a lower risk (*Obstetrics and Gynecology*, 2009).

Less metabolic syndrome

Research suggests that breastfeeding discourages metabolic syndrome. Also called "pre-diabetes," this condition greatly encourages diabetes, heart disease, and strokes; affects one in five adults; and is defined by having three of these factors: a lot of "belly fat" around the waist, high blood pressure, high blood fats, low HDL-cholesterol (the protective sort) and insulin resistance.

- Observations and tests over 20 years of 1,399 of the women in the US CARDIA study found metabolic syndrome was only half as likely in those whose total breastfeeding duration during that time was more than 9 months, as in those in whom it was less than a month or none. In those women who developed pregnancy diabetes, the later development of metabolic syndrome was 6 times less likely in those whose total breastfeeding duration was more than 9 months, as in those in whom it was less than a month or none. The risk reductions remained after ruling out other factors known to encourage metabolic syndrome, such as having less physical activity or gaining weight (*Diabetes*, 2010).

Fewer heart attacks and strokes

The longer a woman's lifetime duration of breastfeeding, the lower her risk of a stroke or heart attack may be

- A study of 139,681 postmenopausal women, at the University of Pittsburgh in the US, associated having breastfed for more than a year with a lower risk of a heart attack or stroke (*Obstetrics and Gynecology*, 2009).

- A study associated breastfeeding for at least 24 months with a 23 percent lower risk of coronary heart disease (*American Journal of Obstetrics*).

Can reduce stress and boost motherly feelings

Breastfeeders benefit from increased prolactin, the milk-producing hormone that encourages calmness. They also have a less intense response to the stress hormone adrenaline. What's more, the oxytocin they produce as they let down milk may discourage anxiety:

- Oxytocin facilitates the release of serotonin and reduces anxiety-related behavior, according to a Japanese study of mice (*Journal of Neuroscience*, 2009).

Closer bond with your baby?

The physical intimacy involved in breastfeeding might encourage a closer bond with your baby. Breastfeeding also stimulates the release in the mother of two hormones. One is oxytocin (page 110). Not only does this stimulate the milk glands to let down milk, but it also promotes the development of maternal behavior, and bonding between mother and baby. The other is prolactin, which can engender feelings of happiness and tranquillity.

Such emotions may be boosted by an increase in hormone-like substances called endorphins that are also stimulated by breastfeeding. Endorphins help reduce the effects of stress in lactating rats, and this may be true in humans too.

Satisfying?

There's something wonderful about nourishing your baby yourself. Giving him the pleasure of being at your breast is rewarding too, as is being able to comfort a crying baby. Many women who breastfeed successfully for as long as they want report being very satisfied even if they are unaware of the health benefits to their babies and themselves.

Enjoyable?

Most breastfeeders find breastfeeding enjoyable. There's something very special about a baby staring up at you and perhaps stopping sucking every now and then to give you a gummy smile. And the sight of a baby's tiny, dimpled, star-shaped hand resting on the breast as he feeds is among the magic moments of mothering.

Many women enjoy talking to their baby, especially toward the end of a feed when he isn't concentrating so much on drinking. And breastfeeding mothers around the world love speaking to their baby in "baby talk." Researchers note that their voices all have a similar lilting, adagio rhythm. This is a delightful interlude when the levels of endorphins (natural "feel-good" chemicals in the blood) are high and those of stress hormones (such as adrenaline and cortisol) are low.

Fulfilling?

Another common feeling is that breastfeeding is one of the things only a woman can do. In today's push toward gender equality this feminine fulfillment is valued not only by the naturally maternal but also by career women who see their enjoyment of breastfeeding as symbolic of their womanliness.

The oneness many breastfeeding women feel with their babies is often quoted as the major advantage to breastfeeding mothers. Certainly they often seem particularly at ease with their babies.

Empowering?

A woman who breastfeeds for as long as she or her baby wants may gain in confidence and self-esteem. One US study (1993) found that women of low economic means who breastfed had more confidence in their mothering and their ability to meet their children's needs.

Possible disadvantages to you

It would be foolish to pretend there are no drawbacks to breastfeeding. But many perceived disadvantages can be overcome and certain other concerns disappear when well aired.

No one else can feed the baby

This isn't true. A breastfeeding woman can leave expressed or pumped milk for someone else to give her baby if she collects enough after each of several feeds.

Expecting to return to work

One in twenty pregnant British women plan to formula-feed because they expect to return to work soon. But very few actually do return to work when their babies are very young. If they do, they often continue breastfeeding (page 317).

Friends aren't doing it

A woman's friends have a big influence on her choice of infant feeding. If she has a lot of formula-feeding friends, she's more likely to formula-feed. It takes a confident or courageous person to break out of line.

Can't see how much he's getting

Our society is obsessed with measurement, and we've been brainwashed into thinking it's important to know how much milk a baby takes. But it very rarely matters, especially if he is healthy and thriving. No two infants are alike, and each needs different amounts of milk at different times. Well-managed breastfeeding is a perfectly balanced demand and supply system, with the emphasis on the supply. The more and better you stimulate your breasts by breastfeeding (or expressing or pumping), with no long gaps and with the baby feeding well, the more milk you'll make.

If ever you fall into the trap of test-weighing your baby to find out how much he's getting, remember that breastfed babies thrive on smaller volumes of milk than formula-feds, partly because breast milk is perfectly digested.

Broken sleep

Breastfeeding helps babies get off to sleep, but breastfed babies tend to sleep less on average than bottle-feds and also tend not to sleep quite as long, especially if they sleep with their mothers and feed at night.

Embarrassing?

Our society equates breasts with sex, and some people think women who reveal their breasts while breastfeeding are immodest or provocative. Yet the idea that women should breastfeed only in private is untenable.

Babies need nourishment when they need it. Women need to go out. And breastfeeding is a human right.

In public, most women choose to breastfeed discreetly, partly for personal reasons, partly to avoid anyone staring or making comments, and partly out of concern for other people's feelings. It's easy to learn how to feed without exposing your breast. A few babies, though, tend to attract attention by making sucking noises when breastfeeding, by kicking in delight, or by choking or spluttering when the milk lets down.

Breastfeeding in public is accepted without question in many developed and developing countries. Public acceptability always advances when a celebrity talks about her breastfeeding or a TV soap or drama, or a film, features a breastfeeding actress.

However, fear of embarrassment deters many women. They may feel anxious not only at the thought of feeding in front of strangers but even (or, sometimes, especially) in front of relatives. For some this is the main thing that puts them off. It's no good telling a woman she needn't be embarrassed, especially if she's breastfeeding for the first time, or is shy and retiring by nature. But perhaps she could use her confidence that she's doing the very best for her baby to strengthen her resolve.

We should all have the courage of our convictions and explain to anyone who makes things difficult for a breastfeeding woman that what she's doing is normal, natural, and best.

Tying?

Some women choose not to breastfeed because they don't want to be tied down. Certainly if a woman is to breastfeed successfully and exclusively, she'll find it easier if she's with her baby than if she has to leave expressed or pumped milk for someone else to give (by cup, spoon, or bottle) while she's out. Some otherwise exclusively breastfeeding women let their babies have the occasional bottle of formula—though this isn't wise for a very young baby (page 144). It isn't wise for his mother either, unless she maintains the stimulus to her milk supply by expressing when she skips a breastfeed.

Outings other than to people's homes may have to be limited in the first few weeks because very young babies can't last long between feeds. This can be overcome if you feed in the car, on a park bench, or in a cafe with sympathetic staff.

Some breastfeeding support groups have lists of shops and other public places that support breastfeeding (For example, the UK food retailer Sainsbury's, among others, provides facilities for breastfeeding customers.) If no such list is available, why not consider compiling one and sending it to your local paper or baby clinic? It could be good publicity for supportive shops.

Rather than worry about never being able to leave your baby, it helps to be positive about taking the baby with you when you go out. There are very few places you can't take a baby, especially a very young, easily transportable one. Even a woman brought up to believe anyone can take her place as a mother may decide to think of her baby as an extension of herself for a few months at least. A baby loves being with his mother, and once this becomes a reality for you, you may not want to go out alone.

Painful?

Some women imagine breastfeeding will be painful. Many breastfeeding women do indeed occasionally have sore nipples, especially early on, and a few have other painful breast conditions. But such problems are usually preventable. And if they do occur they are temporary and easily dealt with.

Unfashionable?

To a certain extent humans have a herd instinct and like to copy each other's behavior. Midwives often remark that if one mother in a postnatal ward is breastfeeding successfully, others tend to copy her. But if she fails, they're likely to stop too.

When formula-feeding first became fashionable, only the relatively wealthy could afford it, but gradually the practice spread, with the middle classes leading the way. But today, women in low-earning families and those with the least education are the ones most likely to formula-feed.

In many hospitals the majority of women start breastfeeding. Once back at home, though, many stop within a few weeks.

Unsexy?

Some women imagine breastfeeding will make them less sexy in their eyes and those of their partner (page 310). But many find the opposite.

Your breasts will sag?

A change in the breasts' shape can happen just as easily to formula-feeders as to breastfeeders. But if you look after your breasts in pregnancy (page 101) and while breastfeeding (page 173), then although when you stop breastfeeding and the milk-producing tissues shrink, they may end up temporarily smaller than before your pregnancy, they'll fill out again with repositioned fat over the next few months.

You won't be able to diet to lose your excess?

A healthy weight-loss program approved for breastfeeding mothers would be okay. But many breastfeeders lose excess "baby-weight" more easily than many formula-feeders anyway (page 184).

Disgusting?

A few women are disgusted by breastfeeding and either refuse to do it or give up after a day or two because it seems "animal-like." One way to help prevent girls growing up with such deep-rooted feelings is to introduce lessons at school mentioning breastfeeding as a normal, natural and beautiful part of child-care. In some schools teachers ask a woman and her breastfeeding baby along to these classes so children can watch and ask questions directly.

Fear of failure?

Unfortunately, disturbing notions of failure are embedded in many young Western women today. And not just about breastfeeding. Not only are most girls raised to fear failure in general, but they have been groomed to see themselves as higher achievers and grade-attainers than boys.

They then observe or otherwise learn that many women stop breastfeeding because they think they haven't enough milk. And it's true that this is by far the most common reason for women to stop breastfeeding (page 199). So they get the idea that failure is almost inevitable.

So at a time in society when potential breastfeeders most fear failure, they absorb the idea that it's hard to succeed. It's scarcely surprising that many decide not to bother even starting.

But even if such a young woman does decide to breastfeed, her very fear can make her fail. She's then likely to be deeply disappointed. This is tragic because babies are denied their natural food and women something they could thoroughly enjoy—and all for nothing, because failure can almost always be avoided. Nearly every woman can breastfeed for as long as she wants if she understands how to make enough milk and has enough help. Taking steps to increase the milk supply generally works within a few days.

Having said this, a very few women are indeed unable to breastfeed fully, whatever they do and whatever help they get. Thankfully they can give their baby formula as well as any breast milk they can make.

four

Breast Milk:
The Perfect Food

O ver scores of thousands of years, each species of mammal has developed milk unique to its own young. Human mothers, of course, are no different. Mammalian milks differ mostly in their content of protein, fat, and carbohydrates. This table shows which milks resemble breast milk most closely:

Fat, protein, and lactose in different mammalian milks

Fat %	Protein %	Lactose %
Donkey 1.2	**Human** 1.1	Rabbit 1.8
Horse 1.6	Donkey 1.7	Whale 1.8
Bison 1.7	Monkey 2.1	Deer 2.6
Goat 3.5	Horse 2.7	Seal 2.6
Monkey 3.9	Goat 3.1	Dog 3.7
Cow 4.5	Cow 3.6	Goat 4.6
Human 4.5	Camel 3.7	Sheep 4.6
Camel 4.9	Bison 4.8	Cow 4.9
Sheep 5.3	Sheep 5.5	Beaver 5
Mink 8	Mink 7	Camel 5.1
Dog 8.3	Dog 9.5	Bison 5.7
Rabbit 12.2	Deer 10.4	Monkey 5.9
Deer 19.7	Rabbit 10.4	Horse 6.1
Whale 34.8	Seal 11.2	**Human** 6.9
Seal 53.2	Whale 13.6	Donkey 6.9
Beaver 56	Beaver 33	Mink 6.9

Compared with other mammalian milks, breast milk contains a moderate amount of fat, extremely little protein, and a very large amount of lactose (milk sugar, a type of carbohydrate).

Animals whose milk contains large amounts of fat and protein, such as rabbits and seals, feed their young much less frequently than animals whose milk has much less fat and protein, such as donkeys and monkeys.

Protein is vital for rapid growth. A young rabbit, for example, doubles its birthweight in about six days. In contrast, this takes a breastfed baby—whose mother's milk has extremely little protein—about 140 days!

Fat in milk helps form a protective layer of fat under the skin. Whale milk, for example, is so high in fat that it's richer than double cream. This is because a baby whale must form a thick layer of blubber very quickly to guard against the cold.

Certain mammals sometimes suckle the young of another species. And over the years there have been a few reports of human young being fed by another animal.

People in various countries over the years have fed their babies with cow, goat, donkey, buffalo, sheep, llama, reindeer, horse, and camel milk, but the first time we used another mammal's milk to any great extent wasn't until early in the twentieth century, when cows'-milk formula became increasingly popular. Today most infant formulas are made from modified cows' milk.

Why was cows' milk chosen as our preferred substitute for breast milk? After all, it's by no means the nearest in composition—a donkey's, for example, is much more similar in its content of protein and lactose.

It happened because the great move toward artificial feeding started in the West, where cows were already being reared for meat and dairy products. Cows are also easily milked. And they produce large volumes of milk, so their milk is cheap.

Differences between breast milk and cows' milk

Cows' milk—whether pasteurized, raw, full-cream, semi-skimmed, skimmed, liquid, or dry—contains three times as much protein but only around two-thirds as much lactose as breast milk. This meant the early modifications of cows' milk to resemble breast milk more closely involved diluting it with water and adding sugar.

However, over the years more and more differences between cows' milk and breast milk have emerged and companies have made repeated modifications in their never-ending and hopeless quest to replicate the unique contents of breast milk.

What breast milk contains

Milk, or "white blood" as it's called in parts of India, is a fascinating fluid that's as much a food as a drink. It contains water, proteins, fats, carbohydrates, minerals, vitamins, anti-infective factors, hormones, growth factors, anti-inflammatories, enzymes, white cells, good bacteria, and trace amounts of whole food protein molecules the mother has eaten, perfumes or medications she's used, and environmental contaminants she's been exposed to.

Water

Water makes up the bulk of breast milk. Other constituents are dissolved or suspended in the water, making the milk white, creamy, translucent or yellow, depending on their proportions. The proportion of water is just right for babies, even if the milk looks "watery."

A thirsty baby given enough breast milk automatically gets enough water, so a breastfed baby who drinks enough breast milk never needs extra water. In very hot weather, a breastfeeding mother needs to drink more so neither she nor her baby becomes dehydrated. In contrast, a thirsty bottle-fed baby who drinks a lot more formula than usual risks getting too much of certain substances, especially if bottle-feeds are made up too strong. This can be particularly dangerous for a baby already dehydrated from diarrhea, vomiting, or a fever. He needs more water, not more formula, and certainly not more extra-strength formula.

Proteins

Breast milk's protein comprises casein, serum albumin, lactalbumin, immunoglobulin (antibodies), lactoferrin, folate- and vitamin B12-binding proteins, enzymes, hormones, and growth factors. Casein is the protein in the solid part—the curds—of curdled milk, so it's sometimes called curd protein. The other proteins are called whey proteins because they are present in the liquid part—the whey—of curdled milk. When a baby swallows breast milk, the stomach acid separates into curds and whey.

Cows' milk is much richer in protein than is breast milk. Its relatively high protein level is necessary because a calf grows fast, doubling its birthweight in 50 days, whereas this takes at least 180 days in the average breast baby.

Cows' milk also contains six times as much casein as whey protein, whereas breast milk contains one and a half times as much whey protein as casein. This means that cows' milk curds are much bulkier, tougher, and more rubbery than breast-milk curds. And this is why babies get indigestion if they drink unmodified cows' milk. The main reason why formula manufacturers dilute cows' milk with water is that this dilutes the tough indigestible casein. Boiling, homogenization, and the addition of various chemicals also make it less tough and indigestible.

Some infant formulas are manufactured to be "whey dominant," with a whey-to-casein ratio similar to that of breast milk. Others remain "casein dominant," with a whey-to-casein ratio close to that of cows' milk.

Once breast-milk protein is in the stomach, it forms finely separated curds whose small size enables them to pass into the gut after only about one and a half hours. In contrast, cows' milk curds stay in the stomach for about four hours. A breastfed baby's stomach therefore empties faster than that of a formula-fed baby. So a breastfed baby gets hungry faster and needs more frequent feeds.

Clearly then, while four-hourly feeds for a bottle-fed baby make sense, breastfed babies need feeding more often.

A formula-fed baby uses only about half the protein he consumes from infant formula, whilst a breastfed uses 95 percent of that in breast milk. Some of the protein a bottle-fed baby doesn't use is passed out in his stools, making them smelly (unlike those of a breastfed baby) and bulkier than those of a breastfed baby.

Because breast milk produces so little waste, breastfed babies actually need less milk than formula-fed ones.

Amino acids

The proportions of free amino acids differ in breast milk and cows' milk. Breast milk, for instance, contains more cystine; cows' milk contains more methionine. This is important for pre-term babies as they can't yet use methionine. Cows' milk also contains less taurine than does breast milk, which is why it's added to infant formula.

Nucleotides

These molecules are present in breast milk but only in minimal amounts, and in different proportions, in cows'-milk formula. They act as building blocks for genes, and for the "cofactors" that are vital for certain enzymatic reactions. They encourage the growth of "good" bowel bacteria, and participate in "cellular signaling" (communication between cells). And they help induce sleep. Most babies make their own, but pre-term and some full-term babies can't make enough. Although scientists aren't aware of any deficiency problems, nucleotides are added to some formula milks.

Fats

These are the main sources of energy in cows' milk and breast milk and are also needed for many aspects of growth and development. They mostly occur as globules of triglyceride fats but are also present in cholesterol, free fatty acids, and phospholipids.

Fatty acids are the building blocks of fats and are classed as saturated, monounsaturated, or polyunsaturated, depending on their structure. Those in breast milk are mainly unsaturated, those in cows' milk mainly saturated. The proportions of fatty acids in breast and cows' milk reflect the types of fats eaten by the woman or by the cows whose milk is pooled together to make formula, though some fatty acids are also made by breast or udder cells.

The amount of fat in breast milk varies from one woman to another. The fat content of any one woman's milk varies during a feed. In the first breast, there is two to three times as much fat at the end of a feed as at the beginning. Breast milk's fat content also changes during the weeks and months after childbirth.

Polyunsaturated fatty acids (PUFAs)—These are particularly important for various aspects of growth and development. For example, they are vital for the development of the PUFA-rich coverings of certain nerve fibers.

Breast milk contains a higher percentage of PUFAs than does cows' milk. Cows'-milk formula contains enough to prevent overt deficiency symptoms of poor growth and thick scaly skin, but some manufacturers increase the PUFA content of particular formulas by replacing some of the saturated fat of cows' milk with vegetable oil.

There are two groups of PUFAs, the omega-6s and omega-3s. Their amounts and proportions differ in breast milk and infant formula.

However, arachidonic acid (AA, an omega-6) and docosahexaenoic acid (DHA, an omega-3) are found only in breast milk. They are particularly important for brain, eye, and nerve development. Indeed, about one-quarter of a baby's brain is made of DHA and AA! Interestingly, researchers have found that breastfed babies of women whose milk is relatively high in DHA sleep better than those of women with lower levels.

Essential fatty acids—Healthy full-term babies can make DHA, AA, and other PUFAs with long-chain molecules, from the "parent" omega-6 and omega-3 PUFAs. The parent omega-6 is linoleic acid, and the parent omega-3 is alpha-linolenic acid. These "parents" are called "essential" fatty acids because our body can't make them. We have to get them from food.

Breastfed babies get all the DHA and AA they need from breast milk. However, infant formula contains highly variable amounts of essential fatty acids. Indeed, it may contain no alpha-linolenic acid. Even if a formula does contain enough essential fatty acids, some babies can't convert them into other omega-3 and omega-6 PUFAs fast enough.

This explains why some formula-fed babies may not get enough DHA for optimal eyesight development. It also explains why pre-term formula-fed babies may not get enough AA for optimal growth or mental development. Making the PUFA-profile of infant formula resemble that of breast milk is expensive. But some formulas—including most of those for pre-terms—are now enriched with these fatty acids.

Why the amounts of fats are important—Researchers wonder whether the amounts and ratios of saturated and monounsaturated fats and PUFAs in breast milk help protect a baby against arterial disease and, therefore, heart attacks and strokes, in later life. Certainly breastfed babies have lower levels of several heart-disease risk factors in later life. Also, we know there is more of another fat, cholesterol, in breast milk than in cows' milk. It's possible, though unproven, that the cholesterol in breast milk helps accustom babies at handling cholesterol. If so, this might reduce their risk of arterial disease.

Digestion of fats—Gut enzymes called lipases split fats into simpler fatty substances. Splitting cows' milk fat releases palmitic acid, a fatty acid that combines with calcium then leaves the body, along with the calcium, in the bowel motions. In breast milk, palmitic acid is built into fat particles in such a way that when fat is digested, its palmitic acid is absorbed into the blood with part of the broken-down fat particle. So calcium isn't lost, which is important because babies need plentiful calcium to build strong bones and teeth.

Unlike cows' milk, which relies solely on the baby's gut lipase for its digestion, breast milk contains some lipase of its own. But breast-milk fat starts being digested by breast-milk lipase even before it reaches the gut. So fatty acids are available sooner from breast milk than from formula.

The digestion of breast-milk fats and cows'-milk fats produces fatty acids as well as simpler fats that help guard against infection.

If a breastfed baby brings up milk, the smell isn't particularly unpleasant, whereas a formula-fed baby's vomit has a much sourer smell which quickly permeates clothing. The difference results from the presence in formula of butyric acid, a fatty acid that smells nasty when partially digested.

Carbohydrates

These supply sweetness and energy and have other benefits too.

Lactose—This forms up to 95 percent of the carbohydrate in breast milk, which is why it tastes so sweet. Given the choice of breast milk or formula, babies prefer breast milk, probably partly because of its sweetness.

Both breast milk and cows' milk contain lactose but breast milk has much more. In the gut, some breast-milk lactose is split into the simple sugars galactose and glucose (see below). The rest travels through undigested, which improves the absorption of calcium and encourages a healthy balance of microorganisms.

Lactose aids the absorption of magnesium, calcium, zinc, and iron.

Galactose—is an important part of myelin, the fatty coating of nerves.

Glucose—Both breast milk and formula contain glucose.

Oligosaccharides—After lactose and fat, these form the next largest group of substances in mature breast milk. Breast milk contains at least 140 different oligosaccharides, while infant formula contains only a very small amount of some and none of others. Breast milk contains more than 15 g/L of oligosaccharides, whereas formula contains only about 9 g/L. Although oligosaccharides are sugars, they aren't digested in the gut.

Oligosaccharides are prebiotics, which means they encourage a healthy population of bacteria in the gut. A baby's gut contains trillions of bacteria of about 1,000 different types. In a breastfed baby, oligosaccharides aid the growth and activity of "good" (probiotic) gut bacteria such as lactobacilli (see page 77) and bifidobacteria. And they suppress the growth and activity of potentially harmful gut bacteria, by preventing them sticking to the gut lining.

Each mother's milk contains a unique blend of oligosaccharides, so the proportions and types of bacteria in each baby's bowel are unique to that mother-baby pair.

Oligosaccharides in traces of breast milk in the throat during and after a feed prevent bacteria such as pneumococci and *Haemophilus influenzae* sticking to the throat, which discourages respiratory infections. They also help prevent urine infections. What's more, there's some evidence to suggest they aid brain development.

There's evidence that oligosaccharides help prevent flu, poor immunity, inflammation, high blood pressure, and high cholesterol in adults. We don't yet know if they have a current or future protective effect in babies.

Formula manufacturers can't yet reproduce the exact types and proportions of oligosaccharides in breast milk.

Minerals

Cows' milk contains almost four times as much sodium, calcium, phosphorus, iron, fluoride, and magnesium, as does breast milk. Manufacturers reduce the mineral content of cows' milk when making infant formula, so as to prevent an overload damaging a baby's kidneys. But in no formula is the mineral content as low as in breast milk.

One reason why it's better not to give cows' milk to a baby under a year old is because its sodium makes it four times as salty as breast milk. This could mean the kidneys have trouble getting rid of it, which could encourage dehydration.

Iron is exceptional as there's much more in breast milk than in cows' milk.

Sodium—The low level in breast milk is ideal for babies because sodium is closely linked with water and an imbalance can be serious, even fatal. This is why formula-fed babies need particular care if they become dehydrated, and why formula must never be made up too strong.

Calcium—Babies absorb calcium more efficiently from breast milk than from formula. This may be because the high level of lactose in breast milk promotes the absorption of calcium from the gut. The relatively low calcium in breast milk aids the absorption of iron from a baby's gut.

Breast milk has a higher ratio of calcium to phosphorus than does formula. This is thought to aid absorption of calcium from the baby's gut, and the uptake of calcium by a baby's bones.

Formula manufacturers have reduced the level of calcium in formulas but even so, there's a little less in breast milk.

Phosphorus—There's nearly seven times less phosphorus in breast milk than in formula. Breast milk's relatively low phosphorus aids the absorption of iron from a baby's gut. Breast milk also has a higher ratio of calcium to phosphorus than does formula. This is thought to aid absorption of phosphorus from the baby's gut, and the uptake of phosphorus by a baby's bones.

The amount in breast milk changes as a baby grows older, while that in formula remains the same.

Iron—There's twice as much iron in breast milk as in cows' milk, so manufacturers add iron when making formula. Indeed, formula contains more iron than does breast milk. However, vitamins C and E, lactose, and copper, all present in higher amounts in breast milk, encourage more efficient absorption of iron, and breast milk's relatively low concentration of proteins, calcium and phosphorus helps too. So a baby absorbs iron better from breast milk than from formula.

A fully breastfed full-term baby of a healthy mother almost never develops iron-deficiency anemia in the first six months, because breastfed babies absorb about half the iron in breast milk, whereas bottle-fed babies absorb only one tenth of that in formula. However, pre-term babies may need supplements of iron before the age of six months.

Fluoride—see page 23.

Trace elements—These minerals include boron, chromium, cobalt, copper, iodine, manganese, molybdenum, selenium, silicon, and zinc. Many are essential as they form parts of enzymes. There's generally enough of most of them in breast milk, and formula, but breast milk may be low in selenium (an antioxidant) if a woman doesn't eat enough selenium-containing food. It's possible that some formulas could be improved by having more selenium.

Vitamins

Breast milk contains more vitamins A, C, and E than does cows' milk but less vitamin K. Evidence suggests that the fully breastfed babies of women who were well nourished in pregnancy, and who eat a well-balanced diet while breastfeeding, don't normally need any vitamin supplements in their first six months.

Vitamin A and carotenoids—These are present in breast milk and cows' milk. Carotenoids are yellowish substances that the body can make into vitamin A and use as antioxidants to protect cells from damage by free radicals (unstable oxygen particles) during illness and stress, for example. Beta-carotene forms 24 percent of breast milk's carotenoids and 85 percent of those in cows' milk. Other carotenoids in breast milk include lycopene and beta-cryptoxanthine, though many remain unidentified. The amounts of carotenoids vary considerably from one woman to another. They also vary according to how many babies a woman has had, what she's eaten, and the time of day.

Vitamin C—This is concentrated in breast milk. So babies of women with a vitamin-C deficiency don't have a deficiency—it's the mother who needs supplements.

Vitamin D—This enables minerals such as calcium to enter and strengthen bones, helping prevent rickets (soft, bendy bones). Colostrum (breast milk produced in the few days after delivery) contains more vitamin D than mature milk, but vitamin D-fortified formula has much more than either.

Your skin produces vitamin D after exposure to the sun's ultraviolet rays and your body stores it for use in the darker months. The amount in your diet has only a small influence on your vitamin D level.

A baby whose face is exposed to bright outdoor daylight for just 15 minutes a day in the summer months in the UK or countries of similar latitudes, makes enough of his own vitamin D.

But there isn't always enough vitamin D from breast milk or daylight to strengthen a baby's bones, so all pre-term and some full-term breastfed babies benefit from a supplement. A supplement is especially important for babies whose mothers go outside very little, always cover their skin, are malnourished, or eat a vegetarian diet containing a lot of chapattis (because chapatti flour contains substances which prevent calcium absorption).

Vitamin K—Breast milk contains less than cows' milk. Hemorrhagic disease of the newborn results from a shortage of vitamin K. It makes the gut bleed and is more common in breastfed babies. Many doctors recommend vitamin K after birth, by injection and/or by mouth, for all newborns, whether or not the mother breastfeeds.

A woman who breastfeeds frequently is likely to produce

more milk—and therefore more vitamin K—more quickly than a schedule-feeder.

Anti-infective factors

Many factors in breast milk help fight infection in babies, whereas formula has very little anti-infective power: When a baby begins to develop an infection, the breast can sense this, presumably via the baby's saliva. It then instructs the immune system to make more antibodies, and lactoferrin.

The proportions of nutrients—breast milk prevents the growth in the baby's gut of certain potentially harmful organisms, including *Escherichia coli* (a common cause of gastroenteritis in formula-fed babies) and dysentery and typhoid bacteria. Breast milk's high lactose, low phosphorus and low protein are particularly helpful.

Lactoferrin—Colostrum is particularly rich in this important anti-infective, iron-binding whey protein, though it's also present in mature milk. It constitutes up to 25 percent of breast-milk protein and there's 10–20 times more in breast milk than in cows' milk. Lactoferrin

- Activates genes responsible for the body's immune response.
- Inhibits the growth of certain potentially harmful organisms, including *Escherichia coli*, *Staphylococcus aureus*, yeasts, and, perhaps hepatitis-C viruses, by removing iron.
- Makes certain bacteria more susceptible to damage by lysozyme (see below).
- Helps act against a parasite called cryptosporidium.
- Transports iron to where it's needed.
- May prevent cancer cells getting the iron they need for growth.
- Has anti-inflammatory action.

Like antibodies and enzymes, lactoferrin loses its anti-infective activity when milk is heated, so the small amount in fresh cows' milk becomes useless during the manufacture of infant formula.

Lactoferrin can be produced by genetic engineering, in which a human lactoferrin-production gene is introduced into cows or soy beans, for example. Formula manufacturers are increasingly interested in adding lactoferrin to their products.

Immunoglobulins—These proteins are antibodies, of which the most abundant is immunoglobulin A (IgA). Others include IgD, IgE, IgG, and IgM. Breast-milk antibodies coat the gut lining and prevent many infective organisms and large protein molecules from entering the blood. In a baby's early weeks they can also be absorbed into the blood. Colostrum contains especially large amounts.

IgA helps combat bacterial, fungal and viral illnesses from which the mother has suffered (including diphtheria, dysentery, flu, gastroenteritis from *Escherichia coli*, polio, pneumonia, rubella, tetanus, typhoid, whooping cough, and various other viral illnesses). It may also help protect against infections to which she's been immunized, though any such protection is small and unpredictable. And it can protect against certain food antigens (food proteins that can trigger food sensitivity in some babies).

A growing baby gradually begins to manufacture his own antibodies in response to infection or immunization. A full-term baby's gut cells sometimes begin to make IgA at around 12 days, though the concentration of IgA-producing cells in the gut doesn't reach the adult level until he's two years old. The early months of gradually increasing antibody formation is called the "immunity gap." Only breast milk can fill this gap, because although raw cows' milk contains antibodies, the heating involved in formula manufacture inactivates them.

Interestingly, calves reared on heat-treated milk or dried milk powder get more enteritis than those drinking fresh untreated milk. The treatment is fresh cows' milk! A parallel was seen in a nursery of formula-fed babies in Belgrade, where an epidemic of *Escherichia coli* gastroenteritis couldn't be stopped even when the babies were fed with donated and boiled breast milk. It was controlled only when breast milk was given raw.

Lysozyme and complement—These proteins interact with IgA to kill bacteria and viruses. Lysozyme is an enzyme present in breast milk in amounts 300 times greater than in cows' milk. It's a "natural antibiotic" that damages bacterial cell walls. Breast-milk lysozyme levels fall in the first few months, then rise until at six months there's more than there was in colostrum, and at one year there's even more.

Cows' milk has significantly less lysozyme, so manufacturers are increasingly interested in adding it to infant formula.

Anti-staphylococcal factor and hydrogen peroxide—These are present in particularly large amounts in colostrum. Together with vitamin C they help kill potentially harmful bacteria such as *Escherichia* in a baby's gut. Hydrogen peroxide is released by lactobacilli in breast milk (see below). There's some evidence that hydrogen peroxide is an *anticancer* agent.

Lactobacilli and other "good" bacteria—Around 800 types of "good" (probiotic) bacteria are naturally present in breast milk and they are very useful constituents. They get there by by traveling in white cells from the mother's gut to her breasts' milk-producing cells. Breast-milk lactobacilli influence which genes are activated in her baby's gut, thereby influencing his digestion. They also release hydrogen peroxide, which has anti-infective properties. Lactobacilli are destroyed when fresh cows' milk is processed to produce infant formula.

Fibronectin—This protein encourages white cells to mop up harmful bacteria. It also reduces inflammation. The large amounts in colostrum explain why breastfed babies have higher levels in their blood than do formula-fed babies.

Live cells—These white cells are the same as certain white cells found in blood. They make breast milk a living fluid. Fresh cows' milk also contains living cells, but these are killed as milk is processed into formula.

White cells from a breastfeed can stick to the gut lining for 60 hours. Those called lymphocytes make antibodies as well as the antiviral substance interferon. And they can be absorbed into the blood where they continue making antibodies. Researchers believe hormonal and other factors in breastfeeding women send IgA-producing lymphocytes called T-cells from her gut's lymph tissue to her breasts. These T-cells tell her milk's lymphocytes about potentially harmful organisms in her bowel so they can protect her baby. They also "remember" past infections and protect against similar new ones for years. White cells called neutrophils, granulocytes, and epithelial cells are found in breast milk and in even larger amounts in colostrum.

Macrophages are large white cells that can engulf foreign particles such as bacteria. They also produce lactoferrin, lysozyme, and complement; may help transport antibodies; and are thought to protect against necrotizing enterocolitis in pre-term babies (page 27).

Mucins—These substances contain protein and carbohydrate and are probably responsible for half the antiviral activity of breast milk. They can stick to unwanted bacteria and viruses and carry them from the body in the bowel motions. They are especially active against the rotaviruses often responsible for diarrhea.

Older babies make their own mucins in their gut. Cows' milk's mucins are removed during formula manufacture. One researcher suggests that if mucins could be synthesized they would make a useful addition to formula.

Free fatty acids—can damage the protein membranes of "enveloped" viruses, such as the chickenpox virus. This may mean that infections with these viruses are less severe in breastfed babies.

Hormones

Breast milk contains many hormones and hormone-like factors, including corticosteroids, erythropoietin, gonadotropins, gonadotropin-releasing hormone, insulin, estrogens, parathyroid hormone, progesterone, prolactin, relaxin, thyroid hormones, and thyroid-releasing and thyroid-stimulating hormones. Some come from the mother's blood; others are made in her breasts.

Certain of them stimulate the breasts to make milk proteins and enzymes. Others, including insulin, prolactin, thyroid stimulating hormone, and thyroxine, may be important to her baby.

Erythropoietin helps regulate red-blood-cell production, and it's been suggested that it may help protect pre-term babies from anemia.

Prostaglandins—These are hormone-like substances found in breast milk but not in formula. A baby with a good balance of omega-3 and omega-6 polyunsaturated fatty acids makes a healthy balance of prostaglandins. The concentration of prostaglandins E and F in breast milk is 100 times that in a woman's plasma (the liquid part of her blood). One function may be to help a baby absorb zinc from breast milk.

Growth factors

Breast milk contains many growth factors.

Epidermal growth factor, for example, is a hormone-like polypeptide (protein fragment) that stimulates the multiplication and development of several types of cell, including certain gut-lining cells. There's a lot in colostrum, and it's particularly valuable for very-low-birthweight babies. There's very much less in infant formula.

Another important growth factor, especially for very-low-birthweight babies, is called transforming growth factor beta. This helps prevent the spread of harmful inflammation.

Anti-inflammatories

Various substances in breast milk discourage harmful inflammation in a baby. They include lactoferrin, fibronectin, and interleukin-10, as well as substances derived from plant-based foods, such as flavonoid plant pigments and salicylates.

Enzymes

More than 70 enzymes have been identified in breast milk. Some are important for a baby's digestion or development, and most are at their highest concentration in colostrum. Lipase has been mentioned. Lactoperoxidase inhibits bacterial growth. Other enzymes include aldolase, acid and alkaline phosphatases, amylase, anti-trypsin, catalase, glutathione peroxidase, lysozyme, and xanthine oxidase.

Enzymes are destroyed by heat. Most enzymes in cows' milk are destroyed by heating during formula manufacture.

Cannabinoids

Breast milk contains at least five natural marijuana-like substances called endocannabinoids. These are cannabinoids produced by the body, as opposed to coming from food (such as green tea or raw cows' milk), or from smoking marijuana.

Breast milk's endocannabinoids activate cannabinoid receptors throughout the body. This stimulates appetite, stimulates a newborn's sucking reflex, is calming and relaxing, and can reduce pain and inflammation, widen airways, and regulate immunity. Scientists suspect it also discourages vomiting, allergy, and cancer; promotes bone growth and optimal energy metabolism; and helps keep nerves healthy.

Breast milk contains three to eight times as high a level as does cows' milk and the highest level is found on the day after birth. Endocannabinoids apparently aren't present in infant formula

Food traces, drugs, perfumes, and environmental contaminants

Breast milk may contain such things as alcohol, caffeine, and trace amounts of whole food-protein molecules. It may also contain certain drugs taken by a breastfeeding woman, particular perfume ingredients (such as musk), and certain environmental contaminants (page 292).

Colored milk

Breast milk varies in color. For example, colostrum is yellower than mature milk, and milk produced early in a feed—especially from the first breast—tends to be more translucent than later milk. Very occasionally other colors are seen.

Yellow milk

Taking a supplement of beta-carotene (made by the body into vitamin A) can color breast milk yellow. Probably eating a large number of satsumas could too, as they can temporarily color skin yellowish-orange.

Red, pink, brown, orange, or otherwise blood-stained milk

Seeing blood in your milk can be a shock, but it's rarely anything to worry about. Check your breasts and if you are concerned about anything, consult your doctor. A cracked or sore nipple is the most likely cause.

Some women's milk is blood-stained in the first week after delivery with no sign of anything else wrong. This is rare, generally disappears within two to five days, and doesn't harm the baby. You can continue breastfeeding. The most likely cause is leaking of red blood cells from blood vessels. Milk normally contains a few of these cells, though a lot are needed to color it.

Blood in breast milk occasionally comes from a tumor. This is almost always noncancerous, and the discoloration stops once breastfeeding is well under way. Discuss with your doctor whether you need further examination.

Green milk

Milk can go green if a woman takes the iron-containing drug ferritin.

Milk of assorted hues

As milk stagnates in a blocked duct or milk retention cyst (one that develops behind a plug in an untreated blocked duct), it can turn one of many colors, including deep yellow, brown, green, and even blue-black. This results from various substances, including cholesterol, cholesterol 5,6-epoxides, estrogens, and fluorescent compounds (including lipofucsin complexes) from oxidized fats.

A smoker's milk may be darker than that of a nonsmoker.

Breast milk's unique scent

Studies in France and England have found that a baby turns to a nursing pad that's been next to his mother's breast in preference to a clean one that hasn't. However, a baby doesn't turn to a pad soaked in his mother's expressed breast milk. So contact of the pad with the breast skin is more important than any milk getting on to the pad. Babies prefer the smell of their own mother's breast to that of other mothers. What on the mother's breast enables this recognition isn't known, but it could be the smell of natural hormone-like substances called pheromones. One study found that 22 of 30 babies preferred the smell of their mother's breast when it was unwashed rather than washed.

Bottle-fed babies like the smell of a pad soaked in breast milk, whoever it's from, and prefer it to that of a pad soaked in their usual formula.

How breast milk changes

Breast-milk's composition varies according to the time since childbirth and the time of day. It also varies during a feed. And it varies according to whether the baby is a boy or a girl. All this is beneficial to a baby.

A calf feeding from its mother benefits from similar changes in her milk. But a formula-fed baby drinks milk of a highly consistent composition because milk converted into infant formula is taken from many cows at different stages of lactation and removed at different times of day.

Colostrum

This is the first milk. It's made from halfway through pregnancy until up to a week or so after birth. It contains nine times as much protein as does mature milk, but less sugar and fat (though it's particularly rich in docosahexaenoic acid). Most important, it contains large amounts of immunoglobulin-A antibodies, giving a newborn baby resistance to infection when he's particularly susceptible.

Formula-fed newborns don't get colostrum. Yet so valuable is it in protecting against infection that some experts believe every formula-fed baby should have a "colostrum cocktail." Indeed, when farmers take calves from their mothers immediately after birth, they give them cows' colostrum ("beestings") for three days to prevent potentially fatal diarrhea called "the scours."

Colostrum looks yellowish because it's rich in beta-carotene. In a newborn it speeds the passage of meconium (sticky, tar-like early bowel motions) through the gut, reducing the absorption of bile pigments, naturally occurring substances that encourage jaundice.

A few days after birth, colostrum becomes more milky and is sometimes called transitional milk. This gradually changes into mature milk.

The amount of colostrum isn't fixed. Letting a baby suck frequently and as long as he wants in the first few days not only provides more colostrum but also hastens the arrival of mature milk.

Mature milk

This contains only a fifth of the protein of colostrum but more fat and sugar. It's also whiter and thinner looking. A baby grows fastest in the first six months, when breast milk contains its highest levels of protein. The amount of protein gradually falls during the first year.

The contents of mature milk vary according to a mother's diet, the frequency of feeds and her baby's age. After the first few weeks many breast-feeding women produce 25–33 fluid ounces (700–940 mL) of milk a day.

Changes during a feed

Early in a feed from the first breast the milk usually looks rather thin, and white or bluish-white. It is relatively low in fat and contains around 10 calories per 25 mL (1 fl oz). The amount of fat in the milk taken from the first breast gradually increases. Toward the end of the feed from that side, the milk usually has up to two or three times as much fat and up to one-and-a-half times as much protein as at the beginning. This makes it look thicker and creamy-white. It also has a different "mouth-feel" as it is more viscous. It contains around 30 calories per 1 fl oz (25 mL).

In the second breast, the differences in the content, appearance, and mouth-feel of milk at the beginning and end of a feed from that side are less dramatic. This is because milk is let down in that breast as the baby feeds from the first breast, and this mixes with the milk already in the ducts and reservoirs.

The changing composition of milk during a feed means a baby who feeds at the first breast for as long as he wants finishes that side with higher-fat milk. If he then feeds from the second breast, the milk is less fatty at first, but even so has more fat than the early milk from the first breast.

Milk whose let-down (release) from the milk-producing glands is triggered by the strong milking and sucking action of a well-latched-on baby tends to be higher in fat than milk that is let down without being milked by a baby, or that is let down by hand expression a baby. Higher-fat milk stays in a baby's stomach and gut longer, so it satisfies him for longer and means he's likely to need fewer feeds than a baby who may get the same volume but doesn't suck or milk so strongly.

Changes during the day

The levels of various constituents of breast milk change throughout the 24-hour day according to a baby's expected needs. For example, it contains its lowest levels of fat in the early hours of the morning, and its highest level of nucleotides—which induce sleep—at night. This suggests it's better to give expressed milk at the same time of day that it was expressed.

- Researchers in Spain measured the levels of three nucleotides (adenosine, guanosine, and uridine) in milk expressed by 30 women six to eight times a day. The samples expressed from 8:00 p.m. to 8:00 a.m. contained the highest concentrations (*Nutritional Neuroscience*, 2009).

Milk for a boy or milk for a girl?

A woman's milk contains more fat and protein if she's breastfeeding a boy than if she's breastfeeding a girl. This is probably one of Nature's way of enabling faster and bigger growth in a boy.

Monthly changes when periods return

When a breastfeeding woman eventually starts to ovulate again, her milk alters slightly before and after ovulation. At five to six days before ovulation (which is usually between days 10–14 of the monthly cycle, with the first day of the cycle being the first day of menstrual bleeding), the milk changes slightly in composition for about 28 hours. A similar change happens at six to seven days after ovulation and lasts for about 32 hours. In both cases there's temporarily less lactose, glucose, and potassium, and more sodium and chloride. Some experienced breastfeeders believe babies notice these changes. Others report a temporary decrease in milk supply, or a less reliable let-down reflex, around the time of a period.

Toward the end of breastfeeding

As a baby breastfeeds less and less, breast milk dwindles and gradually looks thicker, yellower, and more like colostrum.

Pre-term milk

Mothers of pre-term babies produce "pre-term milk." This has a different composition from mature milk, with around 30 percent more protein and higher concentrations of lipase and many minerals (including calcium, iron, and sodium).

As a pre-term baby grows, his mother's milk gradually changes to meet his changing needs.

While a very-low-birthweight pre-term baby will need extra nutrients, given as human-milk fortifier (page 251), the milk of the mother of a heavier pre-term baby is just right for his particular needs.

five

Preparation and Pregnancy

There's a lot you can do now to prepare for breastfeeding. First and foremost, look after your health and well-being so you feel your best and your baby gets a good start. This is also a good time to learn about breastfeeding, to discuss it with your partner, and to find out who will help when necessary. It's sensible to prepare your home so things run as smoothly as possible when the baby arrives. And you need to choose where to have your baby.

What to eat

Eat a healthy balanced diet with five helpings of vegetables and fruit a day. The B vitamin folate (present in supplements as folic acid), calcium, iron, fiber, and a good balance of omega-3 and omega-6 polyunsaturated fatty acids, are particularly important now.

We'll discuss only calcium, omega-3s and 6s, and vitamin D, as these are particularly important if you're going to breastfeed.

Calcium

During pregnancy you absorb more calcium from food. But if your diet is low in calcium, your bones may release some of their stored calcium to meet your unborn baby's needs. This weakens your bones—albeit temporarily.

Calcium-rich foods—include fish, shellfish, eggs, milk, yogurt, cheese, cabbage, watercress, peas, beans, lentils, whole-grain foods, nuts, seeds, tinned sardines eaten with their bones, and homemade soups and stocks made by boiling chicken or other meat bones in water to which you've added a tablespoon of vinegar (which releases their calcium).

A good balance of omega-3 and omega-6 fatty acids

This discourages postpartum depression, so could mean breastfeeding is more likely to be successful.

Omega-3-rich foods—include green leafy vegetables, broccoli, beans, tofu, walnuts (a particularly rich source) and their oil, pumpkin seeds, linseeds (flaxseeds—the richest source), rapeseed (canola), soy and olive oils, meat from grass-fed animals, fish (especially oily fish), and shellfish.

Omega-6-rich foods—include avocados; beans; corn; seeds; rapeseed (canola), sunflower, safflower, sesame, peanut (groundnut), and soybean oils; spreads made from these oils; cereal and other grain-based foods; eggs; and meat from corn or cereal-grain-fed animals.

Scientists recommend having two to four times as much omega-6 as omega-3. But the average westernized diet provides at least 10–20 times as much. So the average pregnant woman has far too much omega-6 intake for optimal health.

Correct any suspected imbalance by eating

- Less cereal-grain food (such as bread, biscuits, breakfast cereal), grain-fed meat, and spreads and other processed foods containing sunflower oil.
- More green leafy vegetables and fish.

Vitamin D

This vitamin aids calcium absorption. Getting enough in pregnancy enables calcium to strengthen your unborn baby's developing bones, thus helping to prevent calcium being taken from yours. It also fortifies your bones, ready for when breast milk supplies calcium to your baby and draws it from your bones if your diet is lacking.

Vitamin D has various other health benefits for you and your baby, and there's some evidence that it helps prevent preeclampsia.

Your main source of this vital vitamin is from the sun's ultraviolet (UV) rays converting cholesterol in your skin to vitamin D. So spend time outside each day in bright daylight, and without sunscreen. Window glass filters out some UV, the amount depending on the type of glass. In countries far from the equator, such as the UK and parts of the US, bright daylight on your face for a few minutes a day in spring, summer and autumn can build sufficient vitamin D stores to last the winter, when the sun's rays are too oblique to make vitamin D in the skin.

A vitamin D supplement?—It's almost impossible to get enough vitamin D from food. And it can be difficult to get enough from bright outdoor daylight on your skin, especially if you're dark-skinned; cover most of your skin (particularly if you also wear a veil); live in very northerly or southerly climes; live in a city with polluted air; or use copious amounts of frequently applied sunscreen. So a supplement could be useful. The recommendations vary from one country to another. For example,

In the UK, the Department of Health recommends a daily vitamin D supplement of 10 micrograms (400 international units—IU) for all pregnant women.

In the US, the National Institutes of Health says the recommended daily amount of vitamin D for pregnant women is 600 IU (15 micrograms). Most over-the-counter vitamin supplements for pregnancy contain 200–400 IU (5–10 micrograms).

In Australia, the Ministry of Health notes that pregnant women who are regularly exposed to sunlight don't need a supplement. But for those who get little sunlight, one of 10 micrograms/day wouldn't be excessive.

Note, though, that some experts suggest that a low vitamin D level in pregnancy may be normal. However, until more is known, most women prefer to adhere to the official recommendations for the country in which they live.

Vegetarian or vegan?

If you're a vegetarian, make particularly sure you eat enough foods rich in

- Iron (page 178).

- Calcium (page 85).

- Zinc—including nuts, whole-grain foods, peas, beans, root vegetables, and garlic).

- Vitamin B12—including eggs, milk, cheese, and yogurt. Note that whatever its source, this vitamin comes from microorganisms.

If you're a vegan (someone who eats no food of animal origin), you need a supplement of vitamin B12.

Avoid the foods most likely to be infected with listeria bacteria

Many experts recommend avoiding soft cheeses such as Camembert and Brie, blue cheeses, unpasteurized cheeses, and insufficiently reheated cook-chilled foods in pregnancy, because of the risk that they may contain an overgrowth of listeria. This is normally harmless but in some pregnant women causes a flu-like infection that can damage their unborn baby.

Avoid liver and liver paté

Many experts recommend avoiding these because they contain high levels of vitamin A that could, at worst, damage an unborn baby.

Your weight

Most women eat no more than usual in early pregnancy and only about 100 calories a day more near the end. But if you're very active or underweight, you may want, or need, to eat more. If you have "morning sickness" (nausea and, perhaps, vomiting, which can in reality occur at any time of day), you won't feel like eating while you're actually nauseous but you can rest assured that this won't harm your baby. Morning sickness is considered normal because it affects one in two pregnant women. Such women are less likely to miscarry their baby, suggesting that morning sickness may be protective in some way.

The average pregnant woman gains 15–40 lb (7–18 kg), composed of the baby, placenta, amniotic fluid, increased size of the womb and breasts, increased volume of blood and other body fluids, and 4–7 lb (2–3 kg) of extra fat. After childbirth, a bottle-feeder may have trouble losing this extra fat. But a breastfeeder should easily lose it (as long as she doesn't overeat), as it's used to make breast milk. Indeed, fat stores built up during pregnancy contribute up to 300 calories a day to breast milk for three or four months. Since a baby needs only 600–800 calories a day, his mother's fat stores therefore provide up to half his calorie requirements, and she needs to eat only an extra 300 to 500 calories a day in addition to her usual intake to produce breast milk without depleting her body of nutrients.

You don't have to store fat while pregnant to be able to breastfeed, though, as long as you have enough to eat when breastfeeding.

Alcohol

Experts can't say how much, if any, alcohol is safe in pregnancy, but the official guidelines in certain countries, including the US, the UK, Australia, and New Zealand, are to have none.

If you decide to drink, aim to avoid it from when you know you're pregnant (or when you know you're trying to get pregnant) and for the first three months of pregnancy. Then limit your intake to one or two units once or twice a week and take special care to avoid bingeing on alcohol. A "unit" here is a UK unit, which is no more than one small glass of wine, a half-pint of beer, a quarter-pint of strong lager, or a measure of spirits. It's also wise to have two or three completely alcohol-free days a week.

Smoking

If you're a smoker, there's no doubt that it is much better for your unborn baby's health and your own to stop smoking.

If you can't or don't want to do this, and intend to continue smoking, it'll still be better for you to breastfeed than to formula-feed.

Choosing where to have your baby

Once you know you're pregnant, book a hospital delivery unless you plan to give birth at home. Choose carefully, as some hospitals are much more helpful than others with breastfeeding.

To help you decide,

- Ask your doctor whether the hospital you're considering has a "Baby Friendly" status (page 90), or at least encourages baby-friendly policies (page 90).

- Ask friends and local women who have given birth there whether the staff were helpful with breastfeeding.

- Ask the hospital for a copy of its breastfeeding policy, and ask what proportion of women who want to breastfeed manage to do so.

- Ask whether you'll be allowed—and, preferably, encouraged—to labor upright if you want, rather than flat on your back. This could be better for you and your baby, which will benefit your early breastfeeding.

With good information, support, and help if necessary, being in the hospital need not load the dice against successful breastfeeding, though breastfeeding is more likely to be successful after a home birth. A hospital environment, after all, does little to encourage the establishment of the let-down (page 148). For example, one newly delivered American woman reported that 50–70 people entered her hospital room each day. This certainly isn't relaxing! Some hospitals employ midwives whose main job is to encourage and advise mothers how to breastfeed.

Baby Friendly Hospitals

More and more hospitals around the world are changing their policies to become eligible for Baby Friendly Hospital status, instigated by the World Health Organization and UNICEF in 1991.

Baby Friendly Hospitals use "Ten Steps to Successful Breastfeeding."

10 STEPS TO SUCCESSFUL BREASTFEEDING

1. Have a written breastfeeding policy and communicate it routinely to all health staff.
2. Train all health staff in the skills they need to implement this policy.
3. Inform all pregnant women about the benefits and management of breastfeeding.
4. Help mothers initiate breastfeeding within half an hour of birth.
5. Show mothers how to breastfeed and how to maintain lactation even if they are separated from their babies.
6. Give newborns no food or drink other than breast milk, unless medically indicated.
7. Practice rooming-in (when mothers and babies remain together) 24 hours a day.
8. Encourage breastfeeding on demand.
9. Give no artificial teats (nipples) or pacifiers to breastfeeding babies.
10. Foster the establishment of breastfeeding support groups and refer mothers to them on discharge from the hospital or clinic.

Many hospitals are working toward Baby Friendly status. For example, in 2012, in Canada, 18 hospitals were Baby Friendly, compared with only one in 2002.

In Australia, only 4 percent of births are in Baby Friendly hospitals.

The same goes for the United States. The figures vary enormously from one state to another. For example, in Nebraska, 22 percent of births are born in Baby Friendly hospitals, while the figure for Alaska is 21 percent and for Maine 19 percent. However, the following states have no

Baby Friendly hospitals: Alabama, Arizona, Arkansas, Delaware, District of Columbia, Georgia, Iowa, Kansas, Louisiana, Maryland, Oklahoma, Michigan, Mississippi, Nevada, New Jersey, New Mexico, South Dakota, South Carolina, and West Virginia.

In Scotland, the percentage of births in Baby Friendly hospitals is 73; in Wales, 64; and in Northern Ireland, 61. However, England does less well, with the percentage in the South West being 57; in the North West, 34; in the West Midlands, 30; in the North East, 26; in Yorkshire and the Humber, 15; in the South East Coast, 6; in London, 2; and in South Central, 1.

However, in Iran, 80 percent of births are in hospitals; in Cuba, 87; and in Sweden, 100.

Hospitals in the UK wishing to apply for Baby Friendly status can visit www.babyfriendly.org.uk (US: http://www.babyfriendlyusa .org). Hospitals in other countries should write to the UNICEF Baby Friendly Hospital Initiative, Palais des Nations, 1211, Geneva 10, Switzerland.

Make a birth plan

Ideally, discuss and agree your birth plan with the hospital staff during your pregnancy. Include ideas of how you want to give birth, breastfeed, and care for your baby. For example, you might say you'd like to

- *Labor upright,* as this is generally safer for babies and easier and quicker for women. It can increase a baby's oxygen supply; shorten labor by making contractions more efficient; reduce the need for painkilling drugs by making contractions less arduous; and make an episiotomy (a cut to widen the vaginal opening) less likely, as the woman has more control over the speed and angle at which her baby comes down the birth canal.

- *Not have a pain-relieving drug* such as pethidine (meperidine) too close to your baby's predicted arrival, as it might make you and your baby too sleepy for early breastfeeds to go well. This could be dispiriting and could lead to you wanting to give up breast-feeding (though there are ways of encouraging a sleepy baby to feed—page 243).

- *Hold your baby immediately after birth.*

- *Offer the first feed as soon as possible,* preferably within the first half-hour after birth.

- *Give only breast milk* and certainly no formula without your permission.

Each of these is important for breastfeeding, partly because the better a newly delivered mother and her baby feel, the easier it is to get breast-feeding off to a good start. Of course, you may subsequently change your mind about any of the plans you make. Or circumstances may dictate other things. But making such a list will help refine your mind and give you a "best practice" guide to aim for. A good maternity unit will try to satisfy your requests, though they'll always put your safety and that of your baby first.

Pain relief in labor

Two drug options, unlike pethidine, won't make you or your new-born baby sleepy. They include

- *"Gas and air."* The gas is nitrous oxide ("laughing gas") and you can control how much you have.

- *Meptazinol (Meptid).* This is weaker than pethidine and less likely to make your newborn too sleepy to breastfeed for many hours.

An epidural injection helps to prevent pain and won't make the baby sleepy but is associated with more difficulties in breastfeeding, and a shorter duration of breastfeeding.

Non-drug options are preferable and include

- *Laboring upright.* If you're interested in this, tell the prenatal-clinic midwives so they can forewarn the labor-ward midwives.

- *Having light, rapid "butterfly" massage around the base of your spine,* done by a birth companion. The "touch messages" sent along the nerves arrive faster at the spinal cord than "pain mes-sages," which helps to block the pain.

- *Using a TENS (transcutaneous electrical nerve stimulation) machine* to give mild electrostimulation to your lower back. The messages this sends along nerves to the spinal cord arrive faster than "pain messages," which helps block the pain messages. If you'd like to use a TENS machine, you'll need to buy or borrow one to take into hospital with you. Try it out first at home so you're familiar with it.

Plan for when you go home

Women who leave the hospital within 48 hours are more likely to breastfeed successfully than those who stay in longer. This is scarcely surprising as most of us relax better in our own environment and therefore produce more milk and let it down more reliably. Also, the loving, constant emotional support and encouragement you need is usually best supplied by family and friends.

If your baby has been in a nursery in the hospital, once home you can have him with you all the time. This makes it easier to breastfeed on an unrestricted basis day and night, which will give you the best start.

Arrange for someone to be at home to help when you return after the birth. You'll then get the rest you need and have time to enjoy your baby and learn to breastfeed successfully.

Involve your partner

Talk with your partner about breastfeeding and what it will mean to him. Tell him what you know about its advantages and suggest he goes to the prenatal class's fathers' night. He might be interested in reading parts of this book too. Chapter 16 is especially for fathers.

He'll probably be pleased to support your decision to breastfeed, especially once he understands the importance of breastfeeding and his value as a protector and encourager. Researchers have found that her partner's attitude is the single most important influence on a woman's decision on how to feed her baby. Partners of women who plan to bottle-feed usually don't know about the health benefits of breastfeeding. They also tend to imagine that breastfeeding makes a woman's breasts sag (which isn't true—page 243—provided you look after yourself) and will spoil their sex life (though fatigue after childbirth is a far more common culprit, whether or not a woman breastfeeds—and he can reduce this by helping you with various chores).

Discuss practical matters such as how he'll get home from work if you usually pick him up but happen to be breastfeeding at the time; how he can sometimes cook supper or why, if you cook, you'll need to be flexible about mealtimes; and how you'll both get more sleep if the baby sleeps in your bedroom so you can easily breastfeed at night. Your partner may sleep better if he decamps to another bedroom.

Some women choose to formula-feed on the basis that their partner will then be able to enjoy feeding the baby. But no breastfeeding mother needs to feel guilty about depriving a man of this experience! He can cuddle his baby as much as he likes at any time other than actually during a breastfeed. And he can give expressed or pumped breast milk by cup or bottle if his baby needs it and his partner isn't able to breastfeed at the time.

Choosing how to feed your baby

Many factors influence a woman's decision on how to feed her baby. In a large survey of expectant mothers in the UK in 1990, these ideas underlaid their feeding choice.

REASONS FOR PLANNING TO BREASTFEED FIRST BABIES

	%
Breastfeeding is best for the baby	85
Breastfeeding is more convenient	34
Closer bond between mother and baby	23
Breastfeeding is cheaper	21
Breastfeeding is natural	14
Breastfeeding is best for mother	13
Mother loses weight more easily	13
Influenced by medical personnel	4
Influenced by friends or relatives	4

REASONS FOR PLANNING TO BOTTLE-FEED FIRST BABIES

	%
Other people can feed baby with bottle	29
Didn't like idea of breastfeeding	27
Can see how much baby has had	7
Expecting to return to work soon	7
Other reasons	6
No particular reason	5
Would be embarrassed to breastfeed	4

Medical reasons for not breastfeeding	2
Bottle-feeding is less tiring	2

Both tables are from *Infant Feeding* 1990, HMSO. The percentages don't add up to 100 as some women gave more than one reason.

What's fascinating is that many of the women who intended to bottle-feed gave reasons against breastfeeding, not for bottle-feeding. In contrast, most of those who intended to breastfeed were positively for breastfeeding, not against bottle-feeding.

So those intending to bottle-feed gave negative reasons, those intending to breastfeed, positive ones. Interestingly, most women who choose to formula-feed focus more on *themselves* and the effect breastfeeding will have on *them*, rather than on *their baby* and the effect breastfeeding will have on *him*.

Perhaps, then, a more thorough discussion in prenatal classes of the imagined disadvantages of breastfeeding, preferably with input from at least one successfully breastfeeding woman, might help parents overcome their perceived negatives of breastfeeding. Also, as the number-one choice breastfeeders give for doing it is that it's best for babies, this fact must be well aired—and certainly not hushed up to allay the possibility of causing guilt in those who don't choose to breastfeed and the very few who can't. It might also be helpful to discuss in more depth a woman's reasons for choosing to bottle-feed.

Note, though, that pregnant women are generally much more interested in thinking about and discussing pregnancy and labor than anything after the birth, including baby feeding. This is one reason why many pregnant women make a decision about baby feeding only to change their mind when the baby arrives.

Your feelings about breastfeeding

If you strongly dislike the idea of breastfeeding, consider doing some emotional digging to discover why, perhaps using the information on page 190. Becoming more emotionally aware may help you make a freer choice. I have seen a great many women who regretted not having breastfed an earlier baby. This is a "loss" that many are sad about—and it cannot be redressed, though it may make the experience of breastfeeding a subsequent baby feel even more valuable.

Sources of information about breastfeeding

Find out as much as you can about breastfeeding now. Even if you've breastfed successfully before, read about it or discuss it because each baby is different and the way he feeds will be different too. If you understand how breastfeeding works, you'll know what might happen, be more confident, and recognize when to get help. See also page 97.

Your breasts could know whether you're having a girl or a boy before you do!

According to research in pregnant monkeys—and the findings are likely to be similar in humans—the developing milk-producing glands and ducts receive messages via the hormone placental lactogen about whether the unborn infant is male or female. If it's male, her milk glands are programmed to produce higher-fat milk than if it's female.

Prenatal classes

Hopefully the baby-feeding session at an prenatal class will focus on breastfeeding. By making friends with other women who want to breast-feed, you can be "bosom buddies" when you have your babies—encouraging each other, giving information, and generally caring for one another. Facebook and other social networking media can make this easy and fun.

Researchers find that antenatal education about breastfeeding makes it more likely to be successful. Information about breastfeeding and the care of a newborn—including an idea of the large number of breastfeeds, the lack of a predictable schedule, and the possibility of setbacks—gives pregnant women a more realistic idea of their future role as breastfeeding mothers. Women who aren't taught about breastfeeding often blame themselves or their baby for breastfeeding problems instead of focusing on factors under their control. And most are.

Other researchers have found that women are more likely to plan to breastfeed if the prenatal class leader favors breastfeeding. So it's wise for people running such classes to make it clear that breast is indeed best. It's also a good idea for the leader to invite a woman to talk about breastfeeding and demonstrate a feed. This is because many young women have never seen anyone breastfeeding, yet doing so can often be a very potent influence on deciding to go ahead. This is more important for many women than knowing about the health benefits.

Information pamphlets

Be vigilant about the source of booklets and leaflets about pregnancy and baby feeding, such as those available in some clinics, surgeries, and babycare roadshows. The way information about breastfeeding is put across in publications sponsored by milk-formula companies can be much less helpful and encouraging about breastfeeding than information sponsored by noncommercial bodies.

One recent example originating from a major formula company in the UK injects anxiety by suggesting that most breastfeeding women sometimes believe they don't have enough milk. This is clever marketing! All breastfeeding women wonder, at some stage, whether or not they have enough milk. But this is no argument for starting to formula-feed.

Interestingly, one pamphlet sponsored by a large formula company some years ago had a photograph of a woman breastfeeding with her sweater pulled down to expose her whole breast. Few successfully breastfeeding women in developed countries do this in public—they pull their sweater up, so exposing little or no breast. Thinking they might have to expose their breasts puts many women off breastfeeding, so such a photo must make one question the company's motives.

Health professionals

If you live in the UK, you may meet your health visitor at your prenatal classes. She'll be your official breastfeeding adviser once you part company with the community midwife (which happens within the first four weeks after birth, normally after ten days) and her support and advice could be invaluable. You can contact her in person at your baby clinic, or by phone. Ask local women expecting second babies whether the local health visitor's breastfeeding advice is good. If she has a reputation for advising formula-feeding too readily, get in touch with an NCT breastfeeding counselor or an LLL leader (page 341).

Learning together

Some health professionals are wonderful in that they go on learning about successful breastfeeding alongside women doing it. The very best helpers know they can always learn more.

Some breastfeeding women are willing and confident enough to learn about successful breastfeeding independently, and even to teach and encourage their midwife, doctor, and, in the UK, their health visitor. This requires an eagerness to learn, together with intellectual humility on the part of the health professional. Some breastfeeding women and helpers team up with excellent and mutually rewarding results. Many such professionals have gone on to help numerous other women. People with this generosity of spirit light the way for others and deserve warm congratulations and gratitude.

There's a section for helpers on page 333.

Breastfeeding support groups

Many countries have national breastfeeding support organizations with local groups. In the UK, for example, the The National Childbirth Trust (NCT) organizes courses of prenatal classes. An NCT breastfeeding counselor usually gives a talk during each course and you can contact her if you need help once you've had your baby. The counselors are volunteers who are well trained in helping with breastfeeding problems on a mother-to-mother basis, and have breastfed babies themselves. Some NCT branches arrange postnatal meetings and support groups too.

La Leche League International (LLLI) is a worldwide organization of women who are breastfeeding or who have breastfed and want to encourage and help each other with breastfeeding. Anyone interested is welcome to attend local LLL branch meetings. Your nearest LLL leader will suggest you contact her if you need help. League leaders are volunteers with an excellent training in assisting and encouraging breastfeeding women; they have all breastfed babies successfully for long periods and can discuss breastfeeding and mothering on a mother-to-mother basis. LLL group meetings are open to anyone, whether pregnant, breastfeeding, or neither.

Furniture and equipment

You'll probably want your baby near you so you can hear him, so you'll need a crib, a portable bed, or a stroller to use during the day. Similarly, if you want your baby by your bed at night for easy feeding, it's a good idea to have a cot with a removable side so the baby's mattress is level with yours, making it easy to slip the baby into your bed for a feed and back again (page 340). This is known as a "sidecar" crib.

Babies sleep anywhere if tired, warm, and full, and in the early days, before they are old enough to roll over or wriggle and fall, some mothers lie them to sleep on a sofa or easy chair, fenced in by cushions or pillows. But this isn't a good idea. Your baby may spit up some milk on the upholstery; someone may accidentally sit on him; a sibling or pet could interfere with him; and the day will come when he'll roll for the first time. Also, note that SIDS in a baby sleeping with his mother is more likely on a sofa.

Think where you'll sit to breastfeed, since a comfortable place will help you relax and reduce the risk of aching shoulders and arms after a feed. A good chair is low, so your lap is flat enough to support the baby well, and has arms or a place to put cushions to support your elbows at the right height. Experiment before you have the baby. A rocking chair can be pleasant and many women are comfortable sitting on a sofa or a bed with their feet up. You don't have to sit up straight to breastfeed—you may prefer to recline. And lying down flat to feed is the most relaxing of all.

Shopping and housework

Before you have your baby, stock up with canned and dried foods, and, if you have a freezer, fill it with prepared meals so you or your partner can rustle something up quickly if you're too tired to cook. Convenience food is a great help early on, though it's better to eat fresh foods whenever possible.

If you can afford it, buy stocks of disposable diapers or, if you're intending to use cloth diapers, cloth-diaper sterilizing solution and washing powder. Ideally, buy stocks of basic household goods too. Shopping with a very young baby can be a headache as he may want feeding so often in the very early days that there isn't much time to be out for long. You might like to ask whether any local shops or supermarkets accept phone or Internet orders and deliver to the door. Your partner could go late-night shopping, or a relative or neighbor might do some shopping for you until your baby is old enough to go longer between feeds.

The laundry generated by a small baby can be a big surprise. If you don't have a washing machine, see if you can possibly afford one now as it'll make all the difference, especially if you use cloth diapers. Otherwise, think about sending bed linen, towels, and other big things to a laundry for the first few weeks. This is especially important if you give birth at home, or come home after 48 hours, as you may soil bed linen in the first few days. An alternative is to use disposable absorbent mats (such as Pampers Care Mats) in your bed early on. If you don't have a machine, buy a few packs of disposable diapers, even if you intend to use cloth diapers eventually, as washing diapers will tire you in the early days. You may consider disposables too expensive or environmentally damaging to continue after the first week or so, but they'll give you an easy start.

Help at home

Consider arranging for someone to help at home for when you return with your new baby, as you'll need to take things easy for a few weeks. This is even more helpful with a second or third baby because there's more work with a family this size. If you don't have any willing relatives or friends, consider paying for domestic help for an hour or two a day if you can. Many partners take a week or two off work to help, especially if there are other children. Whatever happens, you'll need time if you're to breastfeed successfully, especially at first when the baby needs very frequent feeds. Don't expect to be a superwoman. If necessary, let domestic things go and focus on yourself and your baby in the early days.

Clothes

Good clothes to have ready for breastfeeding include loose T-shirts, sweatshirts, sweaters, blouses, and almost anything you can pull up from the waist. These make for easy breastfeeding and allow you to feed without exposing your breast. Feeding a baby with your top pulled up just enough looks as though you're simply having a cuddle, so you look discreet when feeding in public.

Dresses that undo in front are fine for breastfeeding at home when you don't need to be discreet. If you're wearing a blouse when you're out, pull it up to feed rather than undo the buttons.

Some women alter existing clothes to make them more suitable.

Make sure you have several changes of clothes because being in the same things day after day can be depressing, and you may wet your tops if you leak.

When it comes to breastfeeding at night, wear

- A nightie that unbuttons in front.
- Pajamas.
- A T-shirt and some loose bottoms.
- Or nothing but a bra to support your breasts so as to help keep them looking good.

Clothes should be machine washable because apart from milk leaking, your baby may bring up small amounts and you won't want huge dry-cleaning bills.

Some women use a pashmina or other shawl or cloth to cover their baby and their breast as they feed.

Breast care

When you're pregnant, several things can help prevent unwanted long-term changes in the shape of your breasts.

2 TIPS TO HELP KEEP YOUR BREASTS LOOKING GOOD

1. **Avoid overeating**—as this lays down extra fat in the breasts. This can encourage sagging because their extra size can stretch the skin's elastic fibers and their extra weight can stretch the connective tissue that helps support them.

2. **Wear a properly fitting, supportive bra**, day and night if necessary, to prevent the weight of heavier than usual breasts stretching their skin and connective tissue.

Bras

When your breasts start enlarging, from about the fifth month of pregnancy or even before, you'll need a bigger bra, though you may be able to make do for a while by using extenders to increase the chest size of your existing bras (from the NCT Shop, page 342).

You'll need several bras when breastfeeding, because they'll require frequent washing, especially early on when you're almost certain to leak. Some people think cotton "breathes" better than synthetic fabrics. It's important to wear a bra that supports and fits well, yet doesn't squash your breasts or nipples.

Many women wear an ordinary bra and either undo it or pull it up or down to breastfeed. Only 40 percent of breastfeeding women buy a special bra. Pulling the cup down to free the breast works well if the bra isn't too bulky, but make sure it supports you well enough, is large enough, and doesn't squash any part of the breast when pulled down—as this can encourage a blocked duct. If you have small breasts, you may not need a bra at all.

If you buy a nursing bra, note they can have drop-down or zipped cups. Drop-down cups are easiest to use, but go for ones with one hook per cup, rather than rows of tiny hooks and eyes, which make frequent feeds difficult and are awkward to do up and undo discreetly in company. The NCT Shop (page 342) has a good selection, including a style going up to a J cup size. In the UK, women can be measured and order bras from local NCT branch bra agents. Choose bras no earlier than around 36 weeks of pregnancy. If possible, wait until after your baby is born, so they fit well.

Wearing a bra at night—It's sensible to wear a bra in bed during the last three months of pregnancy as this supports your increasingly heavy breasts and helps prevent their skin stretching. Maternity bras sold as sleep bras are usually too insubstantial to provide much support.

Your nipples

There's no convincing evidence that rolling your nipples; rubbing them with a rough towel; applying lanolin, cream, or alcohol; or expressing colostrum in pregnancy will aid breastfeeding. The only reason for rolling nipples, for example, might be to make them less sensitive or get you used at handling your breasts. But that will happen anyway once you start breastfeeding.

However, some pregnant women find it helps to go without a bra, or to cut a small hole in the center of each bra cup, because nipples that rub against clothing become less sensitive.

Flat, inverted (turned-in), or poorly protractile nipples

These result from having short milk ducts that tether the nipples, or short strands of connective tissue that pull the nipple toward the inner breast, or relatively less dense connective tissue under the nipple.

Some prenatal clinic staff routinely check for flat or inverted nipples with the "pinch test." To do this yourself, pinch your areola (the darker skin around the nipple) between finger and thumb to see if the nipple comes out. If it does, it's unlikely your baby will have difficulty. Also, if your nipples usually come out when you're cold or sexually aroused, you shouldn't have a problem.

Between 7 and 10 percent of pregnant women who want to breastfeed have truly inverted nipples (ones that won't come out at all) or poorly protractile nipples (which don't come out much). The good news is that nipple shape and protractility often improve in pregnancy, probably because of the action of estrogens on the tissues behind the nipple. Inverted or poorly protractile nipples are said to hinder 1 woman in 20 feeding a first baby, 1 in 50 feeding a second, and none who've fed two or more. However, a great many women with such nipples manage perfectly well, especially if a skilled carer helps them position their baby so he gets a good mouthful of areola and nipple, and reminds them not to limit the number or length of breastfeeds or give bottles of formula.

Breast shells—Some people think these help flat, inverted, or poorly protractile nipples, but at least one study disagrees. These hollow, plastic or glass, saucer-shaped devices have a circular hole on the inner surface for the nipple. Wearing them inside a bra is supposed to encourage the nipples to protrude through the holes and gradually improve their shape in pregnancy, but nipples that improve with shells would probably have improved anyway.

Breast shells are more useful after a baby is born, when using them for a short while before a feed helps poorly protractile nipples protrude for a long enough time for the baby to latch on well (get a good mouthful of the nipple and areola). After a few seconds the nipple returns to its original shape, so the baby has to catch hold fairly quickly. The disadvantage is that the pressure of the shell can obstruct milk ducts and encourage engorgement. Also, the skin under the shell can become moist and swollen and more liable to soreness and cracks. You can buy a breast shell (made by Medela—page 339) with numerous openings on the rounded dome to allow more air to circulate around the skin. If ordering or buying breast shells, note that some people call them milk cups, or wrongly call them breast "shields."

Avent Niplettes (page 339)—these suction devices look like little clear plastic thimbles and are said to help bring out inverted or flat nipples by encouraging short milk ducts to lengthen.

To use them, hold one on your nipple, then use the syringe (already attached to a valve) to suck the air from between the nipple and the Niplette. When your nipple comes out, release the Niplette and remove the syringe. You can leave the Niplette on all day under loose clothing, and overnight if you wish—either as well as by day or instead. When your nipples have lengthened to fill the Niplettes, you gradually stop wearing them. Two to three months' use should lead to a permanent result.

Niplettes are designed to be used during pregnancy, not while breast-feeding. One small trial found that each of six pregnant women with inverted nipples had normal looking nipples after two weeks of using Niplettes, and all found them easy to use.

If you still have inverted nipples at the end of pregnancy, your baby may still be able to suck efficiently if you "make a biscuit" of your areola and nipple with your thumb and forefinger and offer it to him. You could also use breast shells. Engorgement is the number-one problem in women with inverted nipples, so avoid this at all costs (page 174).

Nipple cleanliness

The Montgomery's tubercles around the areola produce an oily fluid that keeps the areola and nipple supple and kills bacteria. If you wash this off with soap, your skin is much more likely to become sore when you breastfeed. So avoid soap for the last few weeks of pregnancy and wash your nipples with warm water alone. There's no need to use any ointment or cream to prepare for breastfeeding, because nature's own lubrication is best. Similarly, there's no need to remove the yellowish grains of dried secretions you may see on your nipples—a simple water splash is enough.

Expressing milk

There's no need to express milk in pregnancy to remove colostrum or "clear the ducts."

six

How Breastfeeding Works

Changes in the shape and size of a girl's breasts begin a year or so before her periods start and continue until her late teens. Her breasts increase in size during adolescence as fat accumulates and milk ducts branch and lengthen. There's very little glandular tissue now, but small collections of cells begin to form that will later develop into milk glands. After these changes, if a girl's weight is steady her breasts stay much the same until she gets pregnant.

Humans are the only mammals whose breasts enlarge before pregnancy. Human breasts have a sexual role in courtship that isn't seen with the paps or udders of other mammals, and in the developed world in particular this can color our attitudes to breastfeeding.

Your breasts

A breast has 15–20 segments, each containing a gland leading to a main duct which opens at the nipple. These openings look like little crevices and if you pause while feeding your baby, you'll notice drops or fine sprays of milk emerging from one or more ducts at a time. Sometimes several ducts merge within the nipple, in which case there are fewer openings at the nipple than there are ducts.

Milk-producing glands

In a pregnant or breastfeeding woman the glandular part of each segment of breast looks rather like a bunch of grapes on a stalk. Each "grape" is a milk gland ("alveolus") lined with milk-producing cells, each bordering the tiny duct that joins the "stalk" or main milk duct leading from that segment of breast to the nipple.

Each milk gland is surrounded by a fine network of blood vessels. Their blood supplies the gland's milk-producing cells with the hormones that stimulate milk production and the materials they need to make milk. The milk-producing cells become round and full as they make milk between feeds.

Milk ducts and reservoirs

Milk from a gland's milk-producing cells enters the gland's tiny duct. This joins the main duct of that segment of breast. Toward the end of the main duct, beneath the areola, is a widening called a milk reservoir ("lactiferous sinus"). This empties milk through an opening at the nipple. There are 15–20 milk reservoirs. As each fills with milk its elastic walls expand. A full reservoir's diameter is ¼–½ in (½–1 cm). The milk reservoirs store milk ready for the beginning of a feed. They can store even more after six to eight weeks of breastfeeding. This is why any leaking often stops then. The fullness and slight lumpiness you may feel before a feed is caused by milk glands swollen with laden cells and by the full ducts and reservoirs.

Trickles and spurts

Milk leaves a milk-producing gland in a trickle or a spurt.

Trickling milk—Rising pressure within a milk-producing cell as it gradually fills pushes the milk in a continuous trickle into the milk gland's tiny collecting duct. From here it trickles into the main duct of that segment of the breast and ends up in the duct's reservoir under the areola.

Spurting milk—Contraction of the branching network of star-shaped muscle cells that surround each milk gland squeezes milk from its cells into its collecting duct. From here it rushes through the main duct and its reservoir then spurts from that duct's opening at the nipple. This is called the let-down reflex (page 109).

Breast changes in pregnancy

During pregnancy many women notice tingling and fullness of their breasts as early as their first missed period. Indeed, these sensations are often the first signs of pregnancy. Little prominences called Montgomery's tubercles, around each areola, become more noticeable from around six weeks. Anatomically, each tubercle resembles a tiny breast, and contains glands that produce an oily substance which lubricates and protects the nipple skin. In some women one or more of their Montgomery's tubercles actually produces milk.

By five months, most women need a larger bra. In a first pregnancy the nipples and areolas now begin to darken. And you'll produce milk if you give birth any time from now on.

Inside the breasts, cells called alveolar epithelial cells in the small collections of cells that have been present since adolescence, change to become milk-producing cells (lactocytes).

These changes are caused by hormones, some of them present only in pregnancy.

Breast size

By the end of a full-term pregnancy each breast weighs on average 1½ lb (650 g) more than at its beginning, mainly because of the development of milk glands and the proliferation of milk ducts.

The prepregnancy size of the breasts in a woman of healthy weight has little effect on her ability to breastfeed. Some small breasts contain more milk-producing glands than do some large ones.

However, the large breast size of an obese or overweight woman can reduce her milk supply. One study (*Pediatrics*, 2004) suggests this is because such a woman makes less prolactin (the milk-production hormone). The solution is not to diet in pregnancy or while breastfeeding, but to get good help with your breastfeeding technique.

A woman with very small breasts could have a slight disadvantage early in breastfeeding as her breasts may overfill particularly quickly. This could encourage engorgement and leaking unless she breastfeeds or expresses often enough to prevent her breasts becoming too tense. Overfilling becomes less of a problem as the storage capacity of the milk reservoirs increases in the early weeks.

Whatever your prepregnancy breast size, the increase in size of your breasts in pregnancy is quite a good indicator of your ability to get off to a good start with breastfeeding. You're unlikely to have trouble if you need a bra that is one or two sizes larger by the end of pregnancy.

Indeed, one reason why women having their first baby relatively young tend to produce more milk at first is because they have a larger than average increase in breast size.

Most women's breasts are unequal in size before pregnancy. This doesn't matter, though when they breastfeed they may always have more milk one side. And it won't necessarily be the larger breast that produces more.

Nipples

The nipples become larger and more protractile (able to lengthen) in pregnancy. This makes it easier for a breastfeeding baby to latch on (take the nipple and areola into his mouth). A few women's nipples don't change much so a good "latch" may be more of a challenge.

Hormones and milk production

The fall in progesterone after birth helps trigger copious milk production. This is known as the milk "coming in." Other hormones involved in milk production include prolactin, growth hormone, corticosteroids, thyroxine, and insulin.

Prolactin

The level of this hormone increases from the eighth week of pregnancy, peaks at birth, then decreases over the months of breastfeeding. In pregnancy, prolactin stimulates breast growth, but estrogen, progesterone, and placental lactogen act as hormonal brakes to prevent it producing milk in any volume.

The milk-producing hormone—After the birth, these hormonal brakes disappear, so the high prolactin level can then trigger milk production. Prolactin "turns on the taps." It also stimulates the production of two important breast-milk constituents, casein and lactose.

Prolactin is produced by the pituitary gland in the brain. During a feed, stimulation of the nipple and areola sends feedback messages to the pituitary that tell it to make more prolactin. It's a baby's milking action (rhythmic squeezing and milking, or "stripping") that stimulates the nipple and areola, rather than his sucking. This is why a simple breast pump may not be as good at boosting prolactin. A baby with a strong milking action usually raises his mother's prolactin better than a baby with a weaker one.

The stimulation from milking boosts prolactin immediately. Its production peaks 30–45 minutes after starting a feed and falls to its lowest level over the next two hours. The more time a baby spends at the breast, the more milk a woman makes. Each feed places an order for more milk to be made, ready for the next feed. Waiting longer between feeds doesn't produce more milk because it doesn't increase prolactin.

Early and frequent stimulation of the nipple and areola encourages prolactin receptors to develop on milk-producing cells. These capture prolactin from the blood, which enables the cells to make milk. Poor development of prolactin receptors on milk-producing cells caused by insufficient early stimulation of the nipple and areola may explain why the blood's prolactin level isn't directly related to the amount of milk a woman makes. It may also explain why, if a woman breastfeeds only or mainly from one breast, as a few do (page 129), the milk in the little-used or unused breast gradually decreases or even dries up, despite high prolactin levels in her blood as a result of stimulation of the other breast.

To summarize, nipple stimulation is necessary for breasts to respond to prolactin and make milk. Also, the more frequently a woman feeds from a breast, the more sensitive and responsive to prolactin does that breast become.

The increase in prolactin associated with suckling is at its most sensitive in the first week of breastfeeding, which is partly why it's so important not to restrict feeds then.

Prolactin levels are highest at night and in the early morning. This is one reason why there's often more milk than usual at the early-morning feed.

And, perhaps, a "mothering," "nesting," bonding, contentment-inducing and antianxiety hormone—Research suggests that prolactin engenders greater responsiveness by a breastfeeding mother to her young. It can also encourage "nesting" behavior, in which she wants to stay at home and look after, breastfeed, and cuddle her baby, which aids mother-infant bonding. And prolactin can make her feel more content and tranquil.

The let-down reflex

The sudden squeezing of milk out of the milk glands into the milk ducts is called the milk-ejection reflex, or the let-down reflex. Without it, a baby would get only the milk that had trickled into the reservoirs since the last feed.

The time needed to let down milk varies from woman to woman and also depends on a woman's feelings and surroundings. From when a baby is put to the breast the let-down can take 30 to 50 seconds to begin but often takes longer. Some women need two to three minutes of nipple stimulation before their maximum milk flow occurs. So a hungry or thirsty baby may finish the milk that's trickled into the ducts and reservoirs since the last feed before any new milk is let down. This can be frustrating for him.

Stimulation of the nipple and areola by the milking action of the baby's mouth is the most important trigger for the let-down. It sends messages along nerves to the pituitary gland, which then releases oxytocin. This hormone then travels in the bloodstream to the breasts, where it makes the muscle cells around each milk gland contract and squeeze milk into the milk ducts.

Other let-down triggers

These include hand-expression or pumping of milk; the sight, sound, or thought of the baby (or even someone else's baby); and full breasts. An experienced breastfeeder automatically releases oxytocin when she or her baby is ready for a feed. This is because her let-down reflex is "conditioned" by experience. Sexual stimulation can let down milk too.

What you see and feel

As your milk lets down, you may notice

- *Tingling, tension, and warmth* in your breasts immediately before.

- *Dripping, spraying, or leaking of milk.* Any one let-down consists of a series of spurts of milk, with a gap between each spurt. Milk may spurt from the other breast too.

- *A pleasant whole-body feeling* sometimes likened to a sneeze or an orgasm.

- *A sense of relief* as your baby removes let-down milk and your breast becomes less tense.

- *Any initial nipple pain disappearing* as the milk lets down (as this equalizes the negative pressure created by the baby sucking).

- *Other sensations.* One woman, for example, described letting down in the first few weeks as like cold water trickling down her breastbone; later she had tingling throughout her breasts, and later still, itching beneath each areola.

- *"After-pains"* caused by rhythmical womb contractions in the early days.

- Also, your baby will suck with rhythmical, one-per-second sucks that mean he's swallowing let-down milk. You may hear a "glug-glug" as he swallows.

The sensations you experience may vary from one baby to another. In some women the sensations of the let-down change or disappear over the months or years of breastfeeding. Some women know they are letting down only because their baby settles at the breast or is thriving and growing.

How many let-downs?

There may be up to eight let-downs per feed, each associated with a rise and fall in the blood's oxytocin level. Oxytocin falls very rapidly after the start of a let-down and is gone in about four minutes. The first let-down of a feed is associated with the highest oxytocin level.

The reliability of the let-down

Breastfeeding is said to be "established" when the let-down reflex is so well conditioned by repeated feeds that it virtually never fails. It also means your breasts have adapted their milk production to match your baby's needs. All this usually takes some weeks.

Before then, the let-down is easily disturbed by anxiety, embarrassment, or other stress. For example, if her baby cries and becomes restless, perhaps turning away or "fighting" at the breast, an inexperienced mother may become so anxious that she doesn't produce oxytocin and can't let down her milk.

Different looking drops and sprays at the nipple

During a feed or when expressing milk, you may notice different looking drops or sprays of milk emerging from different duct openings at the nipple. Some look bluish-white and relatively thin, others creamy-white and thicker, and others somewhere between. The reasons for this are

1. The composition of milk from any one reservoir depends on whether it's leaving the breast early or late in a feed. Some drops or sprays contain milk that was already in the ducts and reservoirs at the beginning of the feed, others contain milk let down during the current feed, and others a mixture of let-down milk and the milk already there.

2. A baby empties different reservoirs at different rates, depending on his position at the breast.

3. The segment of breast from which a drop comes may not have been completely emptied by the last feed.

4. Milk ducts sometimes merge within the nipple, in which case there are fewer openings than reservoirs. If some segments of the breast were emptied more thoroughly than others at the last feed, and their ducts merge, the combined milk may look neither thin nor thick.

At the beginning of a feed from the first breast most drops contain bluish-white thinner milk; toward the end, most contain creamy-white thicker milk.

At the beginning of a feed from the second breast, the drops or sprays may look much more similar to each other. This is because as the baby feeds at the first breast, milk is let down into the reservoirs of the second. Here it mingles with milk that has trickled down since the last feed

Leaking

Warmth from a hot environment or the baby's mouth can cause leaking from full breasts. Although the muscle fibers in the nipple and areola are usually contracted, which keeps the openings of the milk ducts at the nipple firmly closed, warmth lengthens them. This releases their tight hold on the ducts, so milk can escape.

Leaking can also occur from full breasts just before a feed, or if you hear a baby cry, or you lean forward or sideways.

Last, leaking may result from milk that lets down without the baby drinking it or you collecting it.

How your baby gets milk

A baby obtains milk by rooting for the breast, holding the nipple and areola in his mouth, sucking and milking the breast, and swallowing.

Rooting, sucking and milking, and swallowing are called feeding reflexes because each occurs in response to a particular stimulus.

Note that a baby sucks, a mother suckles. "Suckling" is the act of breastfeeding, and a baby is sometimes called a suckling.

Rooting for the breast

Rooting is the primitive reflex searching movement a young baby automatically makes in response to something stroking his cheek or lips. His mouth moves toward the stimulus, his head bobbing as he searches for it, with the degree of bobbing lessening as he gets closer. Rooting stops and sucking and milking begin when he finds the nipple and takes the nipple and areola into his mouth, or when his mother puts them into his mouth. Rooting also stops temporarily if she gently puts a finger or a pacifier into his mouth, or if he finds his own finger or thumb to suck. After about three weeks, a breastfed baby stops rooting because he's learned to move his head directly toward the nipple.

Holding the breast in his mouth and latching on

A baby holds the breast between his upper gums and his tongue, with his tongue covering his lower gums. To latch on, he sticks the front of his tongue out beneath the nipple and as far as his lower lip, curls it up slightly, then pushes his tongue up against the nipple and areola. He then sucks to help hold the breast in place.

Sucking and milking

Sucking—When a nipple touches a baby's palate, he automatically sucks with his cheek muscles to draw the nipple and areola well into his mouth and keep them there.

This sucking reflex is instinctive and at its strongest 20–30 minutes after birth. If a baby isn't put to the breast during this time, the reflex weakens, but after 40 hours or so it strengthens again. A delay of eight hours or more before the first feed reduces the chance of breastfeeding successfully. Specifically, a delay of more than 12 hours increases the likelihood of stopping breastfeeding in the first two weeks because of insufficient milk. But if you really want to breastfeed, delays such as these won't stop you.

When milk is flowing fast, a baby sucks slowly, strongly, and purposefully at a rate of about 1 suck per second. When milk isn't flowing, he sucks faster and less strongly, in short, sharp bursts of "flutter sucking" at a rate of about two sucks per second. Both sorts of sucking help stimulate the production and let-down of milk, but stronger sucking is more effective.

One researcher notes that newborns "write their signature with their sucking rhythm," since each has a constant and unique pattern of the number of sucks per minute and the intervals between sucks.

A sucked nipple is about twice as long as usual, and the nipple and areola together form a teat shape in the baby's mouth. As his cheeks suck, they create a vacuum which draws milk into his mouth and encourages the milk reservoirs to refill.

Sucking is obviously a very important way of getting milk, but "milking" is even more important.

Milking—The main way a baby gets milk is by milking the reservoirs beneath the areola with his tongue in response to the stimulus of having the nipple and areola in his mouth.

To milk the breast, he presses his tongue up against the nipple and areola from underneath. He then moves his tongue backward, and, as he does so, its muscle fibers contract with rhythmical transverse waves that squeeze milk from the reservoirs. The further a baby draws the nipple and areola into his mouth, the better he empties the reservoirs. Meanwhile a baby's jaws open and close vigorously to help his tongue compress the nipple and areola.

If you could see inside your baby's mouth, you'd see your nipple and areola go back to the junction of his hard and soft palate. You'd also see a furrow down the length of his tongue's upper surface. The "teat" made from your nipple and areola fills this furrow.

Your baby's milking action stimulates your let-down, which ejects milk from the nipple in fine jets toward the back of his mouth. All he needs do is swallow.

Many babies start a feed with continuous rapid sucking and milking for around 30 seconds. Then they settle into a rhythm of bursts of about 15–20 deep sucks, accompanied by milking, and followed by swallowing. Each burst is followed by a pause. As a baby pauses for three to five seconds between let-downs, his lower jaw drops, releasing the tongue's pressure on the nipple and areola and allowing the reservoirs to refill with let-down milk. He can then use his tongue again to strip the newly let-down batch of milk.

Coordinated contractions of muscles of the tongue, throat, and gullet occur in response to the presence of milk in the mouth and throat and enable a baby to swallow the milk.

Impaired feeding reflexes

Feeding reflexes may be temporarily impaired in a low-birthweight baby, or in one with an infection or jaundice. They may also be impaired by brain damage, or by a cleft palate or other mechanical jaw problem.

Demand and supply

A good let-down reflex is one important factor that's vital for successful breastfeeding. Another is the understanding of the principle of demand and supply.

While a baby feeds, he stimulates the nipple and areola, which boosts his mother's prolactin and oxytocin. In general, the more your baby is at your breast, the more prolactin you'll make and the more milk you'll have. Also, the more often you feed him, the more reliable your let-down becomes.

"Demand and supply" is a better phrase than "supply and demand," because the demand for milk produces the supply of milk, not the other way round. However, there are two reasons why the word "demand" isn't particularly appropriate either.

First, babies let their mothers know they're ready to feed by being restless or nuzzling at the breast. So they make their needs known gently, rather than in a "demanding" way (though they do cry if they aren't fed soon). A mother quickly gets to know her baby's cues that he's ready for a feed, so the term "cue feeding" has been suggested instead of "demand feeding."

Second, a few babies don't make their needs known, especially if they've often been left to cry in their mother's mistaken belief that feeds must be at set times. Such babies become quieter and quieter even though they're in desperate need of milk. Without attention to their needs they can starve. And they learn that the world is an unfriendly place that makes them unhappy.

Every time your baby gives the cue he's ready, you can offer a breast. This doesn't mean you should feed only when he asks—you may want to because your breasts feel full or it's a convenient time for you. Neither does it mean you have to feed at the slightest sign of a cue, since many babies can wait awhile, especially if you distract them.

Successful or natural breastfeeding puts no rules or limits on suckling time, provided a baby is latched on properly—if not, he may keep asking for feeds simply because his poor feeding position means he can't get enough. This is irritating and frustrating for him.

Babies allowed to feed as often as they want, take very variable numbers of feeds during the 24 hours. In the early days some ask for a feed every hour or so. The greatest number of feeds often occurs on the fifth day after birth. In a study many years ago in Sheffield, 29 percent of babies allowed to feed when they wanted had eight feeds on the fifth day and 10 percent had more than nine.

Historically, many hospitals misguidedly recommended a breastfeeding schedule of every four hours for a large baby, every three hours for a small one. Unfortunately, with the increasing medicalization of childbirth and mother and baby care, and the tight control exerted over women and babies while they're at the hospital, this poor and baseless advice remained widespread for decades and is still given in some out-of-date, non-baby-friendly hospitals today.

Women's experiences and scientific research agree that any schedule that restricts the number of feeds produces poor results.

Any woman who wants to breastfeed successfully should discard any schedule restricting the frequency of feeds. She should feed whenever she or her baby wants.

One sure way of reducing the number of feeds your baby asks for (and thus decreasing your chances of breastfeeding successfully) is to keep him apart from you. In countries where mothers carry or hold their babies by day and lie by them at night, the babies spend much more time at the breast. Babies allowed to feed pretty much when they want, day and night, are almost always breastfed fully and successfully and continue for an average of three years until they no longer want to be at the breast.

Researchers in Africa who watched mothers sleeping with their babies found that no baby went longer than 20 minutes between feeds! Contrast these lucky infants with the many in developed countries who are rationed to one feed a night at most until their mother's milk dries up—which usually doesn't take long.

Two words of warning: first, never compare your baby with that of any other woman. Each is unique and we should let them be so. Young babies need very frequent feeds (page 124). Some settle into a self-created routine of six feeds a day within a few weeks (page 125), but this isn't a goal to aim for, just one of many patterns your baby may adopt in time.

Second, note one expert's comment that if a baby has five or fewer feeds a day, the likelihood is that his mother's milk will dry up within a month through lack of stimulation.

Some people wonder whether demand feeding will spoil their baby. But they're using the word "spoil" wrongly. A spoiled child is one whose upbringing has been such that he's unpleasant to be with. As he grows older, he's ill at ease with himself too, because he knows he upsets people. A spoiled child is generally one whose "wants" have been met but not always his "needs." As a child grows older, he may want to do something you don't want him to do, or have something you don't want him to have. Giving in is the real way to spoil him.

But a baby's "demands" are vital to his well-being and survival. Meeting them is not the same as giving in to him!

The challenge here, especially for first-time mothers, is to discern the difference between needs and wants. In a very young baby, this is often impossible. As he grows a little older, you'll probably learn to recognize very quickly exactly what he needs. Later still, you won't always have to respond immediately to every "demand" because he'll trust you and therefore be more capable of waiting. And you'll gradually come to recognize the difference between his needs and his wants.

Remarks such as "If you feed him more often than every four hours, you'll spoil him" tend to come from women who brought up their babies by the clock and as a result probably couldn't breastfeed for as long as they wanted.

It's making him wait to get the attention he needs that can spoil him, not meeting his need for milk (or for comfort, diaper changing, more or less clothing, or your attention) when he requires it. The younger the baby, the more urgently his needs must be met. A baby left to cry for long periods from hunger or thirst can despair. He quickly learns that despite his powerful feelings, other people don't seem to care if he's in trouble. This dashes his self-confidence and trust in others.

Length of feeds

The length of a feed is a matter for each baby-mother pair and shouldn't be dictated by health workers or by baby-care "experts" who don't understand how breastfeeding works. The average time a baby spends at one breast is about ten minutes, but averages come from many babies—and while some get all they need in five minutes, others need 20 or more.

Feeding times vary because

- The let-down may be slow.
- Some babies are hungrier than others, perhaps always, or perhaps because they're having a growth spurt.
- Some babies aren't very alert, especially early on, so need more time to feed.

"Feeds"?

Talking about the time a baby spends at the breast as a "feed" makes us think of it as a time to get milk down in as businesslike a way as possible to obtain nutrients. But many babies, especially early on, like to drink in a leisurely way, snoozing between bouts of sucking and milking. While doing this, they may let go of the breast temporarily, or hold the nipple in their mouth and give occasional gentle, "fluttering" sucks for minutes at a time. It's not uncommon for a young baby sometimes to spend hours at the breast in this fashion, if allowed. Such behavior can be perfectly normal, which makes counting feeds meaningless because many such encounters involve very little actual "feeding" at all. However, such behavior can also result from poor positioning at the breast, so it's wise to check for this.

It's particularly important not to curtail feeds in the first few days, because you could take your baby from the breast before your let-down begins. Short suckling times don't prevent sore nipples but often prevent or delay the establishment of successful lactation and benefit mother or baby only in very occasional circumstances (page 220).

Babies' breasts

The commonly observed enlargement of the breasts in newborn boys and girls results from maternal hormones traveling across the placenta before birth. Sometimes they even contain a few drops of milk. Both swelling and milk eventually disappear, sometimes over several months or longer.

seven

Breastfeeding Your Baby

The moment of birth comes after months of waiting and hours or days of labor. Pride in producing a baby that a few hours ago was a wriggling bump mingles with relief and, for most women, curiosity, excitement, and elation. Not surprisingly, many are tired and a few, exhausted.

But the first few days with your new baby are pivotal for breastfeeding because it's now that you'll both learn how to do it and get good at it. So it's really important to make a good start.

As the weeks and months pass, you'll become increasingly confident.

You'll find more information about several of the techniques mentioned in this chapter—including how to hold your baby and position him at the breast, and how to express (including how to do breast compressions), switch-nurse, pump, collect and store milk—in chapter 8.

The first cuddle—skin to skin

Hopefully, you'll have your precious first cuddle without delay. Cuddling your baby with his naked body against your naked body is an excellent way to start mothering him.

Early skin-to-skin contact is good for him because it provably helps stabilize his heartbeat, breathing rate, and body temperature, and reduce any pain (for example, from having an injection, mucus sucked from his mouth and throat, or other medical procedures) or other stress.

It's also good for you because it provably reduces stress and the risk of the "baby blues" (page 192) and helps stabilize your body temperature.

And it's good for both of you because it makes it more likely you'll breastfeed, as well as breastfeed for as long as you want. What's more, it sets the stage for the intimacy of your relationship.

The benefits of early suckling

It takes a single-minded woman to put her baby to the breast amidst all the activity in a typical labor ward, but it's worthwhile for five reasons.

First, suckling produces oxytocin. This encourages womb contractions, which help push out the placenta and may reduce bleeding.

- A study in Singapore found that breastfeeding immediately after birth makes the womb contract nearly as much as an oxytocin injection (*International Journal of Gynecology and Obstetrics*, 1994).

The usual practice today, though, is for a doctor or nurse to give an injection of Syntometrine (oxytocin plus ergometrine—see page 289) to make the womb contract (and so help expel the placenta) and to reduce bleeding, even though research suggests this can interfere with breastfeeding.

- In this study 168 women received ergometrine after the second stage of labor and an equal-sized group did not. The latter group were more likely to continue breastfeeding for more than four weeks. The researchers recommended not giving it routinely to newly delivered mothers who want to breastfeed (*Midwifery*, 1990).

Second, suckling-induced womb contractions occurring while the umbilical cord is still intact squeeze the cord. This gives the baby an extra helping of blood and, therefore, of iron. Your midwife or doctor needn't cut the cord until the placenta has separated.

Third, putting your baby to your breast within 30 minutes of birth takes advantage of his sucking reflex being at its strongest then. Afterward, many babies become tired and disinterested, and it may be 40 hours or so before they're keen to suck again.

Fourth, waiting for your placenta to come out—which may take up to half an hour—is time well spent on your baby's first feed. Many mothers aren't sleepy and want to be with their baby. And being together now makes a woman more likely to breastfeed successfully and for longer.

Fifth, you're more likely to sleep well later if you cuddle and suckle your baby now and aren't anxious about where he is and what's happening.

What to do

Lean back comfortably against some pillows. Don't lie down flat—semi-reclining is best. Put your baby—clad only in a diaper—with his naked chest against your naked chest. A light blanket over you both is all you need as long as the room is warm.

Let him nuzzle your breast. Some newborns become excited, lick the nipple, and start to feed. Others keep the nipple and areola in their mouth but aren't in any hurry to feed and sometimes simply gaze at their mother. Latching on and feeding properly come later, when they're ready.

Greet your baby and welcome him to the world. This meeting is an intensely special time, so let yourself enjoy it. Have a good look at him. You may not feel a rush of motherly love—this often takes time—but you'll probably be curious to examine and touch him. Newborns have a very distinctive smell, which many mothers find delightful.

After a while, he may slowly wriggle up toward your breast, then root for your nipple and latch on of his own accord. This "self-attachment" is one of Nature's miracles. A newborn doing this may instinctively adopt a similar position to that in which he lay in your womb.

Alternatively, you can give him a little guidance.

Early suckling may feel natural to you. But feeling unsure what to do is normal too, especially with a first baby. Don't be discouraged if he seems disinterested. He'll like the smell of your breast even if he doesn't know what to do with it yet. And if he tastes the sweetness of your colostrum, he may be much keener, so express a drop or two, rub it over your nipple and areola, and touch your nipple against his lower lip every now and then.

If he doesn't feed within an hour or so of being born, express a few drops of colostrum and drip them into his mouth every two hours or so.

Getting comfortable

A semi-reclining position is a particularly comfortable for the first feed and anytime you like afterward. If your perineum is sore—after stitches, for example—sitting on an inflatable rubber ring or a "Valley cushion" (page 340) can make all the difference. It may help to put your baby on a pillow on your lap.

If your breasts are tense, soften the one you are going to use by expressing a little milk, as this makes latching on easier.

How your baby feeds

Your baby won't feed continuously, like a bottle-fed one does, but will pause between bouts of sucking. This is because as your milk lets down, it flows in repeated cycles of several spurts then a short pause. He simply adapts to this milk flow.

Wrapping your baby

If your baby sleeps after a feed and you want to lie him down, wrap him snugly in a shawl or a crib sheet (though not so he gets too hot). This way he'll be less likely to wake with a start. Carrying him in a baby sling has a similar effect. Toward the end of pregnancy, your womb held him fairly tightly, so being wrapped up may feel comfortingly familiar.

A few babies, though, dislike being "swaddled" this way.

Relaxing and enjoying your baby

Relaxing helps you enjoy breastfeeding. If you're in the hospital and would feel happier with the curtains drawn around your bed, ask someone to do this. Be encouraged by positive comments about your breastfeeding.

Your newborn may stare at you from time to time, or all the time. Having him do this can be a wonderful feeling, so relax and enjoy it. Sometimes you may choose to feed with you and him both naked, the room warm, and a diaper ready to soak up any leaks from you or the baby.

Once you're home you might like to cuddle, wash, and even feed him while you're having a bath. He'll probably like it much better than being bathed in a baby bath because you'll be holding him close and he'll feel more secure. Make sure first that the room is warm, the water temperature is suitable, and someone is there to take him from you.

Many women enjoy massaging their baby with warm oil, and babies nearly always enjoy this too. This is safest done on a towel on the floor where his oily body can't slip from you.

There are no limits to the time you and your baby spend together. Babies thrive on body contact, love, and attention.

What's your baby getting?

The earliest milk is called colostrum; the later milk is called mature milk.

Colostrum

At first your baby gets colostrum. He doesn't need much to drink for the first few days as nature intended him to have only small amounts. The small volumes of colostrum you produce are worth their weight in gold. Infant formula can't compare for goodness and protectiveness.

Your colostrum won't look much, but don't doubt your ability to nourish your new baby in these first few days.

Note that a one-day-old baby's stomach holds only about one and a half teaspoonfuls (5–7 mL or 0.1–0.2 fl oz) at most. A three-day-old baby's stomach capacity is only a little bigger, at ¾–1 tablespoonful (22–29 mL or 0.75–1 fl oz). And a seven-day-old is about 1½–2 table-spoonfuls (44–59 mL or 1.5–2 fl oz).

Colostrum's higher protein level enables many newborns to last longer between feeds than when the mature milk comes in. This could be Nature's way of helping a newly delivered mother get some sleep.

Mature milk

After the third stage of labor, once the placenta is delivered, a woman's level of the hormone progesterone falls. This triggers a sudden increase in the amount of lactose in the milk-producing cells. This, in turn, attracts water into these cells, which greatly increases the milk volume. This is popularly known as the milk "coming in." The milk is now called mature milk. Milk usually comes in slowly, but in some women it comes as a deluge.

Mature milk usually comes in between the second and fifth days after delivery, though may arrive earlier in women having a second or subsequent baby. The more often and the longer a baby feeds, the sooner milk comes in. Indeed, it can come in on the second or third day if a woman feeds her baby frequently, but not until four or five days if she feeds infrequently.

When milk is relatively slow to come in—which means it doesn't come in until after 72 hours (three whole days)—this is very often because a woman isn't feeding often or for long enough, or because her baby isn't positioned well enough at the breast and so can't latch on well enough to stimulate milk production.

It's really important to start using effective breastfeeding techniques from day one, and to feed frequently in the first three days after child-birth, because it'll make your milk come in sooner. If you don't do it now, you may get into the habit of feeding infrequently. This could make your milk supply dwindle and your baby gain less weight. So you'd probably give up breastfeeding. *Slow-to-arrive milk is a signal to pay more heed to breastfeeding technique.*

- Delay in the onset of milk production occurred in 33 percent of first-time mothers and only 5 percent of other mothers, according to this US study (*Pediatrics*, 2003).

- A US study of 432 first-time mothers noted delayed onset of milk production in 44 percent (*American Journal of Clinical Nutrition*, 2010).

Other factors associated with slow-to-arrive milk include a cesarean section (C-section), a long labor, age over 30, overweight or obesity, a raised level of the hormone cortisol (which could be associated with stress) and a low-birthweight baby. This is partly because each of these can hinder a woman from using effective breastfeeding techniques.

When to feed your baby

Feed him when

- He gives "feeding cues" that tell you he's ready. He may become fidgety, put his hands to his mouth, make feeding movements with his mouth, root, turn his head to you, nuzzle you, stiffen or cry. Crying is a very late sign of hunger and a sign so acute that it's distressing. If you're sensitive to his cues so you can feed him before he cries, you're likely to be a successful breastfeeder. Unless you always keep him by your naked breast so he can feed when he wants—which is what happens in some parts of the world where, as a result, breastfeeding is very successful—these cues are his only way of telling you he's hungry.

- He hasn't asked for a feed for three hours since the beginning of the last one. If he's asleep, wake him. Too many gaps longer than this could endanger your milk supply. Some babies sometimes go four to five hours, but gaps this long aren't wise until your supply is well established.

- Your breasts are full and you want to relieve their tension.

- You want to go out soon.

How often to feed?

Some newborns want to feed every half hour, others every two hours, and some want to be at the breast on and off for an hour or even several hours. The latter is usually perfectly normal and is sometimes called "cluster feeding."

A young baby needs feeding at least 8–12 times in every 24 hours, with some of them at night. Almost all very young babies need more.

Some women feed their very young babies as many as 30–40 times in 24 hours, others as few as six. However, six feeds a day give breasts very little stimulation—perhaps not enough to produce sufficient milk. Five in 24 hours usually make the milk supply fail. Eight is probably the absolute minimum for very young babies.

The number of feeds a day varies with each mother-baby pair and depends on

- The maturity of your milk—babies need more frequent feeds of mature milk than of colostrum, as mature milk is lower in protein.

- Your baby's age and the length of your pregnancy.

- Your baby's size and health. A small or unwell baby needs particularly frequent short feeds as he lacks the energy to suck and milk well for long.

- Your milk-producing capacity.

- Whether he latches on properly so he can suck and milk optimally. If he isn't well latched on, he'll get only relatively low-fat low-calorie milk which will leave the stomach so fast it won't satisfy him for long. Also, he won't stimulate your prolactin and milk supply optimally, so you may not make enough milk and he could go hungry.

- How strongly he sucks and milks. The more vigorously he does, the more prolactin—and therefore the more milk—you make. A baby who doesn't suck and milk strongly will try to get what he needs by taking longer over each feed.

- Whether you let him feed for as long as he wants at the first breast, and then continue at the second breast if he wants. If you don't, he may not get enough relatively high-fat, high-calorie milk and will be hungry sooner.

- Whether you let your baby be at the breast for comfort as well as for milk. Any stimulation helps increases prolactin, which increases milk production.

125

- Your baby's growth rate—faster-growing babies need more frequent feeds.

- Your baby's preferences.

- Your culture, lifestyle, preferences, and needs.

One reason breastfed babies need frequent feeds is that *breast milk is so well digested that it stays in their stomach for only an hour and a half at most* (compared with nearly two and a half hours for formula).

Babies gain weight better with frequent feeds because these stimulate greater milk production. Frequent feeding by a well-latched-on baby also encourages the development of prolactin receptors on the milk-producing cells in the milk glands. These attract prolactin which allows the glands to make milk.

To put frequent feeding into perspective, remember that your placenta fed your unborn baby continuously. A breastfed baby of under nine months has been dubbed an "exterogestate fetus," implying he's so immature that he has to rely on being fed much of the time, just as he was in your womb.

Ideally, *feed on an unrestricted basis*—when he seems to want a feed, when your breasts are full, and if you have other reasons of your own. This successful, natural way of breastfeeding meets both a mother's and a baby's needs and desires. Women who feed this way aren't bothered when their babies want more feeds some days than others—they simply give them what they want, trusting the baby to know what he needs. Breastfeeding tends to be much more successful in cultures in which women feed frequently. Babies allowed completely unrestricted feeds—for example, those carried next to a naked breast all day in developing countries—don't have to cry before they are fed, and feed very much more often than most Western breastfed babies.

For example, the young babies of modern hunter-gatherers called the !Kung San, in South Africa, are allowed to feed when they like. They consequently choose to feed about four times an hour, for about two minutes or so each time, day and night!

Women who feed as often as their baby wants usually feed much more often and more successfully than schedule-feeders. But this calls for a particular frame of mind. Bottle-feeders nearly always know how many feeds they've given over 24 hours. But successful breastfeeders can't usually say how many feeds they've given. There may even be times of the day when feeds are more or less continuous.

Demand-feeding, done whenever a baby "demands" a feed by crying—can work well. But some babies don't demand enough feeds, so they don't stimulate the breasts enough. This makes the milk supply dwindle and prevents the let-down becoming reliable.

Don't feed on any schedule. The more schedule-feeding there's been over the last 100 years, the less successful breastfeeding has become. The World Health Organization and the American Academy of Pediatrics recommend that the number of breastfeeds should be led by the baby. This is because studies repeatedly show that women who breastfeed in an unrestricted way produce more milk and breastfeed for more months (or years) than those who follow any kind of schedule. They are also only half as likely to get sore nipples and engorged breasts. And their babies put on more weight and are less likely to become jaundiced.

Don't be anxious about conflicting advice from friends, relatives, and health workers, as some people, including certain self-styled baby-feeding "experts," still promote breastfeeding every four hours (at say 2:00, 6:00, and 10:00 a.m., and 2:00, 6:00, and 10:00 p.m.). But this advice is for bottle-fed babies—not you and your baby! Nature has made women so only a very few produce enough milk using such a routine. Most women find their milk supply slowly dwindles with six feeds in 24 hours, as they don't provide anywhere near enough stimulation for their breasts. Women who don't produce enough milk with only six feeds a day are the normal ones! A proportion of mothers who give up breastfeeding because they don't have enough milk are those who give only six feeds a day. As for reducing the number of feeds to five a day, one researcher has found that this causes one in three women to produce insufficient milk.

Women differ as to how much breast stimulation they need to make enough milk, but the vast majority find their milk supply increases if they feed more often.

It isn't sensible to compare how many feeds you give with how many another woman gives, because while this may be interesting, you could find yourself competing over whose baby lasts longest between feeds. The lack of competition at home is partly why many women breastfeed more successfully if they leave hospital soon after delivery or give birth at home.

Frequent breastfeeding is good news for midwives. Research in a hospital in Oxford in the UK found the midwives' workload fell dramatically when they no longer insisted on scheduled feedings.

Anthropologists can predict how often any mammal's young need to be suckled by the amounts of protein and fat in their milk. If there's a lot (as in seal and rabbit milk), the young need infrequent suckling—perhaps only once a day. But if, as with human milk, the milk is low in protein and fat, the young need frequent suckling. Along with other animals with low-protein milk, humans are grouped as "continuous-contact mammals." Given the chance, our babies suck on and off much of the time, which seems to be what Nature intended. We automatically reduce the frequency of feeds our babies ask for by not carrying them next to our naked breasts all day and not sleeping naked next to them at night.

As babies get older, most want fewer feeds and some settle into their own routine of perhaps relatively regular two-, three-, or four-hourly feeds. But not all do, and each is an individual, so don't compare your baby with any other—even with previous babies you've had.

- In a study in Sri Lanka, 58 babies aged 4–6 weeks fed 6–20 times every 24 hours: 5–17 times by day and 1–5 at night (Asia Oceania Journal of *Obstetrics and Gynecology*, 1994).

Asking for frequent feeds is normal as long as a baby is healthy, thriving, and latching on well.

Sometimes feeds are erratically spaced, in which case just stop what you're doing and take them in your stride. Unrestricted breastfeeding means feeds are not occasions that can be planned.

Why he might want more feeds than usual

Sometimes your baby may want many more feeds than usual. This could be because

- He's extra hungry because he's having a growth spurt (below).

- He's hungry because of some other mismatch between your milk supply and his needs.

- He's upset or unwell and needs the comfort of being at the breast (See chapter 10 for how to increase your supply)

- He needs to soothe tender or itchy gums because he's teething.

- He's thirsty because it's a very hot day.

Your milk supply will catch up in two or three days if you let him feed for as often and as long as he wants.

Growth spurts

Babies may suddenly want more feeds because they're growing faster than before. US researchers say some babies grow ½ in (1.25 cm) in 24 hours during a growth spurt! Growth spurts can occur at any time, though common ages for them are three weeks, six weeks, and three months. Babies are often unusually restless because at first there is a mismatch between their mother's milk supply and their need for milk.

The good news is that when a growth spurt begins, your baby will instinctively ask for more and/or longer feeds. This will increase your milk supply. But it'll take two to three days of increased stimulation for you to produce significantly more, so be prepared for him to be unsettled for this long.

If you're already demand-feeding, give at least two and preferably more extra feeds a day. And have no long gaps between feeds at night.

Waking your baby

Some women worry about waking their baby to feed during the day. But this is the right thing to do if it's a long time since a feed. You might also want to wake your baby if your breasts feel full. If you don't either do this or express some milk, they'll become tense or engorged (swollen) and your milk production will slow down. Never go so long between feeds that your breasts feel tense and lumpy. Remember you are part of a nursing pair— sometimes you'll feed for your baby's benefit, sometimes for your own.

One breast or two?

Many women feed from both breasts at each feed. When your baby finishes at the first breast, he'll almost certainly stop spontaneously. This is generally better than switching him to the other breast after some arbitrary time, as it means he's more likely to get a good helping of fat-rich newly let-down milk from the first breast.

Have a short break if you like, then offer the second breast. If he's still hungry, he'll feed from the second breast. Sometimes you may need to switch sides several times during a feed. If he snoozes after coming off the first breast, wait awhile to see if he wakes again and wants the other one.

Many babies drink from only one breast during each feed, which is fine if you

- Let him feed at that breast until he's had enough.

- Alternate the breast you give at each feed.

- Express the unemptied breast to prevent it becoming lumpy or tense. Otherwise it might not produce as much milk as it could. This is partly because of the back-pressure of the remaining milk on the milk-producing cells, and partly because milk contains a hormone-like inhibitory factor that reduces milk production if some is left behind.

Which breast first?

If you fed from both breasts during the last feed, start the next feed with the breast you fed from last, as it will probably be less well emptied. If you fed from only one breast during the last feed, start with the other next time. The let-down is more efficient early in a feed, and a baby sucks more strongly at the first breast, so the first breast is usually emptied better than the second.

Note that your baby may sometimes need to go back to the first breast after finishing the second. Indeed, you may switch sides several times.

Some babies prefer one particular breast. This is often the left one, possibly because the mother's heartbeat soothes them. Most women have one breast bigger than the other. If the difference is mainly caused by fat, a baby may find it easier to feed from the smaller one, but if the difference is in the amount of glandular tissue, he may prefer the larger one. Some women only ever feed from one side. It's then wise—in view of the differing rates of cancer in used and unused breasts (page 47)—to express milk from the unused breast after a feed.

How long should a feed last?

As long as your baby is well positioned and latched on, it doesn't matter how long a feed lasts. *Simply let him feed till he's had enough.* He'll finish more quickly as he gets older (unless he's tired, bored, upset or ill).

Sometimes he may want a snack, at other times, a feast. Researchers in South Africa found that a demand-feeding baby took feeds of very different volumes at different times—one feed sometimes being 10 times as long as another.

He may feed for different times at different feeds, depending on

- How hungry or thirsty he is.

- How much milk is already in your breasts at the beginning of a feed.

- How strongly he sucks and milks. Some babies do it so enthusiastically and strongly that they stimulate several let-downs in rapid succession and thus get what they need very quickly.

- How long it takes you to let down.

- How reliable and strong your let-down is—and therefore how fast your milk flows.

- How much milk your breasts hold.

- Whether he feeds from one breast, or two, or goes from one to the other several times.

- How much he needs the comfort of being at the breast.

- How tired or alert he is.

- Whether he's simply enjoying being at the breast.

Babies differ in how quickly they feed

Some babies feed slowly and sporadically, others speedily. And while some get most of their milk in the first few minutes at each breast, others take longer. In one study, one baby got all he needed in four minutes from just one breast, while another took nearly 22 minutes and fed from both breasts, but most were in between. In my professional experience, many babies take longer—sometimes much longer—than 20 or so minutes for a feed. If your baby does this it's probably normal for him. But it's wise to check that he's well positioned and latched on. There's no reason to stop feeding unless you have something else to do, or have sore nipples.

Some babies soon run out of steam and need to wait a while to muster the energy to suck hard enough to stimulate another let-down. You can help by doing breast compressions (page 163).

Each baby has his own unique pattern of the number of sucks per minute and the intervals between sucks—and therefore his own speed of feeding and his own unique pattern of stimulation of the breast.

You may be told, wrongly, to feed your baby for a set number of minutes each side and to increase this time each day to ten minutes a side on the fifth day. Such restriction is unnatural. It hinders milk from coming in, may not give your let-down time to work and become established, may not allow as many let-downs as there could be, prevents your baby getting as much colostrum as he could, and encourages sore nipples.

All this has been known for years, but a few hospitals and health workers still enforce these outdated guidelines. Ideally, question such rules openly to give unknowledgeable staff the chance to learn. If you find it difficult to question authority, especially just after having a baby, simply go ahead and suckle as long as you and your baby want. Interestingly, a study in the UK in 1981 found that 80 percent of those women who decided for themselves how long feeds should be were still breastfeeding at the end of the first week, compared with only 57 percent of those who were told how long to feed.

How to tell he's had enough

Many babies show they've had enough by coming off the breast. They may fall asleep as they release their latch. Near the end of his feed a baby may relax his fists, smile, or arch his back. Accept your baby's judgment.

Lots of babies, especially in the evening, or if pre-term, like to have frequent small feeds with short gaps of, for example, 10 to 15 minutes between them. Or they may doze on and off during a feed. This can make it difficult to know when they've had enough milk and when they are simply enjoying being at the breast. But after a while you'll get to know how much he's had by feeling your breasts.

One reason a baby may fall asleep only to wake up again soon for more milk, is because the level of cholecystokinin rises during a feed. Made in his gut, this hormone rises in the presence of fat. This signals the stomach to slow its activity so the gut can digest the fat properly. But cholecystokinin is also a "satiety" hormone. And in a very young baby who's naturally taking time over his feed, it may rise enough to signal fullness before his stomach is actually full. During a short sleep, it falls again, and the baby then wakes, rightly feeling hungry because he hasn't had enough yet, and wants another feed. He may sometimes do this two, three, or four times, until he really is full.

What about stopping a feed?

Some babies have to be gently removed from the breast or they'd be there all day. If your nipples are sore you'll probably want to limit the length of feeds for a day or two—but don't do this for too long unless you express some milk after each feed to give your breasts more stimulation, or your milk supply will diminish. And don't reduce the frequency of feeds.

Never pull your baby off the breast while he's feeding as suddenly breaking the strong vacuum in his mouth could damage your nipple. It's better to put the tip of your little finger gently into the corner of his mouth and push the nipple sideways to allow air in. Your baby will then come away easily without hurting you.

Why won't he stop feeding?

Some babies who don't want to stop feeding aren't latched on properly, so they persist in order to get enough milk. Others may have gotten into the habit of using the breast as a pacifier to help them drop off to sleep or provide comfort. This is fine if it's all right with you and you're not getting sore. And it'll certainly boost your milk supply!

Your baby's feeding pattern and behavior

Your baby's behavior at the breast falls depends on his personality, past experience at the breast, and hunger, and on the nature of your let-down. Some babies always take a long time over feeds. Others regurgitate several times during and after. Many snooze on and off. And some drink in a fast, no-nonsense manner.

Many babies behave differently at different times of the day and almost all change their patterns as they grow older.

Tips for daytime feeds

Keep the room warm if you have a winter baby, as cold air can contract the muscle fibers in the areolas and nipples. This constricts the openings of the ducts at the nipple, delaying the release of milk. This, in turn, would frustrate your hungry baby. While his mouth would eventually warm your nipples, it's wise to start off feeling warm.

Keep your cell phone at hand unless you are willing to ignore its ringing while you're feeding. You may even decide not to use the phone, so as not to interrupt the "zen" of breastfeeding. If you like to read while feeding (and don't have another young child needing attention), have something on hand. You could even consider getting a music stand to support a book or magazine and leave your hands free. You may find it relaxing to watch TV or listen to the radio or to music on your portable media player or smartphone. Or you may just love to watch your baby feeding, especially if he stares up at your eyes, as many do. A lot depends on how long a feed takes. If he's a quick feeder, you won't get bored and seek diversion.

Ideally, a feed should be a time to look forward to and enjoy. If you look to your own creature comforts, your milk will let down well and you'll be able to relax and see feed times as oases of peace. Some babies prefer quiet feed times and don't feed well in noisy surroundings. Older ones are particularly easily distracted.

After a while you may find you can even breastfeed as you walk around, enabling you to fetch something you want, for example.

Many women feel very thirsty when feeding, especially in the first few weeks, so keep a drink by you.

Naps

If your baby has naps in a separate room, you may not hear him waking. So unless you are prepared to check every few minutes, have him with you or at least within earshot. If he needs to sleep, household noise is unlikely to keep him awake. If he doesn't need to sleep, it'll be much better for him to watch and listen to what's going on than to lie in a quiet room getting bored and lonely, gazing at the ceiling, then crying.

Many breastfeeding mothers say they know when their baby is about to wake, even if he's in another room. This may be because their breasts are full and ready for the next feed, though it's also possible that some sort of sixth sense is alerting them. Some even start to let down their milk just before their baby makes it known he's awake.

Going to sleep at the breast

The easiest way of helping a sleepy young baby get off to sleep is to let him stay at the breast until he nods off. Some babies do this anyway when they've had enough, while others doze toward the end of a feed, not letting go but waking every so often to nibble or lightly suck. If you gently remove your breast, he may drift into a deeper sleep. If you watch him, you'll notice he makes occasional sucking or mouthing movements as if still at the breast and, from time to time, a smile or a frown may flicker across his face as he dreams. You may notice similar expressions just before he wakes. He may also open his eyes several times as he goes off to sleep, as if to check you are still there. Once he's sound asleep and you've finished cuddling him, put him somewhere warm, safe, and within earshot to sleep.

The only snag with this is that a baby frequently or always allowed to go to sleep at the breast gets into the habit of needing to be at the breast to fall asleep. So some women prefer not to allow this.

What you do depends on whether you

- Enjoy it.

- Are okay with him to rely on it while he's still very young.

- Want to be able to leave him with a sitter. While many babies settle to sleep easily without their mother, some find it more difficult.

- Are content with the idea of him continuing to need the breast to go to sleep as he grows older.

Other ways of getting him off to sleep

Many babies happily go to sleep if put in a warm, comfortable place after a feed. And some regularly nod off in a car, stroller, or sling, lulled by the motion or noise. Rocking your baby in your arms is another time-honored way of inducing sleep.

If you breastfeed while your baby is in a sling, and he then goes to sleep, adjust his position so his head faces up and clears the sling and your body.

How your baby goes off to sleep will vary with the time of day, where you are, and what you're doing. Most babies prefer a familiar place, especially when they're older. If yours is used to having you there as he goes to sleep, he'll tend to expect this every time. This is the norm in many families and in many cultures—some of which consider the idea of putting a baby to sleep in another place, away from his mother, most peculiar.

There's nothing more pleasant if you have the time than going to sleep with your baby alongside you on your bed. You'll wake refreshed and may find he sleeps extra well with the familiar and reassuring smell, feel, and sound of your body.

How long your baby sleeps

He may fall into a pattern of sleeping of perhaps 60–90 minutes between feeds, or he may be an irregular sleeper. Many young babies wake soon after what seemed to be the end of a feed and want to go back to the breast. This is normal—especially in the evenings, and for very young, pre-term, or unwell babies. A few babies fuss and can't get to sleep because they are still hungry after a feed. This could be because their mother took them off the first breast before they'd had enough of the relatively high-fat milk that's available later in a feed at the first breast.

Carry your baby in a sling if he is unsettled but you have things you must do.

Rooming-in at the hospital

"Rooming-in" means that you have your baby in the same room as you. It makes breastfeeding twice as likely to be successful than if he were to be elsewhere. You're also likely to sleep better because you won't worry whether he is crying unattended or being given bottles.

Many women say they remember the agony of hearing their baby crying in a distant nursery. A woman doesn't know the sound of her own baby's voice this soon after birth and may be anxious every time any baby cries that it's her baby. She'll have far more peace of mind if she's with her baby. And her milk will come in sooner if she can pick him up for a feed whenever he "asks" for one, and whenever she wants to relieve the tension in her breasts.

In general it's fair to say that no hospital has enough staff to give a baby the love and care his mother can, so it's scarcely surprising that babies who room-in are more contented than those who don't.

Rooming-in also makes life easier for hospital staff. And it leads to less noise because babies don't have to cry for long, if at all, to get attention. Increasing numbers of hospitals now facilitate this practice.

If you're in a large, open-plan ward, be sure to pick up your baby as soon as he needs a cuddle or a feed to avoid him crying and disturbing other mothers.

If you'd like him in a bassinet by your bed at night and there's no good reason not to, but the hospital staff aren't keen and you don't feel like being assertive, ask your partner or other helper to have a word.

Sleeping and night feeds

It's worth mentally gearing up for night feeds because you'll be doing plenty of them. Night feeds may become less frequent from two months or so, but many babies continue wanting them for a long time.

Young babies have more periods of light, REM (rapid eye movement) sleep than do older children and adults, and are most likely to wake for a feed during these times. As your baby gets older, he'll have longer periods of deeper sleep and will wake less often.

When you feed your baby at night, do so calmly, quietly, and with the light as low as possible. This helps him learn that nighttime isn't for play and talk.

If he goes into a hospital nursery at night, tell the staff on duty that you're a breastfeeder. Although they should know, it's easy for an inexperienced person, a new agency nurse, or a nurse who thinks she's doing you a favor, to give your baby a bottle. Some women tie a card on their baby's bassinet, saying, "I'm a breastfed baby. Please take me to my mother when I cry."

You may be too excited to sleep much yourself soon after giving birth. It's common to want to live through the birthing experience over and over again in your mind, as though "learning" it. However, try to get as much sleep as you can between feeds, as you'll probably be tired and broken nights take their toll. Midwives may suggest you rest on your tummy for an hour or so every day. If your breasts are at all full, make yourself more comfortable by lying with one pillow beneath your head and another below your upper abdomen so there's a "tunnel" for your breasts. Some mothers dream very little in the first few days or even weeks after the birth, probably because their sleep patterns are broken by their baby waking.

Night feeds are essential if young babies in particular are to get the frequent nourishment they need. Night feeds also encourage good milk production and successful breastfeeding. And they can be a very special quiet time for mother and her baby to be together. Understandably, though, most of us are so used to the long sleeps of our pre-baby days that we long for unbroken nights again as soon as possible.

The fact is that night waking is natural and normal. For example,

- Of 3,172 babies aged three months, 47 percent woke once or twice a night and 46 percent woke three or four times, according to a study in Thailand. Waking more than an average of twice a night was more likely in boys, and in babies who'd had more than three sleeps during the day, those who slept in a rocking or swinging cradle, those exclusively breastfed, and those in the habit of falling asleep at the breast (*Sleep Medicine*, 2008).

Babies wake for many reasons. They may be hungry, thirsty, cold, or ill, or be roused from light sleep by noise, light, or some other stimulus. There are several ways of helping your baby sleep. But there's no point in trying to make him sleep for longer than is necessary at his stage of maturity.

Keep things dark

When feeding, don't flood the room with bright light because this will make you both less sleepy and more likely to stay awake for a long time. Put a low-wattage bulb in the light or install a dimmer switch. If your baby sleeps in your bed, don't turn on the light unless you must—to change a diaper, for example.

Keep things quiet, calm, and low key

It's tempting to talk to your baby when you're both awake and everyone else is asleep, but it's best to stay quiet and calm. This way, a feed won't excite him so much, and he'll wake less and less often as night feeds become increasingly unnecessary for adequate nourishment.

Be ready for diaper changes

Your baby may happily go back to sleep without a diaper change if he's warm and comfortable, but it's worth keeping clean diapers on hand so it's easier if you do have to change him.

If using disposables, be sure they fit really well and have plenty of absorbency. If using cloth diapers, put a diaper pad inside, consider using two diapers at once, and insert a one-way liner next to his skin to help keep it dry.

These simple tips will mean he's less likely to wake from feeling cold or otherwise uncomfortable in a single dirty diaper. He'll also stand a better chance of going through the night without a change.

Cut down on caffeine

Coffee, tea, cola, and other caffeinated soft drinks aren't usually a problem, but some babies, particularly pre-term ones whose liver can't yet break down caffeine very well, have trouble sleeping if their mothers drink a lot of caffeine.

Give up smoking

Becoming a nonsmoker might help your baby sleep longer:

- A study of 15 breastfeeders who were smokers, at the Monell

Chemical Senses Center, Pennsylvania, US, found that babies spent 53.4 minutes sleeping after their mother had smoked but spent 84.5 minutes sleeping after a day's abstention (*Pediatrics*, 2007).

Look after yourself

It's easy to believe you need a certain amount of sleep, but most of us experience no ill effects from having less than usual, or from having broken nights. However, if you feel tired, get more rest by going to bed earlier, or napping when your baby sleeps in the day. If you wake at night feeling hot and sweaty, with full breasts, either wake your baby for a feed or express some milk. This is because the longer your breasts remain full, the more likely they are to become engorged and to start to produce less milk.

The advantages of night feeds

When your baby wakes you, enjoy feeling his warm, soft body nestling against you. Some busy women enjoy the luxury of undisturbed time during night feeds to think, plan, or pray. If your baby doesn't mind having the light on, night feeds can even be times for reading, texting, surfing the web, or just looking at your baby. But don't let any of these activities hype you up so much that you don't let down your milk!

Let your baby sleep in your bedroom

Many parents do this, as it makes getting up less disruptive and means you're more likely wake as soon he becomes restless, rather than when he cries. This is less disturbing to both of you and to other members of the household, and means he's more likely to go back to sleep soon after a feed.

If you put his crib by your bed, you won't have to get out of bed to lift him out when he needs a feed. The sides of most cribs don't drop low enough for this to be as easy as it could be. However, a "sidecar crib" (page 340) is more helpful. This attaches to the side of your bed and can be open to it. Your baby is then right by you and on the same level, so it's easy put an arm around him to comfort him, or to slide him into your bed for a feed. Also he'll have his own mattress and bedclothes.

- Research at Durham University in the UK found that babies who slept in a sidecar crib or in their mother's bed fed twice as often as those who slept in a separate crib (*Archives of Disease in Childhood*, 2006).

How long you keep the crib in your bedroom is up to you and your partner. Some mothers move it out when their baby is a year old or more; and some get their baby used to going to sleep and waking in a separate room sooner rather than later.

If you can't or don't want to sleep with your baby in your bedroom, then when he wakes, either bring him into your bed temporarily, where you'll both be warm and comfy, or feed him in his room.

Let him breastfeed in your bed

This is easiest for night feeds, and means you stay (lying down, which disturbs your sleep much less. Also, there's no crying to wake everyone, because you so readily sense his restlessness that you can feed him before he needs to cry. You'll also know he's safe and warm. Your baby will almost certainly feed more often than if he were in another room, and you'll almost certainly be more rested in the morning than if you'd had to get out of bed several times. He'll feel secure nestling against your body, sensing your movements, and hearing the sound of your breathing.

Although most new parents imagine they'll never sleep with their baby, most in fact do. In other words, it's normal. A recent study found that over half the babies in the US spent part of the night in bed with their parents. In some countries most mothers sleep with their babies the whole time. Even if they don't intend to do it, parents sometimes fall asleep with their baby, especially during night feeds.

- A UK study of 1,356 babies aged up to one year found that nearly one in two newborns slept with their parents at some time. On any night in the first four weeks more than one in four babies slept with their parents. And on any one night in the first year one in five babies aged three to twelve months spent at least part of the time sleeping with one or both parents. Bed-sharing was more common in the early months in the most affluent families.

And breastfeeding was strongly associated with bed-sharing, both at birth and at 3 months (*Archives of Disease in Childhood*, 2004).

When you want to feed from the other breast, roll over with him in your arms so he's on your other side. Or just twist your body so he can feed from the other breast. You'll probably find it most comfortable to feed him with your arm crooked around the top of his head, and a hand on him to keep him in place. After a feed you can leave him lying on his back by you, with you on your side, facing him. Or you can put him into a crib.

If he needs burping, sit him up while you stay lying down.

Don't forget to keep something to drink by your bed, as you may feel very thirsty while feeding.

Last but not least, it makes sense to have as large a bed as you can afford and fit into your room.

Sleeping safely together

Some women fear suffocating their baby, perhaps by rolling on him. However, the chances of this are extremely low if you use the tips below.

15 TIPS FOR SAFE SLEEPING WITH YOUR BABY IN BED

1. Don't go to sleep with him until you've checked he's lying on his back. Remember—"Back to Sleep."

2. Don't let him get too hot. He needs about the same amount of sleep-ware as you

3. Don't sleep with him if you or your partner is extremely overweight, takes sleeping tablets or recreational drugs, or is drunk, as all these encourage suffocation by "smothering."

4. Don't sleep with him if you or your partner are a smoker—even if neither of you smokes in bed—because this encourages sudden infant death syndrome.

5. Don't sleep with him if you or your partner are so exhausted or unwell that his wriggling, altered breathing, or cries wouldn't quickly arouse you.

6. If another child sleeps with you, either you or your partner should always lie between that child and the baby.

7. Don't sleep with him if your mattress is very soft, as there's a tiny chance that if he were to roll on to his tummy, this could suffocate him.

8. Put the side of the mattress up against the wall so your baby can't fall out, or put the back of a chair or a cot against the mattress edge.

9. Use a sheet and blankets rather than a duvet, as a duvet could settle around his nose and suffocate him. Make sure he isn't lying near a pillow, as this could suffocate him.

10. Put him between you and the edge of the bed to sleep, rather than between you and your partner.

11. Remove any long ribbons from your nightwear so your baby can't get entangled.

12. Don't sleep with him on a sofa, armchair or reclining chair, as this increases the risk of sudden infant death syndrome.
13. Ban pets from the bed.
14. Don't leave him sleeping alone in your bed as he could wriggle around enough to shift position. This could be a problem if he were to move toward a pillow, for example, or even fall off the edge of the bed.
15. Once he's old enough to roll, put the back of a heavy chair against the side of the bed to stop him falling out when you're asleep.

If you don't want your baby to depend on you lying by him to go to sleep at night, there's a solution. When you give the last feed before you go to bed, don't let him go to sleep at the breast, but when he seems sleepy lay him in his cot so he gets used to going to sleep in his own bed without you lying by him. When he wakes, bring him into your bed for a feed, then take him back to his bed if you want. This means he'll be first in his bed, then yours, then perhaps in his again. Many families who use this approach go through a transitional phase of "musical beds" for some months.

Some women feel uneasy about having their baby in bed. Some dads too are antagonistic, though it should be possible to sort this out if you listen lovingly to one another.

Ask your partner to help

If your baby sleeps in another room and you're tired out, ask your partner to get up and bring him to you in bed, then to put him back into his crib after the feed.

When will your baby give up night feeds?

This depends. Some breastfeds sleep through the night at a few months old, some even earlier, but a great many perfectly normal, healthy babies wake for many months, some even for years. Some wake several times, others just once after their parents have gone to bed, and from time to time a baby might want to breastfeed more or less constantly for a while at night.

Breastfed babies tend to wake more often than bottle-fed ones.

One UK study found that the most significant factor in the history of three-month-olds who woke for breastfeeds was being breastfed more than 11 times over 24 hours in the first week. However, it certainly isn't worth reducing the number of feeds early on simply to reduce the likelihood of night waking later, because—provided your baby is well latched on—frequent feeds are normal, natural and vital for successful breastfeeding. And it isn't worth stopping breastfeeding just to get unbroken nights, because many bottle-fed babies wake at night anyway, and bottle-feds often take much longer to settle after a night feed.

If your baby gives up night feeds early, make sure you breastfeed often enough in the day to maintain your milk supply and stop your breasts overfilling. You may have to express some milk before you go to bed or during the night to prevent discomfort. If your milk supply dwindles, either express some milk or wake your baby for a feed before you go to bed.

Sleep patterns change, sometimes with more waking, sometimes less, but young children grow up and night waking doesn't last for ever—though it may seem it will at the time!

Breast milk only

If your baby must be apart from you, make sure the hospital staff know you want him brought to you as soon as he needs a feed. Also, ensure they know you don't want him to have anything other than your breast milk to drink. They should not give formula, water, or glucose water ("sugar water")—except in the unlikely event that it's medically essential, for example, if your baby has low blood sugar which doesn't respond to more frequent breastfeeds (page 265).

Giving newborn breastfed babies anything other than breast milk is unnecessary for the vast majority. It's also not a good idea in the early days as it can interfere with the establishment of breastfeeding. It's also a fact that mothers who give their breastfed babies bottles of formula are much more likely to give up breastfeeding before they want to.

Don't put off by excuses. He's your baby, and feeding frequently and on an unrestricted basis is the best way to establish successful breastfeeding. If he has anything else to drink, he won't want to breastfeed as often as he otherwise would, so your milk supply will diminish unless you express frequently to make up for him wanting relatively few feeds.

Unfortunately, some hospital maternity units are so out of date that breastfeeding mothers are routinely given bottles of formula to "top o" their babies after a feed.

8 REASONS WHY BREAST MILK ALONE
IS ALMOST ALWAYS BEST

1. The more your baby feeds, the sooner mature milk comes in.

2. Frequent breastfeeds help you make plenty of milk.

3. Colostrum supplies the right nourishment, as well protective antibodies and other substances not present in formula. It also encourages his bowel to expel the sticky early motions (meconium).

4. Formula satiates a baby's appetite for several hours, making him less likely to want to breastfeed. If you give complements or whole feeds of formula, the resulting reduction in breast stimulation will decrease your milk supply.

5. Bottle-fed babies last longer between feeds because it takes longer to digest formula.

6. Formula contains foreign proteins which, especially if your baby has an allergic family history, might increase his risk of allergic and autoimmune diseases in later life.

7. Sugar water is nearly always unnecessary for a full-term, healthy baby, because breast milk provides all the sugar and water he needs. A high-calorie drink satiates his appetite and makes him less likely to want to breastfeed. A sudden slug of sugar is unnatural and best reserved only for when medically essential.

8. Properly and exclusively breastfed babies don't need extra water. Breast milk provides enough even in the early days and in hot countries. Research at the University of Rochester in New York showed that breastfed babies given water, or cows'-milk formula "complements," lost more weight in the first few days and were less likely than exclusively breastfed babies to start gaining before they left the hospital.

In the US, about one in four breastfeeding babies receive formula in their first two days, according to a US government report in 2011.

Is it okay to give occasional bottle-feeds of formula at home?

Giving bottle-feeds of formula is nearly always bad news for a breastfeeding woman and her baby in the early days of breastfeeding. They reduce the supply of breast milk because a baby full of formula doesn't want frequent breastfeeds, yet breast stimulation is essential for milk production.

Women who want to breastfeed successfully shouldn't allow formula feeds. As one mother put it, "How can demand and supply work if you suppress half the demand?"

If formula is recommended because your baby doesn't seem to be thriving, you can almost certainly increase your milk supply (page 204) and give no formula. For example, feed more frequently. If your baby has to have formula, breastfeed as well at each feed. Give the formula by cup rather than by bottle. And either express each breast after the feed or give the formula via a supplementer. This way you'll increase the stimulation to your breasts, which will make more milk.

Doctors and midwives may call drinks of formula "complements" or "supplements." A complement is a drink (in a cup or bottle) of formula given after a breastfeed, and a supplement is one given instead of a breastfeed.

How your breasts feel

Milk-producing cells make and release milk more or less continuously, so the amount in the breast depends to some extent on the time since the last feed. If your baby doesn't wake and your breasts are uncomfortably full, either express some milk or wake him. You'll sometimes need him to relieve your breasts as much as he'll sometimes need you to relieve his hunger. Breastfeeding is a two-way deal.

Hopefully he'll have his longest break between feeds at night, in which case your breasts will be especially full first thing in the morning. You may even wake with your nightwear and bedclothes drenched with milk. The early morning feed is often the most pleasant simply because it's such a relief for tense breasts.

Pacifiers

It's best not to give a pacifier to a baby under four weeks old, because

- Its shape is different from that of the nipple and areola while breastfeeding. This could confuse a baby learning to breastfeed.

- It seems to encourage ear infection, according to one study (*British Medical Journal*, 2006).

- It increases the level of the "satiety hormone" cholecystokinin (page 132). This reduces hunger, so the baby may delay asking for a breastfeed. If he uses a pacifier a lot, your milk supply could theoretically fall, and he could gain less weight.

However, once breastfeeding is going well, having an infant use a pacifier while going to sleep is associated with a reduced risk of sudden infant death syndrome (page 28). But if you're content to let your baby "comfort-suck" at your breast as he goes to sleep, it's likely, though unproven, that this will have the same effect. And it'll certainly be good for your milk supply.

It's better for a child not to go on having a pacifier after a year old.

- A study of 457 children aged 3 years found that pacifier-sucking was associated with a higher risk of dental malocclusion (in which the upper and lower teeth don't meet as they should) than were finger or thumb sucking (*Swedish Dental Journal*, 2010).

In contrast, long-term breastfeeding discourages malocclusion (page 25).

Diaper changing

You may be advised to change your baby's diaper before a feed, because some babies don't feed well with a wet or dirty diaper and others wake if they're changed after a feed. This is all right if he isn't crying, but if he is, wait till afterward, otherwise you may get stressed and not let down your milk. A crying baby may also swallow air, then regurgitate more milk. After a good feed, though, many babies are so content and full that not even a diaper change wakes them. Changing after a feed saves diapers because babies often wet or fill their diaper during one. But if your baby won't feed with a dirty diaper, you'll have to change it earlier. The good news if you have a baby who falls asleep halfway through a feed is that a diaper change may wake him enough to take the second breast.

Your baby's bowel motions

A breastfed baby's motions ("stools" or "poos") gradually change and don't smell unpleasant, unlike a bottle-fed's, which smell foul.

AGE	NATURE OF BREASTFED BABY'S BOWEL MOTIONS IN 24 HOURS
1–2 days	Dark green, sticky meconium
3–5 days	3 or more greenish loose motions

6 days–3 weeks	3–5 or more bright yellow, lookse or liquid motions that may just stain the diaper. Sometimes every diaper is stained
From 3–4 weeks	Possible less frequent, with some babies passina motion only every week or so, some less often. The motions are usually larger than before

Gas

Many breastfed babies don't need burping—they simply bring up any swallowed air spontaneously or pass it out the other end. If you think your baby is suffering from trapped gas, cuddle him after a feed in a fairly upright position, for instance against your shoulder, to let the gas come up. If he doesn't usually burp, lay him down to sleep after a feed if you want. Some people become obsessed with gas, but in many countries women don't see it as a problem and do nothing about it.

Some babies are obviously uncomfortable after a feed but drop off to sleep after bringing up some gas. Such babies sometimes frown or momentarily go cross-eyed. The skin above a gassy baby's upper lip may be slightly blue and he may cry or fidget. If you think your baby is gassy and putting him upright doesn't do the trick, sit him on your lap with one of your hands rubbing his back gently and the other holding his chest. If you then bend him slightly in the middle, some air often comes up, perhaps with a little regurgitated milk. If at night after feeding your baby lying down, he doesn't settle and you think he's gassy, sit him up to help it come up.

Regurgitation

Many babies, especially small ones, regurgitate milk during and after a feed, particularly if the milk flows so fast that they swallow air as they gulp it down, or if they drink too much. Sometimes a baby brings up so much milk that he wants more.

There's no need to worry about any of this if your baby is thriving. However, if your milk flows very fast early in a feed, you could try expressing some before you start, to prevent him having to swallow quickly to keep up.

If the milk has been in your baby's tummy some time, you'll notice it's been changed into fine curds and whey.

Crying

There's a lot going on in the average postnatal ward, with trolley shops, meals, visitors, bed-making, and room cleaning, plus doctors' and nurses' rounds, baths, talking to the person in the next bed, social networking (by hospital phone or, if the hospital allows it, by speaking, texting or emailing on your phone, or emailing on a tablet or laptop) and, if you're lucky, presents, flowers, letters, and cards. Amid all this it's easy to let your baby come second and not feed him when he's ready.

Your baby's cry is designed to alert you to care for him and suggests discomfort or unhappiness. It's not easily ignored, even by a stranger, and a baby who won't stop crying is very disturbing. No woman likes hearing her baby cry, so his cries will probably upset her and could hinder her let-down.

If a baby cries a lot, his mother is likely to think something is wrong with him or his food. If the doctor reassures her that nothing is medically wrong, some women—and, unfortunately, some helpers—believe they must change the baby's feed. For a breastfeeder this means giving formula. But this is almost never necessary. A crying baby's best interests are only rarely served by stopping breastfeeding and changing to formula.

Why is he crying?

Some babies cry much more than others. Midwives and women who've had many children say babies behave very differently and have different characters from the start. Some are quieter, more placid and content, and thus easier to look after; others make much more noise, and are more demanding, less easily satisfied, and more challenging to care for.

Hunger and thirst are by far the most common reasons for crying. Others include a wet diaper; feeling tired, lonely, angry, afraid, tense, or too hot or cold; having gas, colic, a sore bottom, or something poking into or rubbing them; sensing their mother's anxiety or haste; hearing a sudden loud noise; reacting to something the mother has eaten; breathing smoky air; and being ill.

Some babies cry very little, if at all, as their mothers aim—and are able—to recognize, anticipate and meet their needs so well.

If your baby cries at the beginning of a feed—He may be frustrated, afraid or angry if your milk takes time to let down. Try encouraging your let-down before putting him to the breast, and consider waking him and/or offering the breast before he cries, so he doesn't get so hungry he has to cry. If he gets so upset that he can't feed, try rocking him from side to side to calm him enough to settle at the breast.

If he cries after a feed—In a young baby this probably means he's still hungry, either because he hasn't had enough and needs to go back to the breast, or because you didn't let him stay at the first or second breast long enough.

Put him back to the breast and let him feed until he stops spontaneously. If he goes on crying, his tongue will pull right back inside his mouth (look and you'll see this happen), making it harder for him to latch on well. In this case, try to calm him some other way, perhaps by walking around with him. Then when he stops crying, try again.

If your baby often cries in the evening and you think you may not have enough milk for him at that time of day, the first thing to do is to let him stay at the breast as much as he likes. He may be having a growth spurt and needing to increase your milk supply. You could also express some milk after the early morning feed next day, store it and give it from a cup or supplementer if he cries after a feed.

If he won't stop crying—If you leave him crying for long he'll get tired out, because a baby's crying is a very physically active pursuit and uses a lot of energy. After crying for a long time he probably won't feed well because he'll be too exhausted.

The most common cause of continued crying is schedule-feeding. Exhaustion from long periods of crying is one reason why some schedule-breastfed babies don't get enough milk and why their mothers often can't breastfeed successfully. A baby who wakes an hour "early" and is left to cry until the clock says it's time for a feed may not be hungry when feed time arrives. He'll just be tired out and angry or frightened because his tummy hurts and he's been alone. A few days of this and his mother's breasts will lack stimulation and her milk supply will diminish.

Other reasons for continued crying include

- Swallowing too much air while trying to drink fast-flowing milk.

- Being bored, lonely, and lacking attention and cuddles.

- Being sensitive to traces of foods in your milk (for example cows' milk, eggs, peas, onions, garlic, citrus fruit, cauliflower, broccoli, brussels sprouts, beans, cabbage, tomatoes, bananas, apples, oranges, strawberries, rhubarb, spices, chocolate, coffee, or alcohol). Try to avoid eating a lot of any of these.

- Being upset because he senses you're overwrought (perhaps with an evening rush of things to do).

- Reacting to your stress. A Finnish study (*British Medical Journal*, 1993) found that women who'd had stress or physical problems in pregnancy, were dissatisfied with their sexual relationship, or had difficult birth experiences, were more likely to put their baby's crying down to colic. The researchers suggested that learning stress-management and parenting skills might help.

What to do

When your baby is very young, you may know why is is crying, but as the weeks pass some women learn to distinguish between hungry, tired, lonely, angry, and wet- or dirty-bottom cries. In the first few weeks all cries sound much the same to most new mothers. So the only way to decide whether it's a "hungry cry" as opposed to a "wet," "dirty," or "bored" one is to offer the breast. In other words, interpret any cry as a request for food until proven otherwise.

Breastfeed first. Comforting a squalling young baby without delay encourages him to think the world is a good place. It won't spoil him. If you were left to yell for your food, you'd become dispirited or angry. Babies are no different. Many mothers report that babies fed and comforted at the breast whenever necessary grow up to be happy, independent, loving children, not demanding, unhappy, and spoiled.

Being able to comfort a crying baby at the breast is one of the great rewards of breastfeeding.

A schedule-breastfed baby will almost certainly cry a lot because he'll sometimes be hungry before the clock says it's time for a feed and he'll be denied comfort-sucking time. But babies breastfed successfully and on an unrestricted basis scarcely need to cry. And babies whose mothers respond to their needs promptly and feed them as often as they want tend to cry much less than other babies. One study showed that frequently fed babies cried only about half as much at two months old as those fed less often. By four months the difference was slightly less but still noticeable.

Research shows that babies breastfed "on demand" cry much less than schedule-breastfed ones. It's difficult to ascertain the long-term psychological effects of prolonged periods of crying but they certainly make both baby and mother unhappy at the time.

10 WAYS TO CARE FOR YOUR CRYING BABY AND YOURSELF

1. Try breastfeeding (above).

2. Check simple things like whether he has a cold, wet or dirty diaper, or is too hot or too cold.

3. Sit and cuddle him—or get your partner to do the cuddling, as some colicky babies are calmer with someone else.

4. Gently massage his tummy in a warm room, using a little warmed oil and circling his tummy with slow, rhythmic, clockwise movements.

5. Consider whether you've eaten anything that could upset him (for example, cabbage, onions, unaccustomed spicy food, or alcohol) and avoid it or eat less of it in future.

6. Try holding him in different positions after a feed, for example, with him leaning slightly forwards and bending to the right, with your arm pressing against his abdomen. He'll assume this position if you hold him with his back to you, your arm around his right side, and your right hand supporting his crotch.

7. Try carrying him around in a sling while getting on with other things: your movement, warmth, sounds, and closeness may be comforting, and you can talk or sing to him as well. Several types of sling leave your hands free to get on with your work but keep the baby secure and contented as you walk around. One US study (1986) found that babies cried only half as much when carried more by a parent. Other babies are pacified by a ride in a buggy, pram or car.

8. Eat healthy, enjoyable, regular, balanced meals, plus a nutritious snack in each gap between breastfeeds.

9. Relax and rest more and ask for help to ensure your needs are met.

10. If necessary, consult your midwife, health visitor (in the UK), or breastfeeding leader or counselor.

Could it be colic?

Colic is intermittent pain caused by muscle spasm of the bowel wall. It nearly always improves after the first three months.

However, many babies cry for long periods in the first three months, especially in the evenings, for no apparent cause, and this is traditionally put down to colic. It's sometimes called evening colic or three-month colic, though it's highly likely it isn't actually colic at all. Many people assume crying results from air passing through the bowels, but there's no evidence for this. Indeed, X-rays show that colicky babies have no more air in their bowels than do other babies. Having said this, some babies cry less from "colic" if they have a bowel-calming medicine.

The vast majority of studies show that whether a baby is breastfed or bottle-fed makes no difference to whether or not he has colic. However, one study found colic to be more likely in babies who started solids before three months. And some women claim vitamin drops give their babies colic.

Possible causes of colic

- Poor latching on, so the baby doesn't milk the breast properly and encourage the let-down of higher-fat milk; he then goes to the second breast to fill up with even more relatively low-fat milk, so as to get enough calories. A properly attached baby milks the first breast well enough for it to let-down some relatively higher-fat milk, so he gets the necessary calories from a lower volume of milk. Low-fat milk tends to leave the stomach quickly, and because there's such a lot of it, there's a large amount of lactose (milk sugar); this then ferments in the gut and produces gas, or wind, which causes colic and, perhaps, a sore bottom.

- Being switched to the second breast before he's finished at the first one has the same result. This is particularly likely with a mother who makes a lot of milk and is trying to curtail feeds.

- Breathing smoke-filled air, or drinking the nicotine-containing breast milk of a mother who smokes.

- Having a medical condition that can cause colic, such as gastroenteritis or even an obstructed bowel. If you don't know why your baby is crying, if his cry is worryingly unusual, or if there are other abnormal signs, consult a doctor.

Normal weight loss in a baby

A newborn's body has enough fluid to last for the first few days while he's getting small volumes of colostrum. As he uses up this fluid it's normal to lose weight. Most healthy newborns lose up to 7 percent of their birthweight in the first few days of life, and some as much as 10 percent. There's only any need for concern if they lose more than 10 percent, as this suggests the mother's breastfeeding technique is poor or something else is wrong.

- Italian researchers report that 7 percent of exclusively breastfed newborns lost more than 10 percent of their birthweight in the first 3–5 days. In 3 in 4 cases, this was because either mother or baby hadn't yet learned a good breastfeeding technique (*Journal of Pediatrics*, 2001).

A baby's weight gain

The speed at which a breastfed baby regains his birthweight depends partly on how often he is fed. Babies fed frequently tend not to lose much in the first week. After that they gain more rapidly than babies breastfed on a three-hourly schedule. And the latter, in turn, gain faster than those on a four-hourly schedule.

Many babies regain their birthweight by 10–14 days, but some take up to three weeks to do this—and a few perfectly healthy ones take even longer (see above bullet).

The rate of weight gain isn't usually important for a healthy baby who's fed on an unrestricted basis, latches on well, and seems content—as long as he's slowly gaining some weight (or at least not losing any more) and is producing enough wet diapers, and his mother's let-down is working.

Note that a relatively heavy newborn often gains weight at a slower rate than an average-weight or a relatively light baby.

Many hospitals have stopped routine test-weighing (weighing before and after a feed to see how much milk was taken) of all babies because a low or absent gain can worry people unnecessarily. It worries staff who don't understand that breastfed babies don't need as much milk as bottle-fed babies, and makes some women doubt their ability to breastfeed. Test-weighing is best reserved for the very few babies who aren't thriving in spite of excellent breastfeeding support and advice.

Some everyday challenges

A woman at home on her own may have practical challenges to consider when breastfeeding.

For instance, what do you do if the doorbell rings? You might decide not to answer. You could adjust your clothes quickly and go to the door with your hungry baby crying in your arms or left safely behind. You could continue feeding as you answer the door, perhaps with a shawl around you.

What if passersby—or the window cleaner—could see in through the window? Just keep a diaper or shawl near so you can cover up if you want. Or draw the curtains or close the blinds.

As for the phone, you could leave it unanswered. You could take it off the hook or set your mobile (cell phone) to "silent." You could sit near a landline so you can quickly reach it. Or you could keep a roving or mobile phone nearby.

Feeding with other children around

A new baby can be a joy and a misery to his siblings, especially if they are very young. The attractions of having a new member of the family are tempered by not yet being able to play with him, and by their mother having a time-consuming interest that is central to her life and takes her attention from them.

Be extra loving and attentive, especially to the next youngest child as he'll probably be most affected. If he wants to try breastfeeding, let him; he's only trying to compete for your attention and will soon get bored.

Include older children in the breastfeeding circle. For example, as you feed the baby, talk with or read to your toddler. Keep an absorbing toy handy. And spend some time later playing one-to-one with the child who feels left out.

It'll be a huge advantage to your other children to observe breastfeeding. This will make a girl more likely to breastfeed herself one day, and a boy more likely to encourage his partner to do so.

Going out with your baby

You can take a breastfed baby almost anywhere.

When invited to someone's home, ask if they mind you breastfeeding. If they'd be embarrassed, feed in another room. You may prefer to go elsewhere anyway. Ask for a drink, cushions or whatever else you need.

Attitudes about breastfeeding in public are gradually changing for the better, though some countries are becoming breastfeeding-friendly faster than others. Scotland now has legislation allowing women to breastfeed anywhere; indeed, if anyone stops a woman breastfeeding in public they can be fined up to £2,500 ($3,815). In Australia women think nothing of breastfeeding when out and about. But in France, few women breast-feed in public and in China this is thought embarrassing. In the US, most states now have a law allowing women to breastfeed anywhere or at least exempting them from being prosecuted for public indecency or inde-cent exposure (http://www.ncsl.org/issues-research/health/breastfeeding-state-laws.aspx). The Philippines allows breastfeeding in public. But Germany and Canada, for example, have no such law. In Saudi Arabia women breastfeed in public, though they do it discretely.

More than half of new mothers in the UK feel embarrassed to breast-feed when out and about, according to a survey of nearly 7,000 mothers by the National Childbirth Trust (2002).

Another UK study found that 84 percent of people in general think it's fine for women to breastfeed discreetly in public, but 67 percent of mothers worry what people would think if they breastfed in public (UK Department of Health press release, 2003).

Nearly all mothers think that large shops and shopping centers should provide a pleasant and suitable place for breastfeeding.

A particular concern of some young women is breastfeeding in front of a man other than their partner. Some fear that young men will joke about what they're doing, or be rude or off-putting in some other way.

A clever choice of clothing is particularly important in a public place such as a train, bus, park, or restaurant. Do a practice feed in front of a mirror to give yourself confidence.

In a restaurant it's polite to feed discreetly, because while you could argue that other people shouldn't be upset, the fact is that some will be. You'll do more to persuade them about breastfeeding if you are sensitive to how they feel. Choose a corner table where you'll be relatively incon-spicuous. You may prefer not to go to an expensive restaurant if you think you won't let down your milk if you're concerned about other diners, or feel that such a place isn't the right environment for breastfeeding away.

It's generally better not to breastfeed in a cinema, theatre, concert or talk, because gurgles, glugs, goos, cries, and so on can annoy others who've paid to be there and rightly expect no disturbance. But if your baby is young and you can rely on him to let you know he wants a feed simply by wriggling quietly, and not slurping or making other noises, you might try sitting at the back of the auditorium, as long as you leave immediately if necessary.

If you go out without your baby, leave expressed breast milk in the refrigerator for the sitter to warm when needed and give from a cup or spoon or, for an older baby who breastfeeds well, a bottle. An older baby won't be confused by a bottle teat—"nipple"—and find breastfeeding difficult afterward, whereas a young baby might. A hungry baby will probably be fine without you because the milk is his usual brew and tastes familiar.

Travel and holidays

Breastfeeding in a car is easy, though feed only in a parked car, not a mobile one. When on the move your baby should be in a proper infant seat. Breastfeeding in a bus or a train isn't so easy because of the lack of space and privacy. But it's still possible. On balance, you might want to aim to avoid it by feeding before you travel.

If you travel with another adult, ask them to do as much as possible for you or you could become tense and tired and not let down your milk well.

Holidays are simpler with a breastfed baby. There's no bottle cleaning and sterilizing and no boiled water to organize, and the equipment is always at hand. If you fly, consider doing so at night so your baby will be sleepy, the aircraft dark and the chance of privacy greater because more passengers will be asleep. Some airlines have a special seat that can be curtained off for a breastfeeding mother.

eight

Some Useful Skills

The first and most obvious breastfeeding skills are holding your baby so you are both comfortable during a feed, and positioning him at the breast so he can latch on well. Others include expressing milk (including doing breast compressions) and "switch-nursing." Pumping is very useful for some women. And many women need to store their expressed or pumped milk safely. Using a supplementer makes all the difference to some women and their breastfeeding babies. There's also some information here on milk banks.

Holding your baby

The best positions are the ones that are most comfortable for you and the most conducive to your baby feeding well.

Semi-reclining

This is useful at many times and particularly when you are feeding your newborn, or when a feed is likely to take a long time. The good thing is that it encourages your baby's feeding reflexes to operate so he can be something of a free agent at your breast. It also means that your body, rather than your arms and shoulders, takes his weight, so it's more comfortable and sustainable for you. And it leaves your arms free.

Lean back on a bed or a sofa, against pillows or cushions resting against the bed-head, sofa-arm, or wall, and position your baby so his chest is against your chest. This is a lovely restful position.

"Cradle" hold

This is the best known way. Sit in bed or on a chair. If the latter—ideally choose a low chair or raise your feet (on a footstool or a pile of books, for example) so your lap is flat. Support your elbow on the chair-arm or on one or more cushions. Your arm won't then take all your baby's weight, which could make your back, neck, and shoulders ache.

Put him with his head on your forearm and with that arm's hand under his bottom. Lay the palm of your other hand on his back. Position him so his face, chest, tummy and knees face your body ("tummy to mummy") and are tucked closely against you, so he doesn't have to turn his head. Either have his head resting on your arm or support him with your other hand around his shoulder. Some mothers prefer to hold their baby with their other arm, his bottom in the crook of their arm and their hand cradling his head. Some babies, though, dislike having their head cradled and push back, away from the breast.

If necessary, tuck his lower arm around your side to keep it out of the way. His chin should be up and his head not bent down.

Most women don't need to hold their breast. But if yours is big you may need to hold it back so it doesn't interfere with him breathing through his nose. Don't squeeze your breast too much as this could obstruct the milk flow. Some women find it helps to support the breast gently from underneath with the flat of their upturned hand.

Lying down

Lie on one side with your baby lying on his side and facing you. Move him toward you with your hand on his back.

By slightly rotating your upper body one way or the other, you can feed from your lower or upper breast.

"Football hold"

This is useful, particularly for mothers of twins. Its name comes from the practice of running with a ball under one arm when playing football or rugby. It's also called the rugby, underarm, or clutch hold.

To do it, hold your baby so his legs point backwards under your arm the side you're feeding from. Support his body with a cushion if necessary.

"Clockface" positioning

Imagine a straight line superimposed on a clockface. This line could rotate through many positions. Now imagine your baby's mouth as the straight line and your nipple and areola as the clock face, and you'll see that the same goes for his mouth at the breast. With ingenuity you can position yourself and your baby so the "line" of his mouth meets your nipple and areola in any one of a great many different positions. This could be particularly useful if your nipples become sore or you get a blocked duct.

Good positioning and latching on

Positioning your baby well at your breast helps him latch on (attach) properly so he can milk your breast efficiently.

- Move him toward your breast but don't push his head (or his rooting reflex will make him turn his head away from the breast).

- Keep his whole body close to you and positioned so he doesn't have to turn his head.

- Adjust his position so his nose is by your nipple, his chin against your breast, and his head tipped back a bit. If he's to get his upper lip over your nipple and latch on well, he then has to open his mouth very wide.

- As his mouth gapes open, with his tongue over his lower lip, quickly bring him on to your breast so his chin and lower lip meet it first. As your breast lands on his tongue it'll open his lower jaw wider, giving him an even bigger mouthful. His lower jaw should be well away from the base of your nipple.

- If he doesn't open his mouth, stroke its corner, or his lower lip, with your nipple until he does. Check nothing else is touching his mouth, such as clothing, as this could trigger his rooting reflex and make him turn toward it.

- He needs to take some of the areola as well as the nipple into his mouth so his tongue can milk the reservoirs beneath the areola. Otherwise he'll only "nipple-suck." He'd then only suck milk from the reservoirs (or swallow any already being let down). He wouldn't milk them and thus provide the optimal stimulation needed to let down milk. He'd then need to nipple-suck more strongly to get milk, encouraging nipple soreness. And because nipple-sucking doesn't optimally stimulate the breast, less prolactin would be released and you'd make less milk for the next feed.

When your baby has finished he'll automatically come off the breast. You can offer the other one either straight away or after a break, though he may want a break or may even have had enough.

7 POINTERS TO GOOD POSITIONING

1. His head will be tipped back and his chin resting against your breast.
2. His lips will be splayed out around a large mouthful of breast.
3. His bottom lip will be pressed back against his chin.
4. To an onlooker, more areola will be visible above his upper lip than below his lower one.
5. He won't be dragging your breast down.
6. His lower jaw and cheek muscles will be working hard. Hollowed cheeks, however, suggest he isn't latched-on well.
7. He'll start doing slower, deeper sucks within half a minute or so.

If he finds latching on difficult

Aim to relax more as this will aid your let-down, which, in turn, will encourage him to try again. He may like to grip your finger while feeding. To help him latch on well,

- Hold your breast between finger and thumb (or index and middle fingers—the "cigarette hold") to make your nipple and areola a little easier to latch on to. Don't squeeze the breast hard as this could obstruct its ducts. Release this hold as soon as he starts feeding well.

- Aim your nipple upwards in his mouth, toward his nose, so it's less likely to get hurt as he sucks.

Expressing

It's useful to learn how to express because

- If your breasts are overfull and tense, your baby will find it more difficult to latch on, but expressing a little before a feed softens them, which makes it easier.

- If your breasts overfill in the first few days you can express a little before or between feeds to ease the pressure and prevent engorgement.

- If your pre-term baby can't yet take milk from the breast, expressing can provide him with milk to take from a cup or feeding spoon, and can keep your milk supply going.

- If you have a cracked nipple, expressing provides your baby with milk to take from a spoon or cup. It also keeps your milk supply going, and allows the nipple to heal.

- If you're going out without your baby, you can leave expressed milk for someone else to give from a cup.

Expressing is easy once you get the knack but the first few times you'll probably get only a few drops. Even later it's normal to express only from a few teaspoons to a tablespoon or two, though women with a larger milk supply might express two to four tablespoonfuls (1–2 fl oz/28–56 mL). These amounts are fine. Babies absorb energy more easily from breast milk than from formula, so need less of it.

10 STEPS FOR EXPRESSING

1. Wash your hands or, if washing facilities are unavailable, use an alcohol or other antiseptic wipe.

2. Have ready a clean container (page 166) labeled with your name and the date if you're going to store it while you're in the hospital, and the date if you're going to store it at home.

3. Get comfortable.

4. Stroke your breast from the outer part to the nipple for a minute or two to encourage your milk to flow. You can repeat this each time there's an interval between let-downs.

5. Feel for the reservoirs under the areola: in a full breast they may feel like peas or little grapes. Put the flat of your thumb over the upper reservoirs, and the flat of your index finger over the lower ones. Some right-handed women find it easier to use their left hand for each breast and to collect the milk in a container held in their right. Vice versa applies for some left-handed women.

6. Move your hand firmly backwards toward your chest, but don't let your finger and thumb slide over the skin.

7. Press your finger and thumb together and move them away from your chest, so you gently squeeze milk from the reservoirs to the nipple. Don't pull the breast or let your fingers slide on the breast.

8. Rhythmically repeat the movements in (6) and (7). After a while you'll see milk slowly dripping from the nipple or, once milk lets down, dripping faster or spraying repeatedly.

9. Carry on expressing once your milk lets down, even in the intervals between sprays.

10. Reposition your hand occasionally to empty another parts of the breast, and change to the other breast if the flow slows.

Expressing stimulates a woman's milk supply better than an electric pump. Expressing just enough to relieve the pressure in an overfull breast takes only a few minutes. Expressing instead of giving a breastfeed could take 20–30 minutes or so.

If collecting milk to leave a feed for someone else to give your baby, either express after each feed for a couple of days so you collect enough. Or express or pump from one breast while your baby feeds from the other. Leave the container in the refrigerator between tim and the small volumes will soon mount up.

It's best not to bottle-feed your baby with expressed milk if he's less than four to six weeks old. This is because a bottle's teat (nipple) is so easy to drink from that bottle-feeding requires a different feeding technique (page 242) from breastfeeding. A baby used to bottles has to work harder to get milk from the breast, which may put him off breastfeeding. If your baby can't breastfeed, or in the unlikely situation that he needs something extra (for example, if he has low blood sugar or excessive weight loss that doesn't respond to more frequent breastfeeds), it's better for him to have whatever's necessary from a cup or feeding spoon (or, if very premature, a tube). Pre-term babies are particularly likely to have trouble breastfeeding if they've had bottles, as are other low-birthweight babies, babies whose mothers had a difficult labor, and unwell babies. Some women want a babysitter to give bottles of expressed breast milk (or formula), so are keen for their baby to get used to a bottle. But even occasional bottles for a young baby can interfere with successful breastfeeding.

Collecting drip milk from the other side while expressing (or feeding)

Some breastfeeding women collect the milk that drips from the opposite breast while they feed or express. They do this to keep themselves dry (in which case they discard it) or to give to their baby later by cup or spoon (preferably not by bottle).

A tip for collecting drip milk easily is to put a clean breast shell inside your bra, positioned with the tiny hole or spout (if there is one) uppermost, so you don't get drenched! Pour the collected milk into a clean container you can cover. The amount will be small but could be invaluable.

Breast compressions

Expressing milk into your baby's mouth when he's at your breast but not swallowing is sometimes called breast compression. To do it, gently compress your breast between your thumb and fingers (placed some way from your nipple and areola). The aim is to squeeze the milk that's already in the ducts and reservoirs into his mouth. This should encourage him to start sucking and milking again. When he stops swallowing, release your hold, so more milk can enter the reservoirs. Then repeat this maneuver several times with your thumb and fingers in a different position each time, so they empty other ducts and reservoirs.

Reverse-pressure softening

This can be useful if your breasts are overfull or actually engorged, because it can soften the part of the breast below the areola for long enough to enable the baby to latch on more easily.

To do it, put the fingertips of one hand in a circle around the base of the nipple then gently press them into the breast for about a minute. This temporarily pushes milk backwards out of the reservoirs into the milk ducts, and tissue fluid away from the part of the breast beneath the areola. Removing your fingertips may leave a ring of little pits, but these disappear within a minute or so.

Alternatively, use reverse-pressure softening by placing your fingers below your areola and your thumb above then gently pressing your breast back toward your chest wall.

"Switch-nursing"

This involves swapping from one breast to the other, perhaps several times during a feed. Each time you switch sides, milk is immediately available in the "new" breast's reservoirs. So your baby will probably suck and milk more enthusiastically. This is likely to stimulate more let-downs and make your let-down reflex more reliable. It also boosts your prolactin so you make more milk.

Switch nursing is a well-tried way of coaxing tired, jaundiced, pethidine-doped, ill, or pre-term babies, or other weak feeders, into sucking more strongly and milking the breast more efficiently. It's also useful for increasing your milk supply.

To do it, change your baby from one breast to the other as soon as his sucking slows down and you hear or see him swallowing less often. So instead of giving first one breast, then the other, then stopping, you carry on feeding by switching back to the first, then perhaps to the second again.

Pumping

Some mothers prefer to pump rather than express. But however good a pump may be, it's not as effective as a healthy baby at milking the breast and stimulating the milk supply. But it can be a godsend in certain situations.

Electric pumping is less tiring than expressing or using a hand pump. But expressing stimulates the milk supply better than does an electric pump.

You might need a pump if your baby

- Is too immature or unwell to get any (or enough) milk from the breast.

- Is in the hospital without you (or vice versa).

Or if you

- Have inverted nipples. Using a pump for a minute or so before a feed helps makes the nipple protrude.

- Want to collect milk to leave for your baby if you're going to be apart—for example, if you're at work.

- Are taking medications that might pass into your milk and harm your baby. Discard this pumped milk and keep your supply going by pumping and expressing until you're off the drugs and can breastfeed again.

- Have an infection that precludes your baby having your milk. Discard the pumped milk but keep your milk supply going by pumping and expressing until the infection is under control and you can breastfeed again.

- Are building up your milk supply after giving your baby bottles of formula.

- Have let your milk dry up but have changed your mind and now want to breastfeed.

- Work away from home and want to pump and/or express while away so you can take milk home and/or keep your milk supply going.

- Are building up your supply to feed an adopted baby.

Using a pump

Before using a pump, sterilize the parts that come into contact with milk.

Aim to start letting down before you begin pumping. Do this by gently massaging your breasts and stroking them toward the nipples. Position the pump's flange (funnel-shaped receiving end) so your nipple rests inside its upper part. Pumping draws your nipple in and out, and contact with the flange encourages let-downs. Spread the first few drops of milk over the skin in contact with the flange so it slides over the skin easily. Don't press the flange too tightly against you as this could obstruct the underlying milk ducts or reservoirs. Massaging your breast while you pump will aid milk flow and encourage let-downs.

Switch breasts when the milk flow diminishes. Do this several times, just as you might when expressing or breastfeeding. At first you'll probably collect only very small amounts of milk—perhaps only 1½ teaspoons (¼ fl oz or 7–8 mL). It's a good idea to finish a session by expressing the last bit of milk, as this will be the most calorie-rich, especially in the first breast.

Pump frequently, because your breasts need frequent stimulation, and because pumping doesn't stimulate your milk supply as well as does breastfeeding. Aim for eight to ten sessions a day—which means pumping two to three times hourly. As long as your nipples don't get sore, try to increase your milk supply by pumping for longer as they days go by, as the increased stimulation will boost your prolactin.

Ideally, pump both breasts in a session, as this saves time and produces more milk.

Women often use pumps unnecessarily when they're in the hospital. This is because the pumps are there, because intervention in nature's process can be attractive if you don't understand how breastfeeding works, and because many women have learned a poor breastfeeding technique.

Many babies given bottles of formula soon refuse to breastfeed because they've quickly learned to bottle-suck and find it easier. If a mother then gives pumped milk by bottle, it makes the situation worse. If your baby finds it hard to breastfeed, but is mature enough and well enough to swallow, give pumped milk from a cup and keep trying the breast as well. Or use a supplementer as you breastfeed.

Only rarely is it necessary to interrupt breastfeeding because of sore or cracked nipples but, if you have to, it's less painful to express than to pump.

Hand pumps

The cheapest and simplest hand pump consists of a plastic or glass container with a rubber bulb to produce suction. The milk you collect is likely to contain large amounts of bacteria because the bulb inevitably retains some milk and is difficult to clean. Compared with expressing, or using an electric pump, hand pumps aren't particularly effective. You can buy them from pharmacies or online. They are sometimes called "breast relievers."

Electric pumps

Generally, the larger the pump, the quicker it builds up suction. The price reflects its sturdiness and quality. Electric pumps are available for hire or loan from certain hospital maternity and special-care baby units and breastfeeding self-help groups. You can also buy them from medical-supply houses, certain pharmacies, and over the Internet.

Storing milk

Keep all equipment, including refrigerator, freezer, and insulated bag or box, clean.

Wash your hands, then express or pump your milk into a clean plastic container—plastic is better than glass as some of the immunological components of milk stick to glass. Containers made from toxin-free plastic have a number-5 recycling symbol and/or the letters "PP" on their base. If intending to freeze the milk, note that disposable plastic milk-storage bags designed for freezing breast milk take up less room in the freezer. Double-bagging milk or putting the bags into a sealed container prevents freezer burn.

There's no need to use a sterilized container. It simply needs either to have been washed in hot soapy water, rinsed well and drip dried, or washed in the dishwasher. Label the container with the date and, if you or your baby is in the hospital, your baby's name.

Put only 60 mL (2 fl oz) at most into a container, as your baby is unlikely to want more for a feed and the smaller the amount, the easier it will be to thaw. If he is likely to take less, put less into the container. Cover the container.

If intending to freeze your milk, leave about 2.5 cm (1 in) of head-room above its surface as it will expand when frozen.

If it'll be a few hours before you use the milk, refrigerate or chill it as soon as possible (see also below).

Storing at room temperature

Breast milk covered and left at room temperature (66–72°F/ 19–22°C) is ideally best used within four hours of collection.

However, its anti-infective factors mean it's safe to be left for up to six hours. Some experts say up to 12 hours is fine.

Storing in an insulated bag or box

How long you can safely leave milk in a insulated bag or box contain-ing frozen ice packs depends on the temperature inside. So if you intend to store milk for long, keep a thermometer inside.

If the temperature remains at 59°F/15°C, your milk is safe for 24 hours, but is best used within 10 hours.

If the temperature remains at 39–50°F/4–10°C, your milk is safe for three days but best used within 24 hours.

Storing in a refrigerator

You can keep expressed or pumped milk in a refrigerator at less than 39°F (4°C) for up to three days—though this is very much on the safe side. One study found it was safe in the refrigerator up to 5 days, another up to 8 days. If you want to keep it for longer, freeze it immediately you've expressed it.

Storing in a freezer

Freezing has little effect on breast-milk antibodies but can harm its living cells, so don't freeze it unless you have to. However, previously frozen breast milk is better for a baby than formula.

You can store your milk in a freezer at a variable temperature of around −4°F (−18°C) for up to six months, but it's best used within three months.

You can store your milk in a freezer that has a constant temperature of –18ºC (–4ºF) for up to 12 months but it's best used within 6 months.

If using a freezer compartment in a refrigerator, store your milk for up to one month.

If using a frost-free freezer compartment in a refrigerator, store your milk for up to three weeks.

When you remove milk from the freezer, use the oldest milk first.

Thawing frozen milk

To thaw frozen milk, either hold the container under running water—first cold, then gradually warmer; or stand the container in a bowl of warm water; or thaw it in the refrigerator overnight.

You can refrigerate leftover thawed milk for up to 24 hours before using, refreezing, or discarding it.

Warming refrigerated or thawed frozen milk

Gently warm the milk by holding its covered container under hot running tap water or by standing it in a bowl of hot water. Never put it directly into a pan to warm it on the hob. Milk is probably more pleasant at body temperature. Some babies drink cold milk but pre-term babies should never have cold milk.

Microwaving?

Don't thaw or warm breast milk by microwaving it. This is because microwaving it at a high temperature (162–208°F/72–98ºC) reduces its anti-infective properties. And while microwaving it at cooler temperatures (68–127°F/20–53ºC) has no significant effect on the actual amount of antibodies, it reduces the amounts of lysozyme, and antibodies to *Escherichia coli* gut bacteria. What's more, microwaving breast milk alters the structure of certain of its amino acids, which could mean a baby can't digest or use them properly.

Also, don't attempt to sterilize a container intended for breast milk by microwaving it. This is because the temperatures reached in a microwave aren't high enough to kill bacteria reliably. You could use a special microwave steam-sterilizer box or disposable bags.

Combining fresh and previously stored milk

Cool the new milk first by refrigerating it for 30 minutes. Add the cold milk to the refrigerated milk. Or add it to frozen milk—but don't add a larger volume than is already frozen.

Use the combined milk within the safe time recommended for the older milk.

Using stored milk

Breast milk separates into layers as it stands but these disappear if you gently swirl the container. It's best not to shake the container or stir the milk.

Before removing the top from a refrigerated or frozen container of breast milk, dry the container with paper kitchen towel so no drips from condensation can contaminate the milk with bacteria.

Using a supplementer

This simple gadget can be very useful. It's also known as a nursing supplementer, nursing trainer, supplemental-supply line, or a nursing system!

It enables a baby to get milk directly from the breast, plus, at the same time, expressed breast milk, or donated milk, or formula, from a fine flexible plastic tube attached to a bag or a bottle.

The Lact-Aid Nursing Trainer has a disposable sterile bag that you hang around your neck. This, in turn, has a tube you can shift from one breast to the other.

The Medela Supplementary Nursing System has a bottle with two tubes, one per breast.

With either of these, you tape the tube to your breast so its free end protrudes about 6mm/¼in beyond the nipple and enters your baby's mouth, along with your nipple and areola, as he breastfeeds.

A supplementer is useful for

- Teaching a baby who's used to bottle-feeding to breastfed effectively.

- Giving a larger feed to a pre-term who doesn't have the energy to suck for long. You express your milk between and after feeds and put this into the bag or bottle.

- Supplementing an adopted baby's breastfeeds with formula.

- Avoiding the need for a bottle so a baby doesn't learn to "bottle-suck" (page 242).

Some women make a supplementer. Here's how to do it.

10 STEPS TO MAKE A SUPPLEMENTER

1. Buy some very thin, flexible plastic tubing. This is available as naso-gastric ("gavage") tubes for babies, as used in special-care baby units. Number 5 French-size tubing is okay for full-term babies and number 3 for pre-term babies. Number 8 is best for babies with a cleft palate. Tubing will stiffen with repeated use and cleaning, and you'll probably need to replace it every week or so, so buy plenty of it. Buy it online or ask the medical supplies department of a hospital with a special-care baby unit if you can buy some from them, or take the contact details of their supplier. See also page 340.

2. Buy a feeding bottle and nipple, and a syringe to clean the tubing.

3. Make a hole in the flange surrounding the protrusion in the nipple. This should be just large enough for the tubing to go through.

4. Enlarge the hole already in the end of the protrusion. This hole acts as a vent so milk can flow freely without being hampered by a vacuum above the milk in the bottle.

5. Put some of your milk into the bottle and screw on the tea-holder and nipple.

6. Push one end of the tubing through the hole in the nipple's flange and right down to the bottom of the bottle.

7. Tape the tube's free end to your breast so it protrudes about 6 mm/¼ in from the end of your nipple.

8. Put your baby to the breast so his mouthful of nipple and areola includes the end of the tube.

9. Hold the bottle in your hand, or, if it's small enough, tuck it into your bra. It should be upright so the milk's surface is level.

10. To interrupt the flow of milk, raise any part of the tube above the upper surface of the milk. To restart the flow, lower all the tube again.

Sterilizing a supplementer and cleaning it after a feed

This prevents contamination with bacteria that could infect your baby's gut.

Sterilize a commercial supplementer and clean it after each feed, according to the manufacturer's instructions.

As for a homemade supplementer, sterilize the bottle and nipple at least once a day. However, don't boil or steam the tubing. Clean all the parts after a feed by washing each part with hot soapy water, and by using a syringe to force some hot soapy water through the tube. Rinse well in the same way and drip dry.

Milk banks

Women with spare milk can donate it for use by babies whose mothers aren't feeding them fully or at all and who may particularly benefit from breast milk. They include very low-birthweight pre-term babies in their first week, as they tolerate donated milk better than pre-term formula; babies who aren't growing and thriving; those who've had bowel surgery; those with poor immunity; and older babies with diarrhea from severe food intolerance. Donated milk has helped save a great many lives. If you'd like to donate milk, ask the staff at the nearest hospital that has a special-care baby unit what to do.

Donors are screened with questions about their medical history and drug intake, and with blood tests. A donor should not

- Be a smoker.

- Drink more than a small amount of alcohol.

- Have too many caffeine-containing drinks.

- Be on any medication that's potentially unsafe for a baby.

- Have been vaccinated recently.

- Have tuberculosis or Creutzfeld-Jakob disease in the family.

- Have taken growth hormones.

- Have had an organ or tissue transplant or a blood transfusion in the last year.

- Have recently lived in a country with a high prevalence of certain infections (though not all milk banks ask about this).

If a would-be donor passes this screening, she'll have tests for HIV 1 and 2, hepatitis B and C, human T-cell leukemia viruses (HTLV 1 and 2) and syphilis.

If screening is satisfactory, her milk is

- Cultured to make sure its bacteria count is low enough.

- Pasteurized at 144.5°F (62.5°C) for 30 minutes (if following UK milk-banking guidelines) to kill as many disease-causing bacteria and viruses as possible (including cytomegaloviruses, and HIV that hasn't shown up in blood tests). Heat this high destroys live cells, and enzymes including lipase (and because lipase aids fat absorption, babies gain less weight than those given raw milk). But lower heat may not kill certain bacteria, for example, those that cause tuberculosis.

- Frozen for up to six months.

One potential problem is that donated milk is often "drip" milk—milk that drips from one breast while the donor's baby feeds from the other. Such milk contains only two-thirds the calories of expressed milk. But the baby's doctor will take this into account and recommend human-milk fortifier or formula as well if necessary.

In Brazil more than 100,000 donors supply 200 milk banks. Interestingly, their milk is collected from their home and taken to the milk bank by firefighters.

Milk banks in westernized countries give donated breast milk to tiny or sick babies. The US, for example, has 11 not-for-profit milk banks. But in certain countries milk banks sell it to companies that in turn sell it to hospitals, researchers (who might work for formula companies), or formula companies that use certain parts of it in special infant formulas.

In some countries milk banks pay milk donors. Breast milk is available to buy online at about $4 US per ounce, but a buyer should insist on proof that both the donor and her milk have been screened for infection by a reliable pathology laboratory.

One woman in Norway was reported to be providing up to 11 L (more than 19 pints) of milk a week. However, a typical donor provides up to 2 L (3½ pints). And much lower amounts are very useful too.

nine

Looking After Yourself

It's very important to look after yourself and not overdo things. Getting exhausted might interfere with your let-down, and trying to be all things to all people could leave you short of time to breastfeed and thus reduce your milk supply. So take things easy, eat nourishing meals and let the world go by. Leave dish-washing, laundry and shopping to someone else for as long as possible, as you'll have your hands full with the baby. All this is doubly important if you have other children.

> **IMPORTANT REASONS TO LOOK AFTER YOURSELF WHILE BREASTFEEDING**
>
> 1. As a mother you're the lynchpin of your family and if you are well and happy the chances are the others will be too. If you become tired and run down, your state will reflect on those around you.
> 2. A fit and healthy woman is far more likely to breastfeed successfully than one who's exhausted. This is partly because she may produce more milk, and partly because her let-down will be more reliable. An unreliable let-down can frustrate a baby and make him cry because he's hungry. This will add to his mother's exhaustion.

Breast and nipple care

Nipple and breast care for a breastfeeding woman is very simple. There's no need to wash your breasts before a feed. There's no need to wash them afterward either, though you might want to rinse them with water. When you have a bath, don't use soap. This is because soap removes the skin's natural protective oils and chemical attractants, which are partly what make your breast interesting to your baby. If you put salt in the bathwater to help heal an episiotomy, splash your breasts with plenty of plain water to remove the salt before you dry them. Don't soak your nipples in water as this will make them more likely to become sore and cracked. Nipples readily become soggy and liable to crack if left moist inside a bra. Avoid this by changing breast pads frequently and leaving your bra off sometimes to give your nipples some air. This may be easier at night.

There's generally no need to put anything on your nipples. Although lanolin, cocoa butter or vitamin E oil won't do any harm, they are usually unnecessary as the Montgomery's tubercles around your areolas produce a protective oily liquid. Your baby will prefer the taste of you to anything else. And the smell of your milk, though imperceptible to others, will attract him when you next put him to the breast. If he's a reluctant feeder, this could make all the difference to his desire to suck.

Many experienced breastfeeders express a little milk after a breastfeed and rub it gently into their nipples to help prevent nipple soreness.

Nipple soreness and pain

You can help prevent soreness if you look after your nipples as described, feed naturally, and position your baby well. However, a lot of women have sore nipples some time in the first week or later. If you do, see page 173. Unfortunately, poor advice—or no advice—on how to make it better and prevent it happening again leads many women to give up feeding.

Engorgement

It's normal for breasts to swell as they start making mature milk in the first week after the birth. Breastfeeding on an unrestricted basis helps prevent them becoming overfull and engorged. Indeed, research shows that schedule-breastfeeding women are twice as likely to become engorged as those feeding more frequently. See page 225 for how to prevent and treat engorgement.

A woman whose breasts became much bigger in the first week may think her milk supply is failing when they become smaller as the days go by. But this isn't so if she's feeding frequently. It's just that breasts tend to get smaller once their milk supply begins to match the baby's demand.

Leaking

Leaking usually means a woman is letting down her milk without having her baby or a collecting cup there to receive it. Or it means her breasts are full and ready for a feed.

It's perfectly normal, especially in the early days, so don't think you're producing too much milk and decide to breastfeed less often. Don't reduce your fluid intake either, as this won't help.

To relieve fullness, either suckle your baby or express a little milk. If your breasts remain full for too long in the first few weeks, they're highly likely to become engorged.

Clean up leaking milk and prevent it soaking through to your top by tucking into your bra a pad of soft clean material such as a handkerchief or an old cloth diaper cut into squares. Or use commercial breast pads (page 339). Another idea is to use a folded piece of a "one-way" diaper liner.

To avoid soaking your other nipple in soggy material while feeding from the first breast (which encourages soreness and cracking), uncover the second breast and let leaking milk drip on to a cloth diaper or some paper tissues. Pressing firmly over the nipple with the heel of your hand for a short while usually stops leaking like magic.

The leaking of the first few weeks gradually lessens as your let-down becomes more reliable and the storage capacity of your milk reservoirs increases. You'll still leak from the opposite breast during a feed.

Breast pads

Cloth pads tucked into your bra will soak up any leaks. Don't use paper tissues or cotton balls because these dry on to the nipples and can be difficult to remove without washing them off. Some women use squares of soft absorbent material such as pieces cut from an old cloth diaper or towel, or a diaper roll.

You can buy purpose-made paper breast pads from pharmacies, super-markets and babycare shops. The cheaper ones are flat, the more expensive ones cone-shaped. Washable breast pads are also available (for example, from Boots in the UK, and from the NCT Shop, page 342).

Most commercial pads work well because they have a waterproof layer. However, this also has a downside in that they prevent air getting to the nipples, which makes the skin wet, soggy and more likely to become sore or cracked. So spend some time each day without them.

Whichever breast pads you use, change them frequently so your nipples aren't bathed in moisture.

Wearing a bra at night

This prevents leaking over the bedclothes in the early days and makes heavy breasts more comfortable. However, going without a bra in bed discourages nipple soreness, as it lets air get to them; placing a cloth diaper loosely over your breasts soaks up any leaks; and putting a waterproof sheet over your mattress prevents leaks soaking through. It's also much easier to breastfeed at night without a bra!

Sore perineum

There's nothing like the nagging pain of a sore perineum to put the dampers on the let-down. Try having a hot bath and ask the hospital staff for a rubber ring to sit on to take the weight off your most tender parts. If you still need a ring when you get home, buy or hire one from a surgical supplies shop or buy or hire a "ring-doughnut" cushion (such as the Valley Cushion, page 340). If necessary, take some suitable painkillers.

Helpers

Ideally you'll have a relative, friend, or even a paid person to help, and hopefully your partner will have arranged time off work early on. Your mother (or mother-in-law) may be the best person to help but mothers nowadays often don't live nearby.

Practical assistance, as well as support, encouragement, and reassurance from an empathic helper, can be a godsend. Make sure you both understand your roles, though, or there could be a problem if the helper wants to take over the baby so as to free you to run the home and care for the other children. Your helper should leave you with as much time and energy as possible to be with your new baby and carry on with breastfeeding. Be sure to get this priority right. Your milk supply may take several weeks to become established and you need time to recover from your pregnancy and labor. So make the most of any help available, and don't rush the helper's departure, especially if you have other children.

Rest, relaxation, and sleep

If you have only one baby, it's comparatively easy to make time for naps when he sleeps in the day. And if you're waking several times a night (which is highly likely, especially at first), you must make time, even if you're the sort of person who would never previously have considered day-time sleeping. For the mother who comes home after only 24–48 hours in the hospital, or for one who gives birth at home, rest isn't a luxury—it's vital. During the first week after the birth, take as much rest as you need and certainly don't busy yourself around the home as if nothing had happened.

The temptation, especially for an efficient woman who held down a busy job before having a baby, is to cram household and other tasks into the baby's sleep time. But being a "superwoman" is neither desirable nor sensible. If you are rested, cheerful and content, you'll feel far better than if you prepare meals, change bed-sheets, sort out your e-mails, and generally exhaust yourself! Even keeping up with text messages and voicemails could be too much in the first week or so.

Ask someone else to do the housework. Domestic chores will always be there but you'll probably mother a new baby only a couple of times ever, so make the most of them. To paraphrase the American saying, "Kissin' don't last—cookery do" . . . "Babies don't last—housework does!"

Relax whenever you can. The secret is not to let undue muscle tension build up, because this is tiring in itself. Even if you don't actually sleep, lie down and read, listen to music, or turn on the radio or TV.

Breastfeeding on an unrestricted basis will help ensure you sit down quietly for long periods. This is what Nature intends.

At night, accept it'll probably be a long time before you regularly have long, unbroken sleeps again. If you can't go back to sleep quickly after feeding the baby, at least stay lying down so you get some physical rest.

A woman with more than one child needs to be even more careful about getting enough rest. If your elder child still sleeps in the day, aim to get the baby to sleep then as well so you can have a rest at the same time. Otherwise, lie down with your baby. Lie on your bed rather than on a sofa in case you fall asleep, as a bed is safer for the baby. Perhaps sometimes you could ask a neighbor, relative or friend to look after your toddler for an hour or so while you sleep. Or you could arrange with another mother to help each other this way.

Visitors

In the first few days, while you'll want to show your baby to relatives and friends and talk about the birth, you may feel shy about feeding in front of them, yet won't want your baby to go hungry. There are several ways of managing visitors. One is to ask your partner to vet anyone who wants to visit you in the hospital. If you wouldn't feel happy feeding in front of them, ask him to put them off tactfully. When people visit you at home you can go to another room to feed if you're embarrassed or think they will be, or if you're not confident enough yet at breastfeeding to do it in front of them.

Later on, how you deal with breastfeeding when you have visitors depends on your ideas and feelings and the other people's views. If you're happy to feed in company, go ahead. You know breastfeeding is natural, normal, healthy and wonderful, and hopefully your visitors will be unfazed and even delighted. Wear clothes you can pull up easily to feed in a discreet way that doesn't reveal your breast, or cover up with a shawl or a pashmina. If a visitor is embarrassed, they can go to another room or sit where they can't see you.

Sometimes, you may prefer, or feel it's more appropriate, to feed the baby in another room. If so, don't hurry the feed as your baby will be much more likely to be in a good mood afterward if he takes his usual time. The downside of this decision is that you will then lose time with your visitors.

If you give your visitor a meal, choose something that won't be harmed by being left in a warm oven if you have to feed the baby beforehand. Remember that he calmer you are, the calmer he'll be, as babies quickly sense and react to their mother's feelings. With a little practice it's perfectly possible to breastfeed a baby at the table without revealing any bare breast, though it's gracious to be sensitive to your guests' feelings.

Your food

A nutritious diet for you will help ensure that breast-milk production doesn't drain your body of nutrients. The scent of certain foods in your milk will also help accustom your baby to the taste of your family's food.

The nutrients you're most likely to be lacking are calcium, iron, and riboflavin (vitamin B2), so check you eat enough foods containing

- Calcium (page 85).

- Iron (in meat, shellfish, egg yolk, dark green leafy vegetables, peas, beans, lentils, whole-grain foods, nuts, seeds, apricots, raisins, and prunes).

- Eating foods rich in vitamin C (such as citrus and other fruit,

fruit juice and vegetables) along with iron-rich foods helps you absorb iron better.

- Avoid drinking tea with a meal as its tannins reduce iron absorption.
- Vitamin B2—including milk, cheese, eggs, meat, liver, kidney, nuts, seeds, beans, yeast extract, whole-grain foods, and fortified foods (such as certain breakfast cereals).

Be sure, too, to have a good balance of omega-3s and omega-6s (page 85).

Do you need to eat more?

Eat just slightly more. Experts believe the average breastfeeder needs only an extra 400–600 calories of energy a day. Things aren't always clear cut, though, because studies show that some successfully breastfeeding women can eat nearly 700 calories a day more than do bottle-feeders, yet still lose fat stored during pregnancy. And yet others need no more calories than bottle-feeding women of the same weight. A breastfeeder's digestive system seems particularly efficient at getting energy from her food.

Studies suggest a woman's milk supply is more dependable if she spaces her food intake evenly, rather than eating most of her daily calories at one meal.

One study found that stopping breastfeeding because of "not having enough milk" was less likely in mothers encouraged to eat more. Another reported that those who breastfeed for longer tended to have larger appetites while breastfeeding than before they were pregnant.

Vitamin C

Breastfeeding mothers of pre-term babies should be particularly sure to eat enough foods rich in vitamin C, especially fresh vegetables and fruits. Such babies have comparatively low stores of iron and a plentiful supply of vitamin C in breast milk helps them absorb iron better.

Vitamin D and calcium

Your milk will supply your baby with vitamin D, so it's particularly important to get enough of this vitamin yourself. Among other things, vitamin D strengthens bones by aiding the absorption of calcium.

Some of the calcium in your bones will find its way into your milk, which will make your bones temporarily less dense.

- Italian research found that bone density decreased for the first 6 months of breastfeeding, then recovered, and by 18 months was higher than before pregnancy (*Obstetrics and Gynecology*, 1999).

To look after your bones,

- Get some bright daylight on your skin each day (page 74).

- Take regular, moderate weight-bearing exercise (such as walking).

- Eat a healthy diet.

- Be a nonsmoker.

- Consider taking a vitamin-D supplement (see below).

Note that taking a calcium supplement makes no difference to bone-mineral density or the amount of calcium in breast milk.

In some countries, breastfeeding mothers are advised to take a vitamin D supplement.

- In the UK—the Department of Health recommends a daily vitamin-D supplement of 10 micrograms (400 international units, or IU).

- In the US—the National Institutes of Health's Office of Dietary Supplements points out that the recommended dietary allowance of vitamin D is 600 IU (15 micrograms).

- In Australia—the Ministry of Health advises that breastfeeding women regularly exposed to sunlight don't need a supplement, but for those who get little sun, one of 400 IU (10 micrograms) wouldn't be excessive.

A supplement will probably be unnecessary if you get some bright outdoor daylight on your skin each day. If unsure, discuss it with your doctor.

Note that experts recommend a vitamin-D supplement for all babies, beginning in the first few days of life, whether or not a breastfeeding mother takes one herself.

Drinks

You'll be more thirsty than usual, which isn't surprising considering the average older breastfed baby takes 600–800 mL (more than a pint) of milk a day, depending on his age and weight. Drink as much as you fancy, so you don't become dehydrated. But don't force yourself to drink, because drinking more than you need could reduce your milk supply. If your baby is satisfied and you are producing pale yellow urine, you're almost certainly drinking enough.

Many nursing mothers feel most thirsty while actually feeding, and like to keep a drink close at hand.

Milk

Milk and other dairy foods are an important part of the traditional diet in dairying countries. But there's no need to drink more milk than usual if your diet is well-balanced and nutritious. And if you don't like milk there's no need to drink any, since you don't need cows' milk to make breast milk. Indeed, most experts consider it unwise for breastfeeding women to eat or drink a large amount of any one food, including cows' milk, especially if the baby has a family history of allergy.

As cows' milk is so common an allergen, you may want to avoid a large intake while breastfeeding, especially if there's allergy either side of your baby's family.

Coffee?

When a woman has a caffeine-containing drink (tea, coffee, cola, or other caffeinated soft drink), caffeine enters her milk within 15 minutes and peaks within an hour. There's still some caffeine in the milk 12 hours later (and even longer in some women).

If taken in large enough amounts caffeine is a powerful drug. A young baby's liver breaks it down only very slowly. Caffeine from a mother who has a moderately high intake (six to eight cups in 24 hours) can accumulate in her baby and cause abnormal activity and sleeplessness. However, this disappears when she avoids caffeine for a few days. Modest drinking of caffeine-containing drinks (such as one to three cups of average-strength coffee a day) is unlikely to cause problems. But if you drink more, aim to have your coffee or other caffeinated drink after you've fed your baby, as this gives your milk's caffeine level time to fall before you feed again. If you suspect you're drinking too much caffeine, try cutting out tea and coffee for a week to see if this makes any difference to your baby.

Smoking increases the effects of caffeine.

Alcohol

The occasional small alcoholic drink is acceptable, even though some alcohol will pass into your milk. If you drink larger amounts, correspondingly more gets to the baby. Alcohol raises prolactin in non-lactating women, so it presumably does so in lactators too, though this isn't yet proven. Alcohol flavors breast milk. The intensity of its taste and its concentration in the milk peak half to one hour after drinking it.

Babies tend to consume less breast milk when their mother has drunk alcohol and until it's been eliminated from her body, perhaps because the altered smell of her milk or sweat puts them off. Alcohol in breast milk can affect a baby's behavior, making him want smaller feeds.

- Babies drink about 20 percent less milk during the four hours after their mother had had alcohol, according to a study at the Monell Chemical Senses Center, Philadelphia (*Alcoholism: Clinical and Experimental Research*, 2001).

When babies drink "alcoholic" milk, they have more frequent but shorter sleeps. Some are temporarily uncomfortable and irritable. The type of drink may make a difference too. Drinking enough to make you tipsy could harm your milk supply by affecting your oxytocin output and making your let-down reflex unreliable, or by making you dehydrated. So go easy and take plenty of water or soft drinks along with any alcohol.

Vegetarians and vegans

If you're a vegetarian, check that you have enough sources of vitamin B12.

Vegetarian sources include

- Eggs, milk, cheese, yogurt and fortified foods such as yeast extract, veggie burger mixes, soy milks, and some breakfast cereals.

- The vitamin B12 in certain seaweeds and fermented soy products (such as tempeh and miso) is unlikely to be in a usable form.

Vegans must take particular care to get enough B12. Low levels are most likely in first-generation vegans who haven't the benefit of traditional wisdom in their family on how to prepare nourishing vegan meals. They also need plenty of calcium, iron, zinc, and riboflavin. Below are vegan sources for the following vitamins:

- Vitamin B12—vitamin-B12-fortified foods (including some plant milks, soy products, and breakfast cereals), and vitamin-B12 supplements.

- Calcium—beans, peas, lentils, nuts, seeds, and whole-grain foods.

- Iron—peas, beans, nuts, seeds, whole-grain foods, green leafy vegetables, elderberries, molasses, parsley, and cocoa).

- Magnesium—beans, peas, nuts, seeds, mushrooms, green leaf vegetables, and whole-grain foods.

- Zinc—nuts, peas, beans, whole-grain foods, root vegetables, parsley, garlic, and ginger.

- Riboflavin (vitamin B2)—nuts, seeds, beans, whole-grain foods, and green leafy vegetables.

Is there anything you shouldn't eat?

Traces of undigested food proteins can enter your milk. If your baby reacts badly after you've eaten a certain food, eat less of it or avoid it until you stop breastfeeding. Onions, peas, cabbage, cauliflower, broccoli, and chocolate seem the most likely foods to make a baby fuss.

It's wise to avoid too much saturated fat (in dairy foods, meat, and foods made with butter, lard, hard margarines, or other hydrogenated fats).

- A Finnish study found that breastfed babies of mothers whose diet was rich in saturated fat were more likely to get atopic disorders such as allergic asthma, eczema, and hay fever (*European Journal of Clinical Nutrition*, 2000).

Avoid any foods that look less than fresh. And avoid entirely food past its sell-by date, as there's more chance of it being moldy—even if you can't see it. Fungal by-products called aflatoxins can affect health adversely in animals, and the same may apply to human babies.

If your baby is sensitive to something you eat, the speed of his reaction depends on how quickly the food enters your milk, and on the type of sensitivity. Some mothers notice allergic symptoms in their babies as soon as after the next breastfeed; others report a delay of two or three days.

Have no more than two helpings of canned tuna a week (a helping being 140 g/5 oz of drained tuna) or more than one helping of fresh tuna a week, to prevent the possibility of exposing your baby to too much mercury.

What if you don't eat enough?

Malnourished women can produce very high volumes of good quality milk. Their milk production is extremely robust except in famine or near-famine conditions. Even severely malnourished, starving women can breastfeed their babies for three months before extra food for them is essential if their babies are to continue growing normally. But this is at their own body's expense—they become short of calcium and protein, for example, and the more babies they have and feed over the years, the poorer their physical state becomes. If they eat so little that the level of a protein called albumin in their blood drops below 30 g/L (1.25 oz per 1.75 pints), their milk supply may fall or even dry up completely.

But this situation is virtually never seen in developed countries, where almost every woman has enough to eat, and the only real likelihood of starvation is from the eating disorder anorexia nervosa.

Slimming

Some women find that fat put on in pregnancy slowly disappears with breastfeeding, but this isn't so for everyone. For your sake and your baby's, don't go on a crash diet while breastfeeding. However, a healthy weight-loss diet won't reduce your milk supply, or be detrimental to the quality of your milk or your baby's growth. Nor will slimming release environmental contaminants (such as pesticides) stored in your fat, as was once feared.

If you need help, go to a slimming club that offers a sensible weight-loss diet approved for breastfeeding women, or see a dietitian. Remember too that exercise will help you lose weight and keep it off.

Looking after your breasts

3 TIPS TO HELP KEEP YOUR BREASTS LOOKING GOOD

1. Avoid overeating because extra fat in your breasts could encourage sagging. This is because their extra size could stretch the skin's elastic fibers, and their extra weight could stretch the connective tissue that helps support them.

2. Breastfeed or express often enough to prevent your breasts overfilling, which could stretch their skin and encourage sagging.

3. Wear a properly fitting, supportive bra, day and night if necessary, so heavier than usual breasts don't stretch the skin and connective tissue.

Exercise

Regular, moderate exercise is good for you. It increases your circulation, boosts "feel-good" naturally produced "feel-good" substances called cannabinoids (page 79), and keeps your muscles strong and flexible and your body fit. So choose a type of exercise you enjoy so you won't get bored, make time for it, and find ways of fitting it into your life. Wear a really supportive bra. Some women even wear two at the same time so their heavy breasts don't move around too much.Most studies report that exercise doesn't significantly affect milk volume or quality. However, some babies' feeding behavior alters after their mother has exercised. Researchers suggest this is because of changes in the scent of her sweat. If you think your baby is distracted or put off by you being sweaty, have a shower after you exercise and before you feed him.

Smoking

Being a smoker can reduce your milk supply, because nicotine reduces prolactin production. Smokers also tend to stop breastfeeding sooner than nonsmokers, and heavy smokers (more than 20–30 cigarettes a day) tend to wean earliest of all. What's more, inhaled cigarette smoke increases the effects of caffeine in a baby. And large amounts of nicotine in breast milk can have unpleasant effects on babies, such as nausea, vomiting, colic, and diarrhea.

So cut smoking out or at least down if you can, especially if you're a heavy smoker. Help is available from quit-smoking groups, telephone help-lines, and your doctor.

If you can't or don't want to stop, it's still better for your baby to be breastfed than bottle-fed. But strongly consider cutting down. And don't smoke anywhere near your baby, because inhaling smoke increases a baby's risk of respiratory disorders such as pneumonia and bronchiolitis, leukemia, and sudden infant death syndrome.

Contraception

Unless you don't mind getting pregnant again soon, you'll need to take precautions after the first eight to ten weeks after childbirth (pages 50–51).

When periods return (page 51)

This will happen some time after you cut down on breastfeeding or your baby starts solids (page 297). You may need extra energy and patience a week before and after ovulation, as your baby may find it difficult to settle, probably because your milk tastes different (Most women ovulate somewhere between days 10–14 of their cycle, the first day of their period being day 1). Your baby may be extra hungry around period time, as your milk supply may temporarily decrease and your let-down become less reliable then.

Shopping

You'll have little time between feeds to shop in the early weeks after giving birth. You could do a big weekly shop with your partner, ask someone else to do it, or use shops that deliver. There's nothing worse than going shopping and having to get a hungry, crying baby home when you're tired and heavy-laden. This said, many women with young babies find the outing to shop a pleasant change from being at home.

Seeing friends

Some women feel lonely if they leave their job, have a baby, and don't have many friends in the same situation. But a baby is an excellent conversation opener, and it'll probably be easy to make friends now. It's best not to set times for meetings away from home, though, because you'll probably end up breaking appointments when your baby wants to spend long, unhurried times at the breast. If you ask friends to your home, make him your priority.

Single mothers

The number of unpartnered mothers is increasing in Western countries, and statistics suggest they are less likely to breastfeed. If you decide to bottle-feed, try to identify why, in case this helps you change your mind. For example, if you believe you won't have enough encouragement and support to breastfeed, you could talk to a relative, friend, neighbor, health professional, breastfeeding counselor or leader, or social worker, about the backup you'll need. You may not know what you'll need until you've had your baby, though, so keep an open mind. Mothers who live on their own need to look after themselves especially well.

How you feel

Feelings are often heightened after having a baby. Some women, indeed, feel as if they're on an emotional roller-coaster for a year or so. Others feel low (page 192). None of this is surprising because the changes in lifestyle for most women after a first baby in particular are immense. Every newly delivered mother is different. She has her own relationships, her own unique experiences of pregnancy and childbirth, and her own ideas, beliefs, hopes, fears, and experience of breastfeeding. Many new mothers are thrilled with what's happened, but others aren't. And while most babies are very much wanted, others aren't. Clearly, there's no right way to feel.

As the days, weeks and months pass, how much you enjoy being a breastfeeding mother depends to some extent on how busy you are. If you slot feeds into a packed day, you may not feel calm and your baby, sensing your tension, might be unsettled. If you're very stressed or anxious you may not let down your milk at all. If this happens, try to slow down for the rest of the day and cut out a few jobs the next day.

Many women feel most stretched and tired in the late afternoon and early evening. Not only may they have to feed other children and get them to bed but they might also want to tidy up, feed the baby and think about an evening meal for themselves and other members of the household. The late afternoon and early evening period is a physiologically "down" time for many people anyway.

Feeling under pressure, or overwhelmed, could hinder your let-down. So be your own time-and-motion expert and aim to organize things so they don't all happen at once. "Proper" meals can wait, as long as you and your family have something to eat to keep you going. Older children can be encouraged to help clean up their toys; and you could give them their food and bath earlier. You could also prepare food for the evening in the afternoon, make full use of your refrigerator and freezer, and cook dishes such as casseroles well ahead of time. And, of course, you could enlist your partner's help while your baby is young.

Surprised by joy

Thankfully the overall experiences of having a baby and breastfeeding are usually positive, and sometimes very much so. Many women get satisfaction from knowing that breastfeeding is the best and most natural way to feed their baby. They enjoy its convenience, are delighted by its intimacy and believe it forges a closer bond with their child. They realize it's best for them too.

One large British survey found that the longer a woman breastfeeds, the more likely she is to plan to breastfeed her next baby, which certainly suggests breastfeeding is a positive experience.

New motherhood—A challenging time

Psychologists sometimes call new motherhood the "third childhood," as it's a sensitive time of far-reaching change (Childhood is the "first childhood," the teenage years the "second childhood.") Certainly it's a time when deep feelings, some of them unresolved, are stirred up in every woman.

A woman may find, for example, that girlhood fantasies about the sort of mother she would be mingle with remembered feelings about the mothering she had as an infant, and with her views about mothers in general.

She now has to deal with her feelings about having this baby, with this man, at this time. Her attitude to babies in general and this baby in particular may or may not match her partner's. Her thoughts about her breasts and the rest of her body, and the family messages she's received about breastfeeding and mothering, join to create a complex mix of ideas and attitudes. Some emotional sorting is conscious and rational but a lot goes on unconsciously.

Some women look to motherhood and breastfeeding to answer life's dilemmas. Others fear being a bad mother or an unsuccessful breastfeeder. A woman may feel pressurized into breastfeeding because she wants to please someone, or get them off her back. She may feel at a loss because she doesn't know anyone else who's breastfeeding. Or she may be wary about how breastfeeding might affect her relationship with her partner. If she doesn't have a partner, she may worry how she'll cope with breastfeeding and motherhood on her own. She may have fears about giving up or returning to work, or not having enough money. If she intends to work she may feel anxious about handing her baby over to someone else. The baby may be unwanted. Or he may remind her of someone in the family she particularly likes or dislikes. Last but not least, some women feel totally unprepared to be a mother, let alone to breastfeed.

Stirred-up emotions represent a challenge which, in turn, represents both a danger and an opportunity. They are a danger if unresolved and suppressed. And they are an opportunity if we recognize them and find ways of dealing with them so we grow in emotional intelligence. A loving partner or close friend can be a great help with all this.

Memories of being a baby

New motherhood can stir up memories of a woman's experience when she herself was a baby.

Psychoanalysts believe babies "split" their impressions of their mother according to how she meets their needs. So they may see her as two people: a "good" mother and a "bad" mother. When a baby girl comes to motherhood, recollections of joy and satisfaction at her hunger being satiated by her "good" mother may mingle with memories of frustration, fear, loneliness, anger, envy and despair when she was left hungry, crying and alone by her "bad" mother.

Such echoes from the past are normal, but their power in the here and now can be very strong.

The astonishingly profound intimacy of breastfeeding can stir up such memories even more. For example, a woman's delight at having her baby at the breast may stem as much from her own remembered bliss and feeling of security at having her needs met at her mother's breast (see below), as from the pleasure of her present experience.

On the other side of the coin, fear that her breastfed baby might be under-fed, dismay at being woken yet again at night, or anxiety that her crying baby is unhappy or doesn't love her, may echo her long-forgotten feelings as a hungry, uncomfortable or unhappy baby who feared the breast might never come. Sometimes such emotions can make a woman feel so ambivalent about breastfeeding that she decides to give up and bottle-feed instead.

Personal growth

The challenge of motherhood and breastfeeding can enrich our life and make us more sensitive to our own needs and those of our baby and our other nearest and dearest. But it's important to remember that you don't have to be perfect. All a baby needs is a "good enough" mother who meets most of his needs most of the time.

Perfect or good enough?—A woman who thinks of her own mother as being perfect can easily set too high a standard when she herself reaches motherhood. She expects to cope easily and is shocked if, or more likely when, reality proves different.

Her image of her mother being perfect is likely to result from babyhood, when anger or other painful feelings about her not responding to and satisfying her needs soon enough were too difficult and frightening to accept. So she suppressed those emotions and grew up thinking of her mother only as a "good" or "perfect" mother, instead of accepting that she was, in reality, imperfect but "good enough."

If you idealize your mother (or your memories of her) and believe you should be a perfect mother yourself, it may be better for you, your partner and your baby to learn to accept that it's okay to be "good enough."

A time of golden opportunity

How can you help make this time of mothering and breastfeeding a time of golden emotional opportunity?

Here are a few ideas:

Listen to your feelings—Be more sensitive to your emotions by listening to your inner voice.

When breastfeeding, ask yourself

1. Am I a "good enough" mother?
2. Do I know what I'm doing?
3. What will everyone think of me if I can't breastfeed?
4. Do I like breastfeeding?
5. Will my baby starve?
6. Will it be my fault if my baby starves?
7. Will I feel guilty if I don't breastfeed?
8. Who's really in control if my baby feeds whenever he wants?
9. What will my midwife and doctor (and, in the UK, health visitor) think if I don't breastfeed?
10. Am I comfortable with the sexuality of breastfeeding?
11. Can I bear caring for this demanding baby who never seems to stop feeding?

12. Is my baby the only person who loves me?

13. Does my baby love me?

14. If my baby really loves me, why isn't he happy?

If any of these questions rings bells for you, consider how it makes you feel. For example,

THESE QUESTIONS MAKE SOME WOMEN FEEL . . .

Question	Feeling
1, 2, 3, 5, and 13	Afraid
5	Helpless
6 and 7	Guilty or angry
8, 11, and 14	Angry
12	Desperate longing and needy

If these emotions aren't familiar, either they don't apply or you may have suppressed them. Suppressed emotions frequently stem from unresolved experiences in infancy. We aren't aware of them because we've erected defenses to stop them hurting us. But anything that stirs them up—particularly being with a new baby—can disturb our defenses and allow difficult feelings out.

For example, a woman might feel strongly that she doesn't want to breastfeed, without knowing why. Or she might become depressed or anxious, or develop compulsive behavior (such as overeating or overwork). Such problems can interfere with her ability to respond to her baby and be a "good enough" mother.

However, becoming more self-aware and learning to deal with their feelings helps many women care for their baby more effectively.

Share your feelings—If you'd like to come to terms with the difficult emotions triggered by becoming a mother, positive thinking and the wish to change may not be enough. You may need to discuss things with your partner, a trusted friend, or your postnatal class teacher. Or you could seek help from your doctor (or, in the UK, health visitor), who may suggest you see a counselor or psychotherapist.

Get encouragement and support—these are vital ingredients of successful breastfeeding and if you need more, ask for them from your partner, other loved ones or friends. They may not know your needs unless you ask. Alternatively, get together with someone you met at an prenatal group and who planned to breastfeed, or befriend a woman you see breastfeeding at a mother-and-toddler group. Seeking friendship opens the possibility of mutual encouragement and support.

Or you could contact your midwife, health visitor (in the UK), or doctor; or a breastfeeding counselor or lactation consultant.

Another avenue is to take part in an online mothers' forum, such as is offered by llli.org (La Leche League's website) or the very popular mumsnet.org.

Boost your self-esteem—You are valuable in your own right, and, as a mother, you're caring for your child at a vitally important time in his life. So make time to

- Recognize how valuable you are.

- Focus on things you enjoy and do well (however small they seem). For example, you may love being with your baby (at least some of the time). You may like the change in pace that accompanied leaving work. Or you may simply be pleased you can manage to get to the shops or cook a meal. Allow pleasure from these simple feelings to warm you.

Feeling low?

Many mothers feel weepy, emotional, and, perhaps, actually low, around the fourth day. This is sometimes called the "baby blues." Unlike postpartum depression (see below), it generally lasts for only a few days. It often coincides with the milk coming in, happens just as often, if not more often, in bottle-feeders, and a likely cause is changing hormone levels after childbirth.

But quite apart from these hormonal changes, it isn't surprising if a woman feels particularly emotional now. Giving birth is both a crisis and a rite of passage, and the excitement and loss of sleep could disturb the calmest person. Also, any hospital procedure that institutionalizes, regiments, and infantilizes women—such as insisting on scheduled breastfeeds, or not allowing rooming-in—does little to help a new mother's heightened emotional state.

Unfortunately, if a mother is having any trouble with breastfeeding, feeling low, however temporarily, can be the last straw that makes her give up.

What she needs is thoughtfulness, encouragement, empathy, and plain straightforward kindness from the recovery-ward staff, family, and friends. All this matters a great deal when you've just had a baby. What she doesn't need is the slightest criticism, as this can hurt more than usual.

A few women become depressed in the first year or so of their child's life. In general, whether a woman breastfeeds or formula-feeds seems to make no difference to her risk of postpartum depression. However, one study (1983) found that exclusively breastfeeding women were more likely to get depressed than partial breastfeeders. Another, in Australia (2003), found that women who felt depressed were more likely to stop breastfeeding early.

10 THINGS TO TRY IF YOU'RE LOW OR DEPRESSED

1. Recount your labor and birth experiences as many times as necessary, to make them feel "concrete" and "real."

2. Ask for specific and practical help. For example, you may want someone to stay with your baby for a couple of hours a day so you can get some sleep or get away from your home.

3. Confide in someone you trust and think will be supportive, such as your partner, mother, sister, or another relative, or a friend or neighbor. Tell your doctor, midwife, or health visitor (in the UK), if necessary. They may suggest you see a counselor, join a group of women in the same situation who are working with a trained facilitator and, if necessary, take antidepressants.

4. Eat a healthy diet with plenty of vegetables, beans, peas, whole-grain foods, protein and healthy fats. Supplements of vitamin B complex, magnesium, calcium, and the long-chain polyunsatuated fatty acids docosahexaenoic acid (DHA) and arachidonic acid (AA) might help.

5. Go out in bright daylight for at least half an hour a day to get enough bright light to boost your level of the nerve-message carrier serotonin and help prevent seasonal affective disorder (SAD).

6. Exercise each day, for example with a brisk walk, a swim, an exercise class, or a workout with an exercise video.

7. Stay in touch with friends, however tempting it may be to shut yourself away.

8. Do something enjoyable each day, such as going for a walk or massaging your baby.

9. Brush up your empathic listening (page 327) and perhaps ask a partner or friend to practice with you. Being able to recognize, name, and express your difficult feelings brings them into the open and prevents trouble building up.

10. Accept that every baby is different. A low-birthweight baby, for example, may spend most of his time feeding, or sleeping, and it may be weeks or months before he matures enough to be alert and responsive enough to offer you more reward.

If you lose your sense of reality, have hallucinations or delusions, or fear you're on the verge of harming yourself or your baby, call your doctor urgently. About one or two in every 1,000 new mothers develop postpartum psychosis, usually in the first two weeks after the birth, and need expert help.

Assertiveness skills

Most helpers, especially perhaps your partner, can't be expected magically to know what you most need as a breastfeeding mother. Helpers can be very well-meaning but tend to do what *they* feel you want or need. So it's up to you to enlighten them by asking clearly for what you want or need.

Before your baby is born Practice being assertive without being aggressive. This involves getting your needs met without trampling over the needs of others. To do this,

- Recognize, name, and state your needs as you see them.

- Acknowledge other people's needs and their motives as you see them.

Then learn how to separate the two sets of needs.

You can learn assertiveness ("assertion") skills by copying other people who are pleasant but firm and don't act as doormats. Or you could learn from a book or course.

You'll find such skills useful in many areas of life—including, perhaps, dealing with people who try to put you off breastfeeding or make it difficult for you.

Managing criticism

Adverse comments or stares from people who are unfamiliar with breastfeeding or confused or otherwise challenged by it can be distressing and can leave a breastfeeding woman feeling attacked and deflated. This is especially so if she isn't all that confident about what she's doing, or is struggling with it. While it's best not to take criticism personally or let it sabotage breastfeeding, this isn't always possible.

If it comes from your partner or a parent, sibling, or other close relative, it could be harder to deal with than if it's from someone you don't know. And if it comes from your mother, mother-in-law, sister, grandmother, or grandmother-in-law, it could be particularly challenging.

This is partly because if this person didn't breastfeed when raising you or your partner, or if she tried to breastfeed but stopped early, seeing you doing it successfully may revive painful memories. For example, she may feel sad or a failure. Or she may, at a conscious or unconscious level, think she didn't have good-enough mothering from her mother and may yearn for what might have been for herself. Not surprisingly, this could make her feel awkward when she sees you breastfeeding. She may then act out her feelings by disparaging what you are doing and, by implication, disparaging you. This doesn't mean she's bad or unkind, just that her discomfort makes her insensitive to your needs and feelings as she mixes them up with those of her own.

If you can find time to try to identify the possible emotions behind a barbed remark, you'll be better able to deal with your reaction.

It's now that a loving partner, friend, or breastfeeding counselor could help get you back on track rather than surrender to an inner voice telling you you're a failure.

How to manage downbeat comments

Try one or more of these tried-and-tested techniques:

1. Ignore it. This will be easier if it comes from someone who is unimportant to you.

2. Say, in a pleasant, matter-off-fact way, something like, "There's a lot of research to show this is worthwhile, and I'll share it with you if you like."

3. Use humor for tension relief and diversion. When I was a young mother and people asked how long I was going to go on

breastfeeding, my husband would sometimes quip, "Probably not beyond his teens!" Work out some funny responses that let people know you're not going to be drawn into a PhD on the subject. Unless they're exceptionally insensitive, they'll back off.

4. Be empathic, if you have the time and energy. While our immediate response is to be defensive when attacked, if we listen empathically, we may be able to defuse the situation for both parties. To listen empathically, put your own feelings and concerns to one side. Now try to understand how your critic is feeling. Then say aloud what emotions you sense lie behind their behavior. For example, "It seems as if you're really upset about this." Be more specific if you sense any particular emotions. This could help them feel so understood that they can separate their views and experiences of breastfeeding from yours.

5. Be gentle on yourself as your confidence in breastfeeding and the way you respond to others grows.

A last word

You may, like many women, not feel like your old self for at least a year. This is because having a baby is physically and emotionally demanding and a huge change in your life.

Finally, the insights and experiences you gain from having a baby and breastfeeding him will change and mature you in ways you could never have thought possible.

ten

Your Milk Supply

Many mothers easily produce the amount of milk that matches their baby's needs. Others have too much or too little, especially in the early weeks before their milk supply is well established. Too much milk can be a nuisance but rarely stops a woman breastfeeding. But too little milk is the most common reason for stopping breastfeeding, or adding formula, in the first nine months.

What women who think they have too little need to know is that nearly every one of them can increase her milk supply.

Not enough milk—The most common challenge

You might think women who stop breastfeeding in the first nine months do so because they want to. But this usually isn't so. The vast majority don't stop from choice, but because they think they haven't enough milk.

This was shown in a large survey in the UK (Infant Feeding Survey 2005, published by the National Health Service Information center—see table overleaf).

The message is clear. When a woman stops breastfeeding, by far the most likely reason—unless she wants to stop—is thinking she doesn't have enough milk. This is more important than sore nipples, far more important than going back to work, and beats breastfeeding being "too tiring" by a long way.

The belief of many women that they can't make enough milk is the main disorder of breastfeeding in the Western world. It is increasingly true in developing countries too. Yet a poor milk supply is nearly always preventable or treatable. A woman may not have enough milk today but the odds of being able to meet her baby's needs within a few days are stacked in her favor—if she has enough information and skilled support to take the right steps.

Almost every woman is able to breastfeed. Just think how much sadness, frustration, and disappointment would be spared if this were widely known! Yet the first advice often given to women with insufficient milk is to give complements of infant formula or to abandon breastfeeding. Both are wrong. And there is no excuse for this if the advice comes from a health professional.

MOTHERS' REASONS FOR STOPPING BREASTFEEDING

	By 2 weeks %	By 4 weeks %	By 6 months %	By 9 months %
Insufficient milk	41	48	37	24
Painful breasts/ nipples	29	9	1	2
Baby rejected breast	21	13	11	16
Took too long/ tiring	17	19	5	9
Mother ill	11	8	5	5
Domestic reasons	7	10	3	2
Too stressful	7	4	3	1
Baby ill	7	3	2	1
Baby couldn't be fed by others	5	6	4	3
Didn't like breastfeeding	5	1	1	0
More settled on formula	2	4	8	3
Breastfed as long as intended	1	4	10	6
Baby not gaining weight	1	6	4	3
Baby teething or biting	0	0	3	14
Returned to work/ college	0	8	15	22

(The percentages in each column don't add up to 100 as some mothers gave more than one answer.)

Nine in 10 women who stopped breastfeeding within six months would have preferred to continue. Four in 10 who stopped later said the same.

What these women need to know is how to increase their milk supply. The only exception is if a baby is dehydrated or starving, in which case the mother needs to give complements of formula or, preferably, donated breast milk, while she increases her own milk supply.

Does everyone have enough milk?

Many women think they don't have enough—and at any given moment some indeed may not—but the vast majority can make enough if they know how.

Indeed, with good breastfeeding techniques most women can supply at least twice as much as their baby needs. Most women could easily feed twins.

However, some women are naturally capable of making more milk than others. Some may simply have more glandular tissue. There are many possible reasons for this. For example, high testosterone in pregnancy can reduce the development of glandular tissue in the breasts, according to researchers in Norway. One possible reason is an unhealthy placenta. The placenta normally converts certain hormones from the baby into testosterone and estrogen. But an unhealthy placenta may produce more testosterone and less estrogen. Breastfeeding is less common in younger women, smokers, women who've had preeclampsia or a pre-term baby, and women who have polycystic ovary syndrome or have given birth to a boy. A raised testosterone level might be responsible in these women.

In practice, such women may simply need more breast stimulation, a better breastfeeding technique, or more skilled support than others if they're to produce the same amount of milk.

Women differ markedly in their breasts' milk-storage capacity, so some have to feed more often than others. A few decide they don't want to devote the time and effort it takes to produce enough milk.

No one knows how many of these women are physiologically incapable of breastfeeding. Studies suggest that only 2–5 percent of women in developed countries are unable to produce enough milk. But many can produce at least some milk, especially if they have good information, support, and encouragement. And it's salutary to note that

- A study in Guatemala reported that every one of more than 400 babies who survived their first two days was successfully breastfed.

- Midwives at the Farm Midwifery Center, Tennessee, say that in their experience only one in 800 women has trouble producing enough milk.

- All 20 babies born in a prisoner-of-war camp in Singapore in WWII were fully breastfed. All the mothers then continued to breastfeed until their babies were over a year old.

This suggests to me that excellent-quality assistance and, in the case of the prisoner-of-war camp, dire need, can enable virtually every breast-feeding woman to produce enough milk.

Aim to recognize in advance whether you're at increased risk of producing insufficient milk. Then you can learn how to increase your milk supply if necessary.

One expert suggests such a woman may be more likely to have

1. Produced too little milk for a previous baby (though of course she may not have known how to increase her supply).

2. Close relatives who've failed to produce enough (though they may not have known how to increase their supply).

3. Little increase in breast size during pregnancy.

4. Little or no breast fullness a few days after delivery.

5. Breasts of different size (though this may not matter, as most women's breasts differ in size).

Is your baby getting enough?

This question comes from when four-hourly schedules were enforced, and many breastfed babies didn't get enough milk because they didn't feed often enough to stimulate their mother's breasts as much as necessary.

It is a loaded question that worries some women so much that it hampers their let-down. The pressure of stagnant milk in such a woman's milk-producing cells, and the lack of stimulation from her baby being unable to empty her breasts, then reduce milk production

It's a question that wouldn't need to be asked if women breastfed as Nature intended.

But it must be asked, as breastfeeding is so often mismanaged and so many women are wrongly advised to restrict feeds according to a non-breastfeeding-friendly schedule or routine.

You'll know your baby is getting enough when he

- Sucks and milks well.

- Feeds often—for example, every 1½–3 hours (which is at least 8–12 feeds a day) in the first few weeks.

- Is satisfied after a feed.

- Doesn't cry or fuss much.

- Gains weight (page 153).

- Thrives—has a good color and firm skin, and is active and alert.

- Has 6–8 soaked cloth diapers or 5–6 soaked disposables a day from the 4th day, or from when your milk comes in. During his first 3 days, a breastfed baby usually has only 1–3 damp or wet diapers a day, as he takes only very small amounts of colostrum.

- Has yellow bowel motions from 7 days old.

- Has 3–4 soiled diapers a day from 5 days old.

And when your breasts

- Let down milk.

- Sometimes leak.

- Sometimes feel full.

Knowing what to expect

Many women think something is wrong if their baby wants frequent feeds day and night, or sometimes wants to stay at the breast for ages. Or they worry if their baby stops feeding, has a short nap, then wants to start again. It's easy to think he is dissatisfied because you don't have enough milk. But these behavior patterns are usually normal.

Sometimes this unexpected behavior so disturbs a woman—especially if it's her first baby—that she feels helpless, out of control and hopeless. Her baby wants mothering. And she does too. If this happens to you, ask for more help and support.

False expectations of how breastfeeding babies should behave are common because we compare them with bottle-fed ones. When a mother gives formula, the only limiting factor is how quickly he can drink it. But breastfeeding is different because it's a dynamic process in which both parties give and take and the baby is partly responsible for the amount of milk made.

Weighing your baby

Weighing a baby shows whether he's growing well. Charting your baby's growth is best done using the new Child Growth Standards charts from the World Health Organization (WHO). These are based on children breastfed for a year, exclusively for four months, and with solids started by six months (The children were also born to nonsmokers and in non-deprived circumstances.) Since breastfeeding is the natural way to feed a baby, the growth of breastfed babies is the norm. There are different WHO charts for boys and girls. The charts are suitable for babies of all ethnic groups. They show where your baby's weight is in relation to others of his age. They are intended for health professionals trained in their use.

Charts based on data from formula-fed babies should be avoided. This is because it's normal for breastfed babies to lose more weight than formula-feds in the first week or so after birth and to take longer to regain their birthweight. Breastfed babies also gain more slowly than formula-feds after six months. So using an old chart based on formula-fed babies' weight gain could suggest your breastfed baby isn't growing as fast as he should.

During the first year, the rate of weight gain gradually falls; during the second year it stays steady. A baby sometimes gains no weight in any one week and may sometimes lose some. What's important is the weight gain over several weeks. A low weight gain, or none, is usually of more concern in a baby who's relatively light for his age.

Be reassured that if his weight has previously been steady for some time, a gain of 60 g (2 oz) in a week is very good. And if he's been losing, then staying the same is an excellent result.

The WHO charts plot a baby's weight according to his standing among 100 babies of the same age. Lines called percentile lines indicate the rates of growth for children for particular percentages. So the 50th percentile, for example, shows the rate of growth for the average-weight baby. Doctors and nurses may be concerned if a baby's weight gain falters and slips from one percentile line to a lower one. However, it's actually very common for the rate of weight gain to fall in infancy.

- A study of 10,844 children in California found that the rate of weight gain of 39 percent crossed two major percentile lines in the first 6 months (major percentile lines being defined as the 5th, 10th, 25th, 50th, 75th, 90th, and 95th) (*Pediatrics*, 2004).

If your baby isn't thriving because he isn't getting enough milk, your doctor or midwife (or, in the UK, health visitor) will advise how to increase your milk supply and tell you if he needs temporary complements. You need extra support with breastfeeding if he loses more than ten percent of his birthweight, doesn't start to gain weight by nine days, or fails to regain his birthweight by two weeks.

Why your milk supply may not meet your baby's needs

Several things can cause a mismatch between your milk supply and the amount of milk your baby needs.

Coming home from the hospital—The change in surroundings, the excitement, and the work you may need to do could temporarily reduce your milk supply, making your baby hungry and unsettled.

There's no need to give formula complements or stop breastfeeding. Your milk hasn't dwindled permanently, and you can readily increase your supply by looking after yourself well and checking your breastfeeding technique in case it isn't stimulating your breasts enough or emptying them sufficiently.

For example, if your baby isn't milking the breast properly, all the time in the world spent breastfeeding won't necessarily produce more milk. But it will tire you both and may dispirit you. In contrast, when your baby milks well, you'll let down more efficiently and your breasts will empty more completely, so you'll make more milk.

Changing needs—Babies don't necessarily want the same from feed to feed, let alone day to day. Sometimes your baby will want more than you've made, sometimes less. Don't think you can't make enough just because he's unsettled. Be guided by him, increase your milk supply if necessary, marvel at your body's demand-and-supply system and don't forget he may be beginning a growth spurt.

Growth spurts—see page 129.

Age

Women who have their first baby in their forties tend to produce less milk at first than do younger women.

Does the number of children you've had matter?

Women breastfeeding a first baby tend to produce less milk at first than those who've breastfed others.

- Women breastfeeding their second child produced 31 percent more milk in week one than when feeding their first child, and slightly more by week four, according to a UK study. Those with the lowest production with their first baby had the greatest increase when feeding their second (*Lancet*, 2001).

Remember you can readily increase your milk supply however many babies you've had.

How to increase your milk supply

Never imagine your milk supply is limited to the amount you're currently making. You can always increase it. All you need is information, confidence, and patience.

20 STEPS TO INCREASE YOUR MILK SUPPLY

1. *Check that your baby is well positioned and latched on* (page 159). This optimizes your milk production by enabling him to suck and milk effectively and empty your breasts.

2. *Increase suckling time.* Breastfeed on an unrestricted basis, which means doing it as often and long as your baby wants. If he's well positioned and latched on, then the more he's at the breast, the more readily you'll let down, the more milk he'll take and the more prolactin you'll have, so the more milk you'll make. Breasts respond to milk removal by making as much milk again, and frequent feeds encourage them to make more. Frequent feeds certainly don't "use up" your milk.

   Your milk supply is likely to take at least two to three days to increase, so don't expect instant results! Be prepared for long and frequent feeds—each lasting perhaps 40 minutes and with a gap of only two hours from the beginning of one feed to the beginning of the next. Your baby may sometimes want to stay at the breast feeding, comfort-sucking, and taking short naps for several hours.

Indeed, many a successfully breastfeeding woman reports that her baby sometimes wants to be at the breast for up to one, two or three hours, especially in the early evening. An inexperienced woman may think something's wrong, when in fact her baby is behaving normally by doing this "cluster feeding." If you sometimes haven't the time or inclination to sit with him, no harm will come from curtailing the occasional feed, but in general let your baby stop when he wants to.

Don't think of the time your baby is at the breast only as a "feed." Of course breastfeeding babies do actually feed for part of the time at the breast but they also get comfort and pleasure (and stimulate optimal development of their tongue, cheeks, and jaws). Women in one African tribe were flummoxed when asked how long it took to feed their babies, because they didn't think of the times their babies were at the breast as "feeds." They put their babies to the breast because it made the infants happy.

It's well worth fitting in more feeds than your baby asks for— perhaps even twice as many—waking him if necessary. Once you've increased your milk supply, your baby may eventually want fewer feeds.

Occasionally a woman's milk supply diminishes because carrying her baby around in a sling or carrier, or on a hip, lulls him so well that he doesn't ask for feeds. If this happens, put your baby to the breast more often than he asks for.

Giving juice, water, or solids will probably reduce his requests for the breast. A baby under six months rarely needs anything other than breast milk.

3.   *Feed from both breasts at each feed.* Normally it's fine to let your baby feed from one breast only, but if you're increasing your milk supply, empty both breasts at each feed. Let him stay at the first side until he's had enough, then, after a short break if necessary, offer the second. Be guided by him as to when he's had enough, because if you take him off before he's finished you'll gradually produce less milk.

Emptying both breasts

- Encourages more let-downs, which makes your let-down reflex more reliable and boosts your milk supply.

- Prevents pressure in tense breasts reducing the blood supply to the milk glands and thus making the milk-producing cells less efficient. Normally, the volume of milk in each breast increases between feeds, but repeated over-filling can counteract this effect.

- Prevents pressure from unemptied milk in tense breasts directly harming milk-producing cells and making them temporarily less able to produce milk.

- Enables the muscle fibers around milk glands to contract efficiently so they let down milk well. If the muscle fibers are stretched because the main milk ducts and reservoirs are full and the milk glands swollen with milk, they may not contract efficiently.

- Prevents a hormone-like inhibitory factor in breast milk slowing milk production.

4. *Express during, after, and between feeds.* During a feed, if he stops swallowing for more than a minute or so, express milk directly into his mouth while he's still at the breast (page 162). Immediately after a feed, when he seems to have had enough, express any remaining milk to encourage greater production. Express between feeds too. Do this four to five times a day for two to three days. The extra stimulation will increase your milk supply. Collect the milk you express after a feed or between feeds. You can then store it and see if your baby will drink it from a cup after the next feed.

5. *Check that you let down well.* It's vital to let down efficiently if your baby is to empty the first breast enough to get its high-calorie, fat-rich hindmilk. In the early days the let-down is less reliable than later when your milk supply is established and you're more confident. Fatigue, anxiety, and pain can hinder or even prevent it.

You may let down several times at each breast, especially if your baby stays at the breast for a long time. Stopping him before he's ready may mean he'll miss out on one or more let-downs. In one study, women who believed they didn't have enough milk were given an injection of oxytocin (the hormone that lets down milk) after a feed. The researchers then measured how much extra milk they let down. Most of the women let down as much again as their babies had already taken. So half of the milk their baby could have had remained in their breasts after the feed. If it usually takes two to three minutes of a baby being at the breast to make the let-down work.

So if you were to restrict suckling time to ten minutes, for example, your baby would be drinking for only seven to eight minutes. While this is enough for some babies, it leaves others very hungry.

Watch for signs that you're letting down (page 110). An unreliable let-down is a common cause of a poor milk supply, but if you know this is happening you've every chance of putting it right. Successful breastfeeding depends as much on efficient emptying of the breasts—which partly depends on a well-conditioned let-down reflex—as on the amount of milk you produce.

Several things can help you let down well

Condition your let-down reflex:

- Get into a routine of practical preparations before a feed.

- Remember that night feeds stimulate milk production, so don't hurry to give them up.

- Breastfeed or express whenever your breasts are tense and full.

- Let your baby sleep no more than two hours by day, or three to four hours at night (from the beginning of one feed to the beginning of the next), as your breasts need regular emptying.

- Wake and feed your baby if you let down your milk unexpectedly.

- Have everything on hand that you might need during a feed for you, the baby, and any other children.

- Decide in advance what to do about the phone, front-door bell, and other people (page 133).

- Relax before and during a feed, and try to clear your mind of any worries.

- Consider listening to slow music.

- Enjoy feeds. Instead of thinking of them as times to get as much milk into your baby as quickly as possible, calm down, stop pressuring yourself, and consider feeds as unique and special times together. Babies grow up very quickly!

Try "switch-nursing" (page 163)

Try switching sides three times and giving him ten minutes each time you switch. If you're feeding two-hourly to stimulate your milk supply, this will mean you'll be feeding for about 40 minutes every two hours. Or you could switch from side to side just twice—going, for example, from your left to your right to your left breast again. The time this takes is a small price to pay for increasing your milk supply.

If you usually need several minutes of breast stimulation before you let down your milk, it's worth leaving your baby at the first breast until he comes off spontaneously, or he may have time only to fill up with relatively low-calorie early milk from that side. He may then be too tired and full to go on sucking. But he won't be satisfied for long, and your let-down won't get the stimulation it needs.

Keep fit

Take the time and make the effort to find forms of exercise you enjoy and can do several times a week. Exercise boosts the body's cannabinoids (natural feel-good chemicals) and helps you relax afterward. This helps you let down your milk. It also increases the blood flow through the breasts, which stimulates milk production.

Look after yourself

- Avoid getting over-tired because this might make your let-down less reliable. Have at least one nap in the day and put your feet up when you sit down. Until your let-down is well established, avoid unnecessary chores; make shopping as easy as possible; cut down on social networking; and don't return to work. Also, don't promise to be anywhere at any set time (though there will be exceptions, such as visits to the doctor).

- Get comfortable when feeding because such things as aching shoulders or a draught won't help.

- If you have sore nipples, trigger your let-down before your baby starts feeding. The pain is unlikely to last throughout a feed (page 220).

- See if a hot shower encourages your let-down, though this isn't practical before every feed. Sometimes you might feed in the bath, as its warmth will help you relax and encourage your let-down.

- See also chapter 9.

6. *Encourage your baby to keep alert and awake* (page 243). Help him stay awake enough to feed well by talking, stroking, and switch-nursing. He should then suck and milk your breasts more strongly and avoid getting into the habit of snoozing at the breast.

7. *Help him suck and milk more effectively* (see numbers 1, 5, and 6 above, and page 241).

8. *Get help from your midwife, health visitor (in the UK), doctor, or breastfeeding counselor if your baby isn't gaining weight well, or is losing weight.* They can help you increase your milk supply by improving your breastfeeding technique. They can also check that your baby's health is good.

9. *Avoid formula if possible.* Giving complements of formula to your breastfed baby can diminish your milk supply, especially if it's done in the first few weeks, before breastfeeding is well established. This is because he will then go longer between feeds so won't stimulate your breasts as well as he should.

The good news is that if he's having formula as well as breast milk, then using the tips in this list means you're highly likely to be able to increase your milk supply and stop the formula. *Be reassured that if your newborn has complements of formula in the hospital, you're highly likely to be able to breastfeed fully once you get home.* If he is already having some formula, reduce its amount by 15 mL (about ½ fl oz) at each feed, so he wants more breast milk. Give the formula not from a bottle but with a cup or spoon (or, if necessary, a supplementer, or he may get so used to a bottle that he'll be loath to breastfeed. Check he's wetting and soiling his diapers as he should (page 200) and contact a health care professional or breastfeeding counselor or leader if necessary.

10. *Eat an enjoyable and healthy diet.* And bear in mind you may need to eat slightly more than before you were pregnant. Drink according to your thirst.

11. *Exercise to increase the circulation in your breasts.* Regular whole-body exercise encourages a reliable let-down reflex and also increases the amount of milk you make by boosting the circulation to your whole body, including your breasts and hormone-producing glands. The volume of blood flowing through the breasts is 400–500 times the volume of milk produced, and the greater the blood flow, the more milk you'll make.

12. *Wear a comfortable bra.* Too tight a bra could decrease your milk supply, because constricting the breasts can reduce or even stop milk production.

13. *Be positive.* Women who really want to breastfeed produce more milk. One study found that breastfeeding women who'd previously said they preferred the idea of formula-feeding were three times more likely to find their baby refused the breast, and twice as likely to say he was a bad feeder, compared with women who always intended to breastfeed. This suggests a positive attitude is very helpful. Interestingly, the study also found that more women who always intended to breastfeed were likely to report that their babies refused a bottle of formula. But many women who want to breastfeed fail simply because they believe they haven't enough milk.

Indeed, many a woman's greatest single concern before embarking on breastfeeding is that she won't produce enough. This concern seems ingrained in many modern women.

14. *Come off the combined pill.* The contraceptive pill, unless of the progestogen-only type, usually reduces a woman's milk supply (For alternative contraception, see page 51).

15. *Be a nonsmoker—or at least cut right down.* Smoking can decrease the milk supply by lowering prolactin. It can also hinder the let-down.

16. *Formerly it was believed that using a pacifier might reduce a baby's demand for the breast, and therefore diminish his mother's milk supply. But this may not be so.*

    • A review of four randomized controlled trials (the most reliable sort of research) concluded that giving babies a pacifier had no adverse effect either on the duration of breastfeeding or on the duration of exclusive breastfeeding (*Archives of Pediatric and Adolescent Medicine*, 2009).

17. *Drink more fluid?* Drink only what you want, because drinking more isn't usually helpful. You'll know you're getting enough fluid if your urine is pale yellow.

18. *Consider traditional milk-boosters.* Over the centuries, women around the world have used amulets, potions, herbal remedies, special foods and drinks, chants, and prayers to increase their milk. There's no harm in trying milk-boosters (galactogogues) provided you also use the proven methods above for increasing your milk supply.

Traditional milk-boosters

• Alcohol, especially heavy beers and stouts. These increase prolactin. But babies tend to drink less milk if it tastes of alcohol, so they don't stay at the breast as much as usual, which means there's less stimulation for milk production.

• Vitamin B. This could improve your sense of well-being, which might help if you've been tense and not letting down well.

• Dark green leafy vegetables.

- Corn, peas, beans, lentils, chickpeas, oats, barley, and brown rice, though there's no evidence that these help.

- Walnuts and almonds are said to aid milk production, as are fenugreek, sunflower, sesame and celery seeds. You can add these to your meals, or take a fenugreek capsule. Animal studies suggest fenugreek seeds have an oxytocin-like activity.

- Caraway seeds, dill, and fennel—made into tea or used in your diet—are traditionally considered "warming." This could mean they relax tense muscles in blood-vessel walls, which may boost the blood supply and aid the let-down.

- Borage leaves and seeds, ginger root, coriander and cumin seeds, nettle leaves, and alfalfa sprouts—made into tea or added to meals—have been used for centuries to increase the milk supply. You can take nettle and alfalfa leaf in capsule form, and nettle as a tincture.

- Vitex agnus castus (chaste tree) seeds raise low prolactin. One study found it increased milk production in four out of five women. After 20 days the average production was three times as high in women taking it as in those not. You can use these seeds to make a tea. The homeopathic remedy Agnus castus (chaste-tree) is also said to help.

- Saw palmetto berries are reputed to help the breasts function properly and can be made into a tea.

- Herbal teas made from raspberry leaves, cinnamon or blessed thistle can help if you're feeling stressed, which may help you let down better. But beware of drinking too much. In one report, mothers who drank nearly 4½ pints (2 L) a day of a tea containing licorice, fennel, anise and Galega officinalis found their babies reacted badly, with restlessness, vomiting, floppiness, tiredness, and a weak cry, as well as poor growth.

- Vervain tea is said to boost milk flow.

- Clover honey is reputed to increase the milk supply.

- Geranium and fennel oils can be added to a carrier oil (such as sweet almond) and used for a whole-body massage to boost your milk supply. Add about ten drops of essential oil to one tablespoonful of carrier, but wash the oil off your nipples and areolas before feeding your baby. Cows' milk used to be said to help breastfeeding women make milk but we now know this isn't true. If you're eating a healthy diet there's no need to drink any cows' milk.

19. *Avoid eating mint, sage, parsley or sorrel, or drinking carrot juice.* These are reputed to reduce milk production.

20. *Consider taking prescribed drugs*: Drugs used for increasing the milk supply work by blocking the neurotransmitter dopamine so it can't inhibit prolactin production. But they don't work in all women, including those who already have plenty of prolactin. They can also have adverse effects. Metoclopramide, for example, can cause severe depression, restlessness, fatigue, drowsiness, dizziness, and cramping. It isn't known whether the amounts that enter breast milk can affect the baby. Domperidone doesn't cause depression but can cause headaches, cramping, and a dry mouth. What's more, it isn't available for breastfeeding mothers in the US because although the American Academy of Pediatrics has approved it for this use, the Food and Drug Administration has warned against it. Chlorpromazine, other phenothiazines, and rauwolfia drugs can cause restlessness, tremors, involuntary movements, changes in the breathing and heart rates, and exhaustion. Any of these drugs should be used only as a last resort.

"Happy to starve?"

A few seemingly content breastfed babies are actually very short of milk and are sometimes said to be "happy to starve." They risk brain damage or other problems if no one notices.

The most common reason behind failure to thrive is a restriction in the number and length of breastfeeds by day and night. Four-hourly, ten-minutes-a-side type of breastfeeding works only for those few women with an unusually plentiful milk supply. Most of us need to feed our babies much more frequently and for longer to get the breast stimulation and emptying we need to make enough milk.

If you and your professional advisers are concerned because your baby's weight gain is small or nonexistent for a few weeks, don't be put off breastfeeding but take immediate steps to increase your milk supply (page 204). If "complementary" feeds of formula are recommended, discuss whether it's possible to delay them for a few days while you increase your milk supply instead. If your doctor or midwife (or, in the UK, health visitor) agrees it's safe to wait, it's highly likely that your baby won't need formula at all. If he's so under-nourished that he needs formula fast, give it by cup after each breastfeed while you spend the next few days increasing your milk supply. Once you're making more milk you'll almost certainly be able to stop giving formula.

If you don't feel confident, ask a breastfeeding counselor or leader for support. She'll have helped many women with this problem before.

Failure to thrive

If you've taken steps to increase your milk supply but your baby still isn't growing well, something may be wrong (page 270).

What if I can't breastfeed?

Even with the very best motivation and help, a tiny percentage of women are unable to breastfeed fully or at all.

If you're among them, there are several things you can do:

- Be grateful you have an alternative.

- Focus on the positive aspects of your experience and count them as successes. One example might be the enjoyment you and your baby have had during some of the breastfeeds you've done. Another is that the breastfeeding you have done is definitely better than none. Your baby is lucky to have a mother who has tried her best. No-one can expect "straight A's" for everything!

- Forgive yourself. If you later discover you might have been able to breastfeed had you known more, received more support and done it differently, don't blame yourself or others but work out what to do if there's a next time.

- Take time to recognize, name, and come to terms with your feelings about being unable to breastfeed as you'd wished. You may experience conflicting emotions, perhaps with sadness, disappointment, guilt, anger, frustration, and helplessness mixing with a degree of relief that you no longer have to worry that you can't breastfeed fully or at all.

- Consider writing, or talking to someone who's prepared and able to listen, about what's happened and about your feelings. Or paint or do something else creative. This could help you move on and enjoy your baby without dwelling unproductively on what might have been.

- Don't lay any disappointment, anger, or guilt on your baby. It isn't his fault and isn't yours either. Your love for your child is more important than your milk, so don't allow difficult feelings to harm your unique relationship.

- When you bottle-feed your baby, hold him as you did when breastfeeding, not like a doll, at arm's length.

- If you still have some milk, consider giving the occasional breast-feed—perhaps in the early morning. If you put your baby to the breast before or after each bottle-feed, you might find the relief of bottle-feeding after worrying about not having enough milk improves your let-down so you produce more than you thought you could.

- And if you have some milk, try a supplementer. This enables your baby to get what breast milk there is while also receiving formula through a fine tube alongside the nipple. It allows his sucking and milking to stimulate the milk supply and gives both of you the pleasure of breastfeeding.

Wet nurses and donated milk

In olden times, women who didn't want to breastfeed, or had trouble doing so, arranged for another woman to breastfeed their baby. This "wet nurse" might have been a relative, or someone paid to do it as a job. However, from the early nineteenth century on, in Europe and America, wet nursing became less common as formula feeding became more popular.

Today, wet nursing is rarely heard of in developed countries and in some countries is frowned on, or even illegal. Many mothers and health professionals don't know about it or, if they do, may not like the idea or know it's safe. If a potential wet nurse is screened by a licensed pathology laboratory to check she isn't carrying an infection that could harm the baby, it could make sense to go ahead. If you want a wet nurse, and if you can find one, she needs to be screened in the same way that potential donors to milk banks are screened (page 170).

Milk banks (page 170) offer donated breast milk generally only for newborns who need it and whose mothers can't provide enough. However, there aren't enough milk banks, especially outside the Western world.

If you find a source of donated breast milk on the Internet, be warned that such milk may not have been properly screened.

Try again next time

If you've failed to feed a first baby, try again when you have another. Many such women breastfeed second or later babies successfully. You'll be more confident and experienced next time. Remember that not breast-feeding for as long as you wanted the first time may mean you'll need more encouragement, practical backup, and skilled support now. It's up to you to make sure you get it.

Too much milk

In the early days, before your supply matches your baby's demands, you may have too much milk. The supply will adjust over a few days but their initial abundance can cause problems, especially toward the end of the first week. A newborn can be bewildered and almost choked by it. He'll turn his head away, cough, sputter, and be reluctant to go on feed-ing. Any excess air swallowed as he tries to drink from this "fire hydrant" may then give him colic.

Manage an overabundant milk supply by

- Expressing before a feed or allowing milk to leak if you start let-ting down before your baby feeds.

- Feeding from only one breast at each feed. The presence of milk in the unemptied breast, together with its pressure as it accumu-lates, stops the milk-producing cells making so much. But don't let the unemptied breast overfill before the next feed. When nec-essary, express just enough milk to prevent lumpiness or tension. Also, express a little just before the next feed so your baby can easily take the breast into his mouth.

- Reduce your milk production by not letting your baby comfort-suck and snooze at the breast. Allow only "nutritive sucking." This is the sort done while actually swallowing milk. You can recognize it by its rhythm of one suck per second.

- Help prevent strong sprays of milk tickling his throat by holding him facing you on your lap and guiding his head on to your breast, holding your nipple if necessary.

- If your breast is very tense, try reverse-pressure softening.

As your baby grows, he'll be better able to cope with an exuberant let-down without choking.

You could think about donating surplus milk to a milk bank so it could go to pre-term or sick babies whose mothers don't want to or can't breastfeed. Ask your doctor or midwife (or, in the UK, health visitor) for details.

When you want to stop (see also page 306)

Cut down the number and length of feeds over several weeks, if possible, as more rapid weaning can cause engorgement or blocked ducts. As your baby receives less breast milk, he'll need other drinks and, perhaps, foods, instead, the choice depending on his age.

A woman who decides to stop because she finds breastfeeding time-consuming, tiring or annoying can reflect that it's better for a baby to have a happy mother who bottle-feeds than to have an unhappy breastfeeding one. But practical help could make all the difference to her decision, so she shouldn't be too proud to ask for what she needs.

Drying up milk after childbirth

If you bottle-feed, your milk will still come in and your breasts could feel very full or become engorged. Whenever they feel this way, express or pump only just enough milk to make them comfortable. Restricting drinks or taking diuretics (prescribed drugs that remove excess body water) don't dry up milk. And Epsom salts are best avoided as they can cause diarrhea. Neither heat, nor ice, nor a tight bra is useful, but some women report that putting a refrigerated cabbage leaf inside each bra cup eases discomfort!

Herbalists say eating plenty of mint, parsley, sage, or sorrel helps dry up milk. Indeed, a traditional aid for French women who want to stop breastfeeding is to eat parsley omelets (See also page 227 for herbal remedies that reduce engorgement).

No provably safe medicine is available for drying up milk. Doctors once prescribed estrogen (stilboestrol). But this sometimes had potentially serious side effects, such as a blood clot in a vein. And stopping it often increased milk production. The synthetic estrogen chlorotrianisene may be safer.

Bromocriptine suppresses prolactin within a few hours but is expensive, and possible side effects include headache, nausea, heartburn, dizziness, and, rarely, high blood pressure, a temporary stroke-like illness, or even a heart attack.

If, like many women, you change your mind and decide to continue breastfeeding, it'll be much easier to build up or maintain your milk supply if you haven't taken a suppressant drug.

In South India women traditionally put strings of jasmine flowers on their breasts to dry up their milk. Research has shown these are as effective as bromocriptine.

Restarting your milk supply

You may want to restart your supply days, weeks, months or even years after stopping feeding. Doing this is called relactation.

If your baby has been on formula for several weeks and your milk supply has dried up, you can start it up again by putting him to the breast frequently. He may be frustrated at first by feeding at an empty breast, partly because the shape of the nipple isn't such a strong stimulus to sucking as the shape of a rubber teat ("nipple").

Either let him have some formula from a bottle to satisfy his initial hunger, then let him feed from you. Or, to avoid the stimulus of a bottle's rubber teat, give him some formula from a cup or spoon then let him feed from you. Once you start producing milk, get your let-down working before you put your baby to the breast. You may find a supplementer helps.

The more often your baby breastfeeds, the sooner you'll produce milk again and the more you'll make. After each feed, express or pump to build up your milk supply. After about two weeks you'll probably be producing enough milk to do without formula.

The keynote to success is confidence. The experience of women all over the world is that their breasts are capable of producing milk again even after several years of being dry, if they have enough stimulation.

eleven

Other Common Challenges

Nearly every challenge to successful breastfeeding passes in time, given good enough information and support—so hang on in there! You're doing a great job. If you need extra help, contact a breastfeeding counselor, La Leche League leader, certified lactation consultant, or a skilled doctor, midwife or, in the UK, health visitor.

Sore, cracked, or blanched nipples

Sore nipples are very common, a cracked nipple much less so. A "blanched" nipple is another possible source of discomfort.

Sore nipples

Up to nine in ten breastfeeding women have sore nipples at some time, especially early on and particularly in the first week. About a quarter develop severe soreness or a crack (page 223). Prevention isn't always possible, but several things can help, and soreness almost always improves with time and care.

Usually the skin is rough. There's reddening and swelling of the small projections on the top of the nipple. There may be a crescent-shaped stripe across the nipple, composed of tiny blood spots in the skin, and occurring where's there's maximum suction. Any broken skin may be crusted too.

Soreness hurts most as the baby starts feeding. But this generally lasts only a minute or so provided the skin isn't too damaged, because as soon as the milk lets down he no longer needs to suck as strongly. This explains why the pain is always less in the second breast.

In women who breastfeed on demand any soreness is usually worst on the third day after the birth. In women who breastfeed on a four-hourly schedule it's worst on the fourth day. Schedule-fed babies tend to damage nipple skin more, probably because they feel hungrier before a feed, so they suck more strongly. Large babies may cause more soreness for the same reason.

Rarely, a sore nipple bleeds. This can look horrifying if blood is regurgitated, but it won't harm your baby, so just treat the soreness and carry on feeding.

Possible explanations for soreness—

- Your nipples aren't used to being sucked. The good news is they will toughen as the days go by.

- Your baby may have been poorly positioned at the breast (page 159). He must then suck particularly strongly to get milk and keep the breast in his mouth.

- You may take a long time to let down your milk because you're stressed or anxious. Your frustrated baby then sucks especially strongly until your milk lets down.

- Your baby could be sucking and milking the breast very strongly out of frustration during the first 3–5 days or so before your milk comes in. Once it does, it's highly likely there will always be some foremilk in the reservoirs when he starts to feed, so he won't be frustrated. If not, this could be because you're cold; if so, put on more clothes, heat the room, or have a warm shower or bath before feeding.

20 STEPS FOR TREATING SORE NIPPLES

Steps 1–10 are for everyone, but you can pick and choose from the rest. The cardinal rule is, DON'T STOP FEEDING.

1. *Change your baby's feeding position several times a day* so no one part of the nipple takes the full suction force each time.

2. *Position your baby well.* If your nipple is striped, your baby is probably sucking very strongly just to hold on. He's unlikely to have enough areola in his mouth. So the nipple endures the full force of his sucking and milking. This draws it in and out of his mouth, soon making it sore. A poorly positioned baby doesn't stimulate the breasts well, so milk production and flow are poor and the let-down unreliable. Milk can't flow into his mouth quickly enough to fill the vacuum created by sucking and reduce the suction on the nipple. Some experts believe nearly all nipple soreness results from poor positioning.

3. *Feed your baby frequently.* This encourages mature milk to come in sooner and makes your let-down more reliable. You may get sore nipples sooner than a schedule-feeding woman, but your soreness will disappear before hers, your breastfeeding will probably be more successful, and you'll be less likely to get a blocked duct or breast infection.

4. *Don't limit drinking time but limit total suckling time.* Taking your baby off the breast (see Step 10) when he's finished actually drinking may help. It isn't always easy to know when a baby has finished drinking, because he'll often pause between bouts of sucking. But if yours is spending a lot of time at the breast without frequent bouts of regular swallowing and purposeful sucking at about one suck per second—even though you're trying to keep him alert and interested by encouraging your let-down—then it's time to stop. As soreness eases over the next day or two, go back to letting him suck for as long as he wants, or your milk supply may diminish.

5. *Encourage your milk to let down before putting your baby to the breast* by preparing for the feed, keeping warm and gently massaging your breast. He then won't have to suck and milk so strongly and for so long to stimulate your let-down. It's also wise to do this because a slow-starting let-down leaves you feeling sore for longer and the fear of pain and actual pain can delay the let-down.

6. *Offer the less sore nipple first* so when you offer the other one, your milk should be flowing well and you may have little or no pain.

7. *Distract yourself* to take your mind off the pain early in a feed when your nipples feel most sore. Try reading, watching TV, or doing breathing exercises.

8. *Care for your nipple skin well* (page 173).

9. *Express some milk after each feed, and rub it on your nipples and let it dry.* This successful and traditional tip helps soreness heal. Various factors in breast milk are soothing and anti-infective and encourage cells to grow.

10. Or *apply lanolin cream.* This encourages "moist healing," which is provably better for sore skin than keeping it dry. Lanolin comes from sheep wool; choose a brand (page 339) free from residues of pesticides used on sheep to prevent blow-fly infestation.

11. Or *apply a warm moist compress* to soothe any soreness between feeds.

12. Or *apply a hydrogel dressing* (see page 339, or from pharmacies) to encourage moist healing, though not if you suspect any infection.

13. *If you interrupt a feed, break the suction by putting a fingertip into the corner of his mouth and pushing the nipple to one side.* Pulling him off might increase soreness.

14. *Treat any engorgement.* A baby finds it difficult to get a good mouthful of an engorged breast, so he is more likely to chew the nipple.

15. *If your nipples don't stand out well, try breast shells for half an hour before a feed.* This lets your baby take a bigger mouthful of breast and thereby avoid sucking on the nipple alone. Clean the shells after use so they can't infect damaged skin next time.

16. *Cool your nipples before feeding your baby to relieve the pain.* Splash them with cold water, or apply a cloth-wrapped cool-pack (from the refrigerator) or a polythene bag of crushed ice or ice cubes. But get your let-down working first, as coldness could otherwise hinder it.

17. *Have a small alcoholic drink, if you do drink alcohol,* 20 minutes before a feed if you think pain hinders your let-down. But don't repeat this if you think it makes your baby less eager to drink your milk.

18. *Consider whether your skin could be over sensitive.* If your nipples are sore throughout a feed, you could have contact dermatitis, for example, from sensitivity to laundry detergent, fabric softener, soap, shampoo, deodorant, a sore-nipple remedy, food particles in your baby's mouth, or a plastic breast shell or pump. Either stop using suspects one by one for a week at a time each so you discover what's to blame, then avoid it in future, or avoid all suspects then reintroduce them one by one when the soreness has gone. Sometimes a teething baby's saliva is to blame. Soreness can also result from thrush (page 235), eczema, psoriasis, or seborrheic dermatitis. These need special treatment. If your doctor prescribes a topical treatment, wash it off before your baby feeds and reapply it after.

19. *Avoid antiseptic sprays.* Some women use an antiseptic chlorhexidine spray, thinking it will prevent sore nipples, nipple cracks, and mastitis. But there's no evidence that it's useful.

20. *If all else fails, try a nipple shield.* Made of ultra-thin silicone, this
has a firm nipple (teat) that gives a good stimulus for the baby
to feed. If you or your baby is in the hospital, wash it well in hot
soapy water and sterilize it before each use. If you're at home and
your baby was full-term and is healthy, washing it with hot soapy
water or in a dishwasher on a hot cycle is fine. Dry it, then store
it in its box or other sealed container. When applying it to your
breast, turn it nearly inside out first. Then smooth it on, stretching it over your nipple. Rocking the tip of the shield's nipple will
help it pop out. Moistening the edges of the shield will help keep
it in place. Express a few drops of milk into its nipple or drip
expressed milk on to its nipple to encourage your baby to feed.
Note that a shield can reduce the milk supply because producing
milk and establishing a reliable let-down depend on the baby stimulating nerve endings in the nipple and areola skin. It can also prevent
a baby from getting all the milk; the thinnest shields keep back 22
percent, thicker ones up to 65 percent! And some babies get so used
to a shield that they won't feed without one. So try slipping it off once
your baby is feeding well. And stop using it at all as soon as possible.

Nipple crack

This usually follows poor treatment of nipple soreness and is very
painful during a feed, especially at first. It usually develops along a stripe
caused by the baby's maximum suction pressure. So if you have sore nipples and see a red or white stripe across your nipple during or after a
feed, it's vital to adjust your breastfeeding technique so the stripe doesn't
crack open. Some cracks become infected by thrush. Cracks are the most
common cause of bleeding from the nipple. Other causes include a benign
tumor called an intraduct papilloma. Unless you're sure blood is coming
from a crack, consult your doctor.

- A Turkish study comparing three groups of women for 10 days
  after childbirth found that those who kept their nipples dry and
  clean were less likely to have developed a crack than those who
  applied breast milk after feeds, or used warm moist compresses
  four times a day (*Professional Care of Mother and Child*, 2000).

There's no need to stop your baby feeding. When the crack heals,
prevent it reopening by varying your baby's feeding position regularly.

Treat it as for sore nipples—Change your feeding position several times a day, and limit your baby's time at the breast if he isn't drinking, to help speed healing.

Skin is more likely to crack if it contains insufficient moisture, and cracked skin heals better if it contains sufficient moisture. So apply cream, ointment, oil, or a hydrogel or non-adherent dressing to it to increase its moisture content and help it dry more slowly and gently. Rapid drying and scabbing won't then create tension on either side of the crack that would separate its edges and so delay healing.

However, it's worth removing surplus surface moisture after a feed, or after leaking, or it could make the skin soggy and more prone to infection.

Consider using a nipple shield (page 223) during each feed until the crack has healed.

If a crack doesn't heal in a few days—or if it's very painful, consider taking your baby off the breast, in which case either express your milk or use a pump. Give the expressed or pumped milk from a cup.

You may need to wait for up to four or five days as the crack heals and before you can breastfeed from that side again, but it's more likely it'll be only one or two days. Gradually resume breastfeeding, starting twice a day and continuing to express or pump regularly between feeds.

Blanched nipple

Nipple pain sometimes precedes whitening and numbness caused by a sudden reduction in the blood supply. The pain resembles cramp, begins during a feed and continues afterward. The blanching and numbness begin during a feed or soon after. The problem sometimes persists for half an hour or more. When the blood supply returns, the pain goes and the nipples may turn blue or red before returning to their usual color. The symptoms are a type of Raynaud's phenomenon, which more usually affects the fingers during sudden cooling.

Warmth (for example, from a covered hot water bottle) may ease the pain.

To help prevent it, keep warm, avoid sudden temperature changes, check your baby is well latched on, and eat foods rich in calcium (page 85) and magnesium (green leafy vegetables, beans, peas, lentils, nuts, seeds, whole-grain foods, and "hard" tap water); or consider taking calcium and magnesium in supplement form.

If the problem is serious you could discuss with your doctor whether to take the prescription drug nifedipine (a calcium-channel blocker), which encourages blood vessels to widen.

Breast pain

Possible causes include engorgement, a blocked duct, and, less often, a breast infection or thrush.

Breast pain makes some women stop breastfeeding but identifying the cause has a very good chance of enabling successful treatment.

Engorgement

Swelling and tension of the breasts is common, especially as the milk comes in after childbirth, but it's usually easy to treat.

Mild engorgement—results from increased milk volume and blood-flow, as well as congestion caused by fluid leaking from lymph and blood vessels pressed on by swollen milk glands. With good management, and as your milk production adjusts to your baby's needs, it should lessen within 12–24 hours. But it could reoccur any time if you don't feed (or express) frequently enough, or if your baby wants fewer feeds. In contrast, in for-mula-feeding women, engorgement after birth tends to last for 1–5 days.

Without good treatment, or if you were to suddenly stop breastfeed-ing, the symptoms could worsen.

Severe engorgement—results from swelling and congestion building up so the breasts become painful, tender, hard, tense, hot, red, shiny, and lumpy, with their skin pitted like orange peel and easily bruised. Swollen ducts and reservoirs may stand out as lumps and "cords," leading some people to describe the breasts as "stringy."

You'll probably feel hot and shivery, you may have a low fever, and you may sweat profusely. You'll also be thirsty. Some women feel weepy because of the discomfort or because it coincides with the "baby blues."

Tension in the breasts flattens the nipples, making it difficult for a baby to get a good enough mouthful of breast to latch on to and milk well. It also squashes and flattens milk-producing cells, which reduces milk production. While this may be good in the short term, in that reduced milk production reduces further build-up of pressure, it's bad in the long-term because the cells' ability to produce milk can be damaged. Also, milk contains a hormone-like factor that can inhibit its production if the breasts remain full for long. This is why persistent engorgement dries up milk.

While you might imagine you have plenty of milk, you're actually on the way to having too little. If you limit the number of feeds, you'll eventually relieve engorgement because your milk production will diminish, but it might never again regain its former potential. Continuing engorgement also encourages mastitis, infection, and blocked ducts.

Poor management of engorgement is one of the most common reasons for a poor milk supply in the early days. Yet women whose milk dwindles this way could almost all have breastfed successfully had they known what to do. One leading American specialist believes engorgement is a problem caused by poor advice!

15 TIPS FOR ENGORGEMENT

1. *Feed, express, or pump frequently,* at least every two hours by day and every three at night, for at least long enough to remove fullness and lumpiness. Offer your breast even if your baby hasn't asked for a feed, or is asleep. He shouldn't have bottles or a pacifier. If you don't want to wake him, take off just enough milk to bring relief. Any more will increase your milk supply.

2. *Encourage your milk to let down before you feed* (or express or pump).

3. *Circle your arms vigorously before you feed,* first one way 20 times then the other 20 times, as this might help relieve congestion.

4. *Soften your breast before a feed by expressing a little milk; or by using reverse-pressure softening.* Either of these makes it easier for your baby to take a big mouthful of nipple and areola. If he sucks only your nipple, it'll get sore. Also, he won't drain the milk reservoirs. And pain from a sore nipple may inhibit your let down so he'll get very little milk, and you'll produce less. If you're badly engorged, an electric pump will be more comfortable than expressing or using a hand pump.

5. *Position your baby well so he sucks and milks effectively.* You'll know he's doing this if he swallows regularly and purposefully and is satisfied by feeds, and if your breasts are softer after a feed. Use breast shells for half an hour before a feed if you need to make your nipples stand out better.

6. *Gently massage your breast toward your nipple* when your baby pauses between bouts of swallowing.

7. *Express or pump after a feed to remove any remaining lumpiness.* Such lumpiness is most likely if your baby is too tired or unwell to suck and milk effectively for long. There's no need to empty your breasts fully.

8. *Wear a supportive and comfortable bra that doesn't press into your breasts.*

9. *Cool your breasts* after a feed for 20 minutes to reduce congestion if they remain uncomfortable. Don't do this before a feed, as it might hinder your let-down. Try applying a packet of frozen peas, an ice-filled plastic bag, or a chilled gel-filled cool-pack (any of these cloth-wrapped to protect your skin), or a refrigerated cabbage leaf or a wetted and wrung-out washcloth. Or splash your breasts with cold water. Don't have a hot bath or apply hot flannels because although warmth encourages the let-down, it also encourages congestion.

10. *Eat nourishing foods,* including a variety of vegetables and fruits for anti-inflammatory antioxidants.

11. *Drink freely*—there's no need to limit fluids as once suggested.

12. *Consider a painkiller.* They usually aren't much help for this pain, but you could try ibuprofen or paracetamol.

13. *Consider aromatherapy.* Gently smooth in 2–3 drops of rose essential oil mixed into 1 tablespoon of carrier oil (for example, sweet almond). Don't get it on your areolas or nipples as its taste could put your baby off feeding, or even be dangerous for him. Or you could try applying an aromatherapy compress. Put a few drops of pure rose, lavender, geranium or fennel essential oil into a bowl of hot water. Cut a round hole in the center of a large handkerchief then lay the handkerchief on the surface of the water so it picks up the film of oil. Now apply the handkerchief to your breast, with the hole over your areola and nipple. Cover it with a towel and wait five minutes Repeat every few hours. The hole prevents oil getting on your areolas and nipples.

14. Consider using a herbal remedy. You can buy herbs from a medical herbalist or herbal supplier. Make cleavers tea by pouring 600 mL (1 pint) of boiling water over 30 g (1 oz) of dried cleavers (Galium aparine) leaves, stems, and flowers. Cover, steep for 10 minutes, then strain. Wring out two washcloths in the tea, and apply to the breasts. Repeat several times a day. Cleavers is said to be cooling and to relieve congestion. Make a poke-root decoction by grinding 30g (1 oz) of dried root with a pestle and mortar, covering with 600 mL (1 pint) of water in a pan, simmering for 10 minutees, then straining

and using as for cleavers tea. This is a traditional remedy. If it's summertime and you have jasmine flowers in your garden, or know someone who has, copy those women in southern India who relieve engorgement by covering their breasts with jasmine flowers!

15. Give yourself a pat on the back. You're doing really well by breastfeeding and taking steps to overcome this temporary problem. Keep going.

Burning or shooting pains

Some women get these in one or both breasts after a feed.

Triggers include thrush, an ill-fitting bra, muscle tension from an uncomfortable feeding position, and trouble from old scars or other problems in the breast. Other possibilities are particularly forceful let-downs, or the baby sucking and milking very powerfully. This could temporarily make one or more milk ducts collapse or become unduly sensitive, or make the breasts refill particularly rapidly after a feed.

Blocked duct

This causes a red, tender lump in the breast that may progress to inflammation (mastitis) that makes you feel flu-like and achy. If the block—or "plug"—is near the nipple, you may see a swollen milk reservoir bulging under the areola and looking rather like a varicose vein.

A block in a duct prevents milk emptying from it. The main causes are engorgement and pressure from a badly fitting bra. Milk builds up in the duct behind the blockage, causing a lump. The ongoing trickle or the repeated let-downs of milk from the milk-producing glands that supply the duct further increase the build-up of milk and therefore the tenderness and size of the lump.

Early and effective treatment, started at the first hint of anything wrong, usually makes the symptoms subside quickly.

But if you do nothing, the surrounding breast tissue will probably become inflamed. This results from fluid and certain other constituents of the dammed-up milk escaping from the duct. This inflames the local breast tissue, reddens the overlying skin and increases your body temperature. Such inflammation has been known to raise a woman's temperature to 104°F (40°C)!

Treatment is urgent because of the risk of infection in stagnant milk above the blockage, in the glands supplying that duct, and in the surrounding breast tissue.

Some women notice a little white spot on their nipple. One possible explanation is that it's a plug of dried milk at the end of a duct. Some people call such a spot a "bleb." It may disappear during a feed one day, though it might stay for many weeks. You could gently squeeze it, when some white matter will emerge. Or you could soften the bleb by putting a a cotton ball soaked in white vinegar over your nipple and inside your bra; the vinegar will have a softening effect that may enable you to squeeze out the bleb more easily. If this doesn't work and if you find the bleb painful or unsightly, you could try to remove it carefully with a needle and a pair of tweezers sterilized in a candle or other flame. Or you could ask your doctor to remove it.

10 TIPS FOR A BLOCKED DUCT

As soon as you realize you have a blocked duct, go flat out with the first nine suggestions:

1. *Empty your breast thoroughly each feed,* as the lower the tension inside, the better your chance of clearing the block. Position your baby well, let him feed as long as he wants and express the remaining milk afterward.

2. *Vary your feeding position at each feed.* This simple tip is one of the most helpful. If possible, position your baby with his chin over the block so the milking action of his tongue and lower jaw helps clear it.

3. *Feed more often to keep the tension in the breast low.* Fit in as many extra feeds as you can, even if already feeding on demand. If your baby doesn't want to feed, express instead.

4. *Offer the affected breast first* to ensure the best possible emptying.

5. *Gently but firmly massage the lump toward the nipple* during a feed (and after, if it's still there) to help release the block. If you persevere you may eventually express a very small "plug" of white or yellow, cheesy or granular matter from the duct's opening at the nipple. This is milk that dried out as its water was absorbed. Many women release a block without seeing a plug. Once the block is released, the milk that lay behind it can be expressed. It's often thick and may flow slowly and spontaneously. Once the milk you express looks normal, you know all the dammed-up milk has escaped.

6. *Check that your bra isn't to blame,* especially if it leaves a band across the top of your breast when its flap is open, or has an underwire that presses on your breast, or you pull down the cup of an ordinary bra to feed.

7. *Relieve pain by applying a hot wet compress or a covered hot water bottle.* Immersing the breast in a basin or bath of hot water for a few minutes before a feed may help too.

8. *Get more rest and relaxation.* Going to bed will make you feel better and may boost your resistance, which will help prevent any inflammation spreading. It's possible that stress may encourage a blocked duct by boosting adrenaline. This increases blood fats, enabling more fat to enter milk. Extra fatty milk is thick and may encourage a blockage by forming a sticky coating on the lining of milk ducts— much as extra fatty blood encourages blood clots by forming a sticky coating on the lining of arteries.

9. *Exercise more*—to increase the flow of blood and lymph in your breast. Do whole body exercise to boost your general circulation and the blood-flow in your breast. And do shoulder, arm and upper-body exercises to boost the circulation of lymph in your breast.

10. *Take antibiotics if the lump persists after 24 hours.* This will prevent infection, and your doctor can prescribe ones suitable for a breast-feeding woman. Don't stop feeding.

Kinesiology—This extremely unusual—and unproven—therapy is said to reduce congestion by increasing lymph drainage. There's no apparent medical explanation, but it can do no harm and might help. Do it yourself or ask someone to do it for you.

Put one hand very lightly over the lump. With three fingers of the other hand, massage the outside of the same-side leg along a line from just below the knee to the hip (think of the side-seam of a trouser leg). Use a firm circular motion for about 10 seconds, and gradually move your fingers up the line. Repeat if necessary with your other hand on another lumpy area of the breast.

Repeated blocked ducts—Various factors can make milk unusually sticky, or encourage fat to stick to the lining of the milk ducts—so narrowing them and encouraging blockages.

Several measures are worth trying:

• Eat a healthy diet—Have at least five daily helpings of vegetables and fruit each day. Avoid too much saturated fat (in meat, dairy food, and margarines, spreads, white cooking fats, and other products containing hydrogenated fats), as it might make your milk more sticky. It may also help to eat more foods rich in omega-3s (page 86). Include onions, garlic (about three cloves a day), pineapple, ginger, avocados, and foods rich in vitamins B1 and B6 (meat, fish, egg yolk, whole-grain foods, green leafy vegetables, peas, beans, lentils, avocados, bananas, nuts, and seeds), vitamin C (green vegetables, potatoes, and most fruits) and vitamin E (nuts, seeds, soy products, lettuce, and vegetable oil), flavonoid plant pigments (vegetables and fruits), and salicylates (vegetables, fruits, and seeds). All these emulsify blood fats (disperse them into smaller globules), so it's reasonable to suppose they do this with milk fats too.

- Consider taking a supplement of omega-3s or lecithin from a health store or pharmacy. Either can make milk less sticky. And omega-3s reduce inflammation.

- Manage stress effectively—since it could interfere with your production and balance of omega-3 and omega-6 fatty acids. Stress is normal and necessary. But you may need to learn how to deal with it better so it doesn't get to you so much.

- Be a nonsmoker—If breast milk behaves at all like blood, which is likely, then smoking (and passive smoking) will make it stickier. Smoking is known to encourage the type of breast inflammation called periductal mastitis.

- Sleep on your back or side—sleeping on your front increases the pressure in your breasts, which could encourage a blocked duct.

- Consider homeopathy—The homeopathic remedy Phytolacca is said to help. The dose is one tablet of 30C or 12C two or three times a day. Don't take it within 15 minutes of eating, drinking, or cleaning your teeth.

- Consider a herbal remedy—Medical herbalists recommend drinking dandelion-root tea (no more than a cup three times a day) and smoothing linseed oil combined with a few drops of geranium or rose essential oil into inflamed breasts. If you do this, wash the oil from your nipples and areolas before the next breastfeed.

Mastitis

This means that part or all of the breast is inflamed. It's most likely to begin in the upper part of the breast, near the arm. Untreated, it can spread and the inflamed area might become infected.

Many people wrongly assume every inflamed breast is infected. But only one in two women with mastitis has an infection. The other has engorgement or a blocked duct. However, engorgement makes infection more likely, as does a blocked duct.

It's important to distinguish breast infection as it's potentially serious and needs antibiotics. Fortunately, tests in a pathology laboratory (page 232) resolve any doubt.

Breast infection—Inflammation associated with infection is variously called mastitis with infection, infected mastitis, or breast infection. It occurs in one in 40 breastfeeding women, most often two to five weeks after childbirth. Infection can begin in the tissue around the milk glands and ducts, or in the ducts.

Infection can affect a part or the whole of the breast. The infected area is red, swollen, hot, painful, and tender, the overlying skin is shiny, and the woman feels shivery, achy, and flu-like, with a fever of 100.4°F (38°C) or higher. The woman may feel nauseated and might vomit. Sometimes pus can be squeezed from the nipple.

Infection can follow poor or delayed treatment of engorgement, a blocked duct or a cracked nipple. Researchers also think infection can enter via the nipple from a baby who picks up the bacteria in the hospital and carries them in his nose without getting any symptoms himself.

The infecting organism is usually *Staphylococcus aureus*. Less often, *Staphylococcus epidermidis* or streptococci are responsible.

Diagnosing infection—It can be difficult to distinguish inflammation caused by infection from inflammation caused by engorgement or a blocked duct.

If only a part of the breast is infected, the symptoms are like those of a blocked duct, but worse.

If the whole breast is infected, it may look as if it's badly engorged. But mastitis due to breast infection usually affects only one breast, whereas severe engorgement almost always affects both.

If there's a lump, it could result from a blocked duct or from an abscess that began with an infection.

Your description of how the trouble started should help identify the cause.

It's best to have a sample of milk sent to a pathology laboratory before starting an antibiotic. If initial tests show your milk's white-cell and bacteria-colony counts are high, this suggests you need antibiotics.

These tests suggest

- **Engorgement**—if your milk has a normal white-cell count (less than 106 per mL) and a normal bacteria-colony count (less than 103 per mL), indicating it's either sterile or contains normal amounts of skin bacteria.

- **A blocked duct**—if your milk has an increased white-cell count and a normal bacteria count, indicating it's either sterile or contains normal amounts of skin bacteria.

- **A breast infection requiring antibiotics**—if your milk has an increased white-cell count and an increased bacteria count.

The lab will inform your doctor and begin culture and sensitivity tests to see which bacteria are responsible and which antibiotic is best. These tests take several days.

If you have obvious signs of infection, and initial tests suggest you need an antibiotic, your doctor will prescribe the one most likely to help. If culture and sensitivity test results show another is more appropriate, it's worth changing, because the wrong antibiotic encourages continued or recurrent infection.

Could it be thrush?—Ideally the lab should test your milk for thrush (Candida albicans, page 233) as well as bacteria. One survey showed that one in two women with mastitis had candida, though this doesn't necessarily mean it caused the inflammation, as it's often a normal inhabitant of the skin. If candida is the likely culprit, you need anti-fungal treatment, not antibiotics.

If you have a bacterial infection—

- Take antibiotics. Start with flucloxacillin (500 mg four times a day) if you aren't allergic to penicillin. If you are, take erythromycin (500 mg twice a day). Tetracycline, ciprofloxacin, and chloramphenicol can harm a breastfed baby so aren't suitable.

- Check your feeding technique and, in particular, keep your breasts well and frequently emptied by feeding, expressing, or pumping. This maintains your milk supply and helps healing. If you let your breasts remain too full—or try to dry up your milk—you risk getting an abscess.

- If you have a blocked duct, see page 228. If you're engorged, see page 225. If you have a cracked nipple, see page 223.

- Rest more. One study showed that women with a breast infection slept less at night than other women, and were less likely to take daytime naps. Take special care when life is extra busy.

- Treat the pain by applying hot wet washcloths to your breast.

- If in the hospital, clean your hands frequently with disinfectant hand-wash solution or alcohol wipes. The staff should do this before touching you or your baby.

- Manage stress effectively, as feeling over-stressed depresses immunity.

- Check your diet is good and contains plenty of fresh fruit and vegetables. Also, consider taking supplements of vitamins C (at least 100 mg a day) and E (10 mg of tocopherol acetate daily).

- Try gently smoothing in vitamin-E cream, or a simple cream scented with three drops of geranium essential oil to each tablespoon. Avoid getting cream on your nipples and areolas. If you do, wash it off before a feed.

- If you smoke, cut down or give up. If you can't, eat more vitamin-C-rich foods and take a vitamin-C supplement (at least 100 mg a day), as smoking reduces your levels of this infection-fighting vitamin.

Can your baby have your milk?—It's almost always better if your baby has your milk. But if the initial lab tests show particularly large counts of dead or alive bacteria, there's a very small possibility that your milk could give your baby gastroenteritis or even septicemia. So he shouldn't drink it even if it's sterilized. Instead, either feed only from your unaffected breast, or give donated breast milk, or formula. Pump or express your infected breast and discard the milk. It's perfectly possible to supply your baby with enough milk from one breast, so don't panic. When the bacteria count of the milk in the affected breast drops, you can breastfeed again.

If it doesn't get better—If, despite excellent treatment, your breast remains inflamed and infected, yet there's no abscess, your doctor should change the antibiotic to co-amoxiclav (taking care to monitor your baby for jaundice). If necessary, he'll refer you to a breast specialist.

Thrush

This infection with the yeast-like fungus *Candida albicans* sometimes coincides with a bacterial infection. Most researchers think candida is present only on the skin; a few believe it can enter the milk ducts.

Thrush can make the nipples and areolas very sore and, perhaps, flaky or shiny, with burning pain. Some women report sharp burning pains that shoot into their breast during a feed, worsen immediately afterward, and sometimes continue between feeds. You may have itchy nipples with flaky pink, red, or purple areas. There may be fine cracks on your nipples, perhaps with white matter inside. The areola may be shiny and slightly swollen, and have a red ring around it. Very occasionally there are adherent white spots on the nipples.

Candida is a normal inhabitant of the skin and bowel but in certain circumstances can multiply, causing infection. If a mother has thrush (for example, in her vagina) or her baby has thrush (for example, in his mouth or on his bottom), they can pass it between each other. Thrush in a baby's mouth may show up with white spots or patches inside his cheeks or on his tongue or gums. These bleed if gently scraped. A diaper rash infected with thrush may look shiny or have a bright pink raised edge.

Candida thrives in warm, moist situations and likes milk, so a baby's mouth and a mother's nipples and areolas (particularly if she wears a bra and uses breast pads) are good breeding grounds. You're more likely to become infected if you've recently taken antibiotics, have sore or cracked nipples, or are on the pill.

Rule out other conditions that can cause nipple soreness and breast pain. If your doctor diagnoses thrush, you and your baby need simultaneous, prompt, and vigorous treatment. This is best carried out for two weeks even if the infected area seems better earlier. There's no need to stop breastfeeding.

Anti-thrush medication—A pharmacist or doctor can recommend an anti-fungal cream or ointment (such as miconazole or ketoconazole) for your nipples and miconazole gel for your baby. If miconazole doesn't work for the baby, use nystatin oral suspension.

Rinse your baby's mouth with water after each feed and put a few drops (1 mL) of nystatin into his mouth. Wash your nipples and areolas after each feed, dry them well, then apply antifungal cream or ointment. Continue the therapy until the symptoms have been gone for at least ten days.

If you have vaginal thrush, this needs treatment. Your partner may need treatment too if you've returned to having sex.

If the thrush still doesn't clear, your doctor may prescribe 1 percent aqueous gentian violet solution for your nipples and your baby's mouth. Apply it once a day and for no longer than three days. It will color your nipples and your baby's mouth a dramatic purple. Oral fluconazole for at least two to three weeks can be prescribed if there's a definite diagnosis of thrush in a mother or in a baby over six months old. Note that fluconazole can worsen symptoms for the first couple of days as the thrush organisms die.

Home remedies—Research shows that treating thrush on the nipples by applying a vinegar solution (a teaspoon of vinegar in a cup of water) after each feed, and treating thrush in a baby's mouth by applying a baking-soda solution (a teaspoon of baking soda in a cup of water) can reduce itching but doesn't cure thrush.

Ultraviolet (UV) light from sunshine or a sunlamp could help get rid of thrush on your nipples, but take care not to get burnt, and protect your eyes with suitable goggles if you use a sunlamp. Expose your breasts for half a minute on day one, one minute on days two and three, two on days four and five, and three on day six. Reduce the exposure time if your skin reddens.

Everyone living with you should take strict precautions, including washing their hands after changing the baby's diaper, or using the bathroom. Keep a separate towel for each person; have a clean bath towel each day; launder towels frequently at 140°F (60°C); launder your bras in water as hot as is safe for the fabric; and put a cup of vinegar into your bathwater and into the final washing machine rinse.

Ideally, don't use breast pads as they encourage infection. If you do use them, change them after each treatment.

Eat a healthy diet, with little or no sugar, foods containing white flour or other refined carbohydrate, or yeast-containing foods and drinks, including alcohol. Eat some live yogurt each day.

Avoid giving your baby formula as thrush is more likely in formula-fed babies.

Other measures—A baby can be reinfected by anything that's been in his mouth. So if he uses a pacifier, boil it for 20 minutes each day.

Breast abscess

This usually results from poor or delayed treatment of breast infection and often shows up as a non-tender lump. One survey showed that *abscesses occurred only in women who stopped breastfeeding because of breast infection.*

Treatment is as for breast infection. If the abscess doesn't resolve, repeated aspiration (drawing off of pus through a needle) or, as a last resort, surgical incision and drainage (usually under local anesthetic) are necessary.

You can feed your baby from the affected breast if you and your doctor are reasonably sure the infection is contained within the abscess (which is usually so). Otherwise, feed entirely from the other side and express and discard the milk from the affected breast until the abscess has gone.

Breast lump

A breast lump can occur at any age and any stage of your reproductive life, so always be "breast aware"—so familiar with the feel and appearance of your breasts that you can report anything unusual to your doctor without delay. It's more difficult to feel a lump if your breasts are large and firm, so feel your breasts after a feed, rather than before. The lactating breast is often lumpy, though such lumps are usually "here today and gone tomorrow," whereas a significant lump stays put.

In a breastfeeding woman the causes of a lump include those that can occur at any other time. They also include those related to milk production. Not surprisingly, these come highest on the list:

- A blocked duct causes a lump that should disappear in a few days with suitable treatment.

- A milk-retention cyst (galactocele) is a non-tender, smooth, rounded lump filled with milk. It's thought to be a blocked duct that never reopened. In such a duct, the dammed-up milk gradually thickens and becomes creamy, cheesy, or oily. It can form an abscess if it becomes infected. If a cyst doesn't respond to the tips for treating a blocked duct, it's no good for a doctor to empty it via a hollow needle because it will refill. But it can be surgically removed under local anesthetic.

- An abscess has usually been preceded by breast infection.

- A fibroadenoma is common and may appear for the first time during lactation. It contains fibrous and glandular tissue. If necessary it can be removed (preferably under local anesthesia) and breastfeeding continued.

- A breast cancer. If you have this, you'll probably be advised to stop breastfeeding because chemotherapy drugs will enter your milk and harm your baby. The type of cancer that develops during pregnancy or breastfeeding is more likely to be aggressive, so never ever delay seeking advice about a lump unless you are sure of the cause and know what to do.

Overweight and obesity

If you're overweight or obese, learning good breastfeeding techniques is particularly important. This is because

- Women who are overweight or obese, or who gain more than advisable when pregnant, are less likely than other women to start breastfeeding. And if they start, they are likely to breastfeed exclusively for a shorter time and stop breastfeeding sooner (*Journal of Nutrition*, 2006).

Possible reasons for problems include difficulty positioning the baby and enabling a good "latch" (especially if your breasts are naturally large, as well as obese), and concerns about body image. In obese women, other possible reasons are their increased risk of pregnancy- or birth-related problems that can affect breastfeeding, such as preeclampsia, cesarean section (C-section), and early pre-term delivery, and the likelihood that their milk will come in later.

With the proportion of overweight and obese women increasing in many countries, it's vitally important for such women to have skilled assistance with learning to breastfeed, particularly in the first 24 hours after birth, and also until breastfeeding is well established.

Challenging feeders

Some babies take to the breast within a few minutes of birth and have no trouble breastfeeding. Some seem disinterested, perhaps feeding briefly, then letting go and crying. And some almost battle with the breast.

Virtually all babies breastfeed eventually with the right help. But an unenthusiastic baby won't stimulate your milk supply well, so you'll need to express or pump after each feed, perhaps for some weeks.

Before labeling your baby as a difficult feeder, deal with any engorgement and check he's well positioned. Then try to identify the reason.

Flat, inverted, or poorly protractile nipples

Some babies have difficulty latching on because their mother's nipple doesn't stand out well enough for them to draw it well back into their mouth. This situation tends to improve after several weeks.

Help your baby latch on by taking your nipple and areola between your finger and thumb and "making a cookie" for him to take into his mouth. Hold it parallel with the line of the baby's lips, not at right angles. Release your grip as soon as he's feeding well because otherwise you could obstruct the reservoirs and ducts and stop the milk flowing.

It may also help to wear breast shells for a few minutes before each feed, as this makes a nipple stand out for just long enough for the baby to take a good mouthful of breast. Using a breast pump for a short while before a feed has a similar effect. Once he latches on, your nipple should stay out for the duration of the feed. When he stops feeding, it'll probably go back in.

Baby kept from you after birth

The best time to start suckling is within half an hour of birth. After this your baby's urge to feed temporarily diminishes, and you may need more patience to get him interested.

Baby affected by drugs you had in labor

The painkiller pethidine (meperidine) is a common offender and in the US many babies are affected by barbiturates. A baby may be drowsy and apathetic about feeding for up to five days, though the effects usually wear off sooner.

Keep your milk supply going by expressing or pumping after each feed. You can also give him expressed milk from a cup or spoon when he's finished at the breast, and offer him the chance to go back to the breast if he wishes. Wake him often for a feed—every two or three hours at least—as the sooner he learns to breastfeed, the better. While you or a nurse may be able to bottle-feed him, this isn't a good idea as he'll be less likely to take to the breast once the sedation wears off.

Another possible culprit is synthetic oxytocin (trade names Syntocinon or Pitocin) often given in labor by intravenous (IV) drip to induce labor or make labor contractions more effective. It's probably needed most often by women who aren't relaxed, so aren't releasing enough of their own oxytocin during labor. It's also given to women who've had an epidural for pain relief, and to those who have a cesarean (C-section), as it reduces uterine bleeding.

However, natural and injected types of oxytocin act differently. Natural oxytocin is effective because it is released in pulses, whereas an IV drip gives a continuous level, so to be effective it has to be given in a high dose. But the concern is that high levels might desensitize oxytocin receptors on the breast's milk-producing cells, make the let-down reflex unreliable, and therefore discourage successful breastfeeding.

- A study in Malaga, Spain, of babies followed up after 5–6 years found that IV oxytocin interferes with breastfeeding, and that this effect is greater with larger doses. This is the first study of the effects of IV oxytocin on breastfeeding (Presented at the Mid-Pacific Conference on Birth and Primal Health, Honolulu, in 2012).

Baby has difficulty sucking and milking well

He may be tired, jaundiced, or full. There may be practical problems such as poor positioning at the breast, poorly protractile nipples, or engorgement. He may have learned to bottle-suck, which involves a different technique from breastfeeding. Painkilling drugs given you in labor, after-effects from a lack of oxygen in labor, or being pre-term could also be to blame.

Such a baby usually fails to gain enough weight despite feeding frequently, sometimes hourly or even more or less non-stop. He probably gets only the relatively low-calorie milk present early in a feed, because his poor sucking and milking don't stimulate the first breast to let down its higher-calorie milk. The lack of stimulation decreases milk production and slows the establishment of the let-down.

His mother may feel tired and desperate. The baby may become disinterested in feeding, sleep a lot, and lose weight. A very few appear "happy to starve."

If there's no apparent reason, if the cause is untreatable, or if it's been treated successfully yet your baby still has problems, use these ten tips to help him get your milk.

10 TIPS TO HELP YOUR BABY SUCK AND MILK MORE EFFECTIVELY

1. *Check your feeding position.*

2. *Offer your nipple and areola "attractively."* Soften a very full breast by expressing a little milk. Encourage your nipple to erect. Put some of your milk on your nipple so your baby can smell and taste it. Encourage your milk to let down before he feeds. Consider using a supplementer so he can get milk easily. Hold your breast as if on a shelf, with your opposite hand supporting it from below, or use a "cigarette hold" to make a "cookie" of the nipple and areola that you hold parallel with his mouth. Gently touch his lower lip with your nipple, and when he opens his mouth, draw him closer to the breast.

3. *Change sides each time he stops swallowing.* This "switch-nursing" encourages better suck and milking and stimulates your let-down. As you switch, try to burp him (bending him at the waist is a good way).

4. *Rouse him,* if necessary, by rocking or jiggling him, or talking or singing to him.

5. *Feed somewhere quiet if noise seems to interfere.*

6. *Encourage him.* Cuddle and praise him after a good session: even a very young baby may respond by doing it again.

7. Experiment with clothing. See if he feeds better firmly wrapped and warm, or unwrapped and not too warm. And try feeding with both of you naked to see if skin-to-skin contact stimulates better sucking and milking.

8. *Feed, express, or pump frequently* and with no long gaps. Aim at first for no more than two hours from the start of one session to the start of the next by day, and three hours at night. Feed sooner if he wants more. If your breasts feel tense between times, express a little, or wake him for a feed, as the pressure in your breasts needs relief so it doesn't suppress your milk supply.

9. *Try breast compressions* (page 163).

10. *Try a supplementer if he isn't gaining weight.* Fill its container with milk expressed or pumped after a previous feed. He'll then get milk more quickly and easily. If you can't produce enough to put in the supplementer, use donated breast milk or suitable formula. As a last resort, give expressed or pumped milk with a cup or spoon.

Jaundiced baby

Such a baby may be sleepy and difficult to interest in feeding. Frequent small feeds are best. As the jaundice clears, he'll become more interested, so be patient and keep your milk supply going by expressing after each feed and more frequently if necessary. Some babies need treatment for their jaundice.

Baby has had a bottle

Don't give a bottle to a young baby because once he learns to "bottle-suck" he'll try to breastfeed the same way. When bottle-feeding, all he needs to do is suck, let milk pour into his mouth, and swallow. There's little up-and-down or in-and-out movement of his tongue and little jaw movement either. But the technique for breastfeeding is different, as both sucking and milking need more effort. Indeed, the muscular effort of breastfeeding is good for his developing jaws.

If he bottle-sucks from you, he'll get very little milk so may give up. With patience you'll get him to feed from you, but it's better to avoid the problem in the first place.

If you're teaching your baby to breastfeed once he's had a bottle, don't muddle him by giving both breast and bottle. Until he can get enough milk by breastfeeding, you can meet his needs by giving expressed breast milk from a cup, spoon, or supplementer.

You can tell whether your baby is bottle-sucking during a breastfeed because

- You'll see his cheeks sucking in. This results from him sucking his tongue; if you pull down his lower lip you'll see his tongue above your nipple instead of below it.

- He may stick out his tongue. This "tongue-thrusting" makes him come off the breast.

- He may do some fast fluttery sucking, at two or three sucks per second, rather than the slower "nutritive" sucking, at one suck a second, that accompanies drinking.

- He won't swallow often. Check by listening for swallowing and watching for the ear movement that accompanies it.

- There'll be long intervals between bouts of sucking.

- Feeds take a long time because poor milking doesn't encourage let-downs.

Once a baby has been breastfed for several weeks, occasional bottle-feeds shouldn't matter if you maintain your milk supply.

Full baby

If your baby has drunk formula since his last breastfeed, he may not be hungry when you next expect to breastfeed. This is because formula stays in the stomach much longer than breast milk.

Rather than give a hungry baby formula, it's always better to breast-feed him—or, if you aren't there, for his carer to give expressed breast milk.

Exhausted baby

If you schedule-feed your baby in the hospital, he may cry from hunger for some time—perhaps as long as an hour—before the next scheduled feed. By the time you feed him he's so exhausted that he feeds for a very short time then goes to sleep, perhaps even before your milk lets down.

This is obviously ridiculous. So while you're in the hospital, insist on feeding him as soon as he cries. The smaller the baby, the more often he'll need feeding and the earlier his crying will exhaust him.

Sleepy baby

A sleepy newborn may be affected by a long labor or by painkill-ers you had in labor. Or he may be jaundiced or tired out from crying between feeds.

It will help if he's alert but not crying when you start to feed him. You may be able to rouse him more by removing his clothes (though don't let him get chilled!), rocking him, or stroking his back. Signs that he's ready for a feed include

- Eyes darting beneath closed eyelids.
- Sucking movements.
- Putting his hand to his mouth.
- Moving in general.
- Making small sounds.

When he's at the breast, encourage him to continue sucking by expressing a little milk into his mouth as he feeds, or gently stroking his cheek near his mouth. If he's too sleepy to get enough milk however much you try to keep him awake and interested, make sure he gets some of the higher-calorie fat-rich late milk from the first breast by expressing after he's finished feeding. Collect the milk and give it by cup half-way through the next feed.

Baby choked or overwhelmed by a strong let-down

Expressing and collecting some milk before you feed your baby should help because the let-down is most powerful early in a feed. Give him this milk by cup after the feed.

Babies who swallow quickly enough to cope with strongly spurting milk often swallow a lot of extra air and get colic or regurgitate after a feed. Some bring up almost a whole feed. If any of this happens to your baby, put him back to the breast and feed him again. He'll keep this milk down because the flow will be much slower and he won't swallow as much air. However, your milk supply will increase because of the law of demand and supply, and your let-down might work even better, making the problem worse at the next feed.

Baby wants feeding very often

How often your baby wants to feed depends on his personality, hunger, thirst, vigor, and contentment.

He's probably asking for what's perfectly normal and desirable for him. Or he may be having a growth spurt. You may be happy to go along with what he wants. But if you'd like a break, try giving him a larger feed when he's particularly needy. This is most likely to be in the evening, when your milk supply is likely to be at its lowest of the day. To arrange a larger feed, express and store milk after each feed earlier in the day, especially after the early-morning one, when you're likely to have most milk. Then, at the time of day when he wants particularly frequent feeds, give this expressed milk from a cup after a feed.

Alternatively, there may be a reason you need to act on. Check that he's well positioned and latching on well. Check too that you're making enough milk and if not, increase your milk supply (page 204). If he's healthy, thriving, and gaining weight, he may have got into the habit of feeding frequently. If you're not happy with this, you may be able gradually to lengthen the gaps between feeds by distracting him or asking someone else to look after him so your presence doesn't make him want to feed.

Excited baby

A baby so excited by the idea of feeding that he "bounces" as he searches and lunges for the nipple, and at the same time waves his arms around, may disturb himself so much that he can't settle.

Try wrapping him firmly but not too tightly in a shawl or cloth to keep his arms by his sides. Encourage your milk to let down before he goes to the breast, so there's milk as soon as he starts to feed. Rub a little milk over your areola to see if its smell helps him concentrate. If his behavior puts you off so you find it difficult to let down, you could try using a supplementer.

"Fighting" baby

A baby who fights at the breast may have experienced being nearly smothered by a full breast and so have learned that getting milk means being unable to breathe through his nose. Check your breast isn't obstructing his nose. It may help to lift your breast gently with your hand from underneath. With your patience he'll forget his early unpleasant experiences.

If a very young baby bobs his head backward and forward and won't take the breast or latch on properly, feeding him in the reclining position often helps.

Don't confuse fighting with the fussing, or playing and butting, some young babies do while waiting for milk to let down. They are happy once milk flows, whereas fighters still may not feed well.

If your baby remains reluctant to take the breast, try popping a rubber nipple (teat), perhaps filled with expressed milk, into his mouth. Once he latches on, withdraw it and substitute your nipple.

Refusing a feed

If your baby uncharacteristically refuses to feed, it could be because you smell different from usual, perhaps because of perfume, a different perfume, or a new soap, cream, or other toiletry. Or your natural scent and the taste of your milk may have changed. The composition of breast milk changes slightly five to six days before ovulation and again six to seven days after ovulation (page 83). Sometimes a baby takes a dislike to the flavor of something his mother has eaten, so it's worth thinking back over your last two meals to see if you've had something unusual.

Babies also sense when their mother is upset, and a few then become reluctant to feed. Some babies go on a "nursing strike" for no apparent reason and all you can do is keep offering your breast and giving expressed milk by cup.

Refusing one breast

Occasionally a baby refuses to feed from one breast. He may be more comfortable one side or the milk may come more easily from that breast. Unusual causes include blindness or deafness one side.

Try beginning a feed from the side he prefers, so the milk starts flowing from the other side. Then transfer him to the other breast without turning him around. If this doesn't do the trick, express milk from the unused breast to maintain its milk supply, and keep trying at each feed. He'll almost certainly come round to the idea of feeding from both sides again. Many babies (and, indeed, many mothers) prefer one side to the other. The less well stimulated side will eventually produce less milk. Any resulting lopsidedness between your breasts will resolve in time.

Baby throws his head back

This is most often seen in pre-term babies and generally disappears by eight weeks. Try gently bending your baby forwards, so his back curls, to see if this more relaxed position helps him settle at the breast. Wrapping him firmly in a shawl will help keep him in this position.

If he also arches his back, try feeding him while holding him firmly in the "football hold." Put his bottom against the back of your chair and bend his legs upward, so his body bends forwards at the hips.

Floppy baby

A floppy baby doesn't feed effectively because his muscles are very relaxed, so feeds are extremely time-consuming. Expressing milk after and between feeds and giving it in a supplementer will help you continue breastfeeding.

Teething and biting

Most babies start teething at around four to six months and their first tooth generally erupts at around six months. Teething involves a tooth pushing up against the gum, then breaking through. As an erupting tooth pushes against the gum, it can inflame the gum, making it sore and, perhaps, itchy. If clamping on to the breast with their gums brings relief, they'll want to do it again and again.

You don't want your breast used as a teething aid. So if you think your baby is feeding only to relieve teething trouble, and the extra time spent "feeding" is taking too much time, or making your nipples sore, try firmly rubbing his gums with a clean finger instead. He'll probably look surprised but it may do the trick. Another idea is to give him a refrigerated gel-filled teething ring or other teething toy to hold and bite on.

If he clamps down on your breast, try not to grimace, cry out, or make a big fuss. If you do, he'll be very interested in your response and may want to do it again. He may think it's a good game. Just take him off the breast at once and say "no" firmly each time. That way he'll learn that clamping makes his time at the breast stop, which might discourage him. An alternative is to pull him closer to you, which will make him let go because he can't breathe.

Some babies bite from frustration if the breast is too full or there isn't enough milk, in which case deal with the underlying problem.

If he has one or more teeth, this shouldn't be a problem while he's actively breastfeeding, as the pressure then comes mainly from the tongue below your nipple and areola, and his palate above, and his upper jaw and therefore the upper teeth don't move. But if he isn't actively nursing, his tongue will slip back into his mouth, and if he then bites, any lower front teeth could hurt you.

One solution to his clamping down on the breast is to learn the signs that suggest he's about to bite, then either distract him, or take him off the breast before he starts. Another is to pop the tip of your little finger into his mouth between his gums.

Other causes of clamping are frustration that the milk is slow to flow, in which case stimulate your let-down (page 109) so it starts sooner.

Low birthweight

About 7 percent of newborn babies have a low birthweight, defined as less than 5½ lb (2500 g). Worldwide, 22 million low-birthweight babies are born each year.

Two in three low-birthweight babies are born early, after less than 37 weeks of pregnancy, and are called *pre-term* or premature. Depending on a baby's post-conception age (the number of weeks from conception to birth, plus the number of weeks since birth), his feeding reflexes—rooting, sucking and milking, and swallowing—may not be present at birth and could take some weeks to appear. His post-conception age gives a good indication of a pre-term's maturity (Note that the usual way in which women calculate their unborn baby's age is from the first day of the last period, but conception is generally around two weeks later than this.)

One in three low-birthweight babies is "small-for-dates," weighing less than expected for the gestational age (length of pregnancy). This is almost certainly because such babies were poorly nourished in the womb. They tend to make a lot of mucus, which can make them gag and regurgitate. At first they may suck poorly and have a poorly coordinated swallowing reflex.

Breast is best

Pre-term babies who are mature and well enough to receive milk do best on their mother's milk because

- • The composition of a pre-term's own mother's milk is designed to meet his needs at his particular level of maturity. It contains relatively more protein, ionized calcium, chloride, immunoglobulin A, lactoferrin and lysozyme, and less lactose. As he grows, the milk's composition adjusts to his changing needs.

- Pre-term babies may not have had enough time in the womb to build up big enough stores of iron in their liver, as such stores increase most rapidly in the last few weeks of a full-term pregnancy. However, pre-term breastfeds are less likely to become anemic than pre-term bottle-feds, because although there's more iron in formula, the iron in breast milk is better absorbed.

- Pre-term babies digest breast milk earlier and better than formula (including pre-term formula) and are less likely to bring it up.

- Breast milk enables a growth rate similar to that at which a pre-term would have grown had he stayed in the womb, or just a little slower.

Pre-term babies given sugar-water and formula complements lose more weight than those breastfed exclusively and frequently.

- It's especially important for pre-terms to get plenty of docosahexaenoic acid (DHA—an omega-3 fatty acid needed for rapid brain growth in the first three months), as they've missed out on the large amounts that cross the placenta in the last weeks of a full-term pregnancy. Breast milk is a good source. Ordinary formula contains no DHA, or virtually none, so most formulas are now fortified with it.

- A pre-term baby particularly needs the protection against infection and allergy that only breast milk provides.

- Pre-term babies breathe better if breastfed than if bottle-fed, and are less likely to have episodes of being short of oxygen, according to studies in Chicago (1999). Some are already short of oxygen (from respiratory distress syndrome, or a heart defect) so bottle-feeding could be more hazardous in this respect.

An advantage to the mother of a pre-term or small-for-dates baby is that she may feel closer to him if she breastfeeds. This is important because bonding can be challenging amid the equipment and busy-ness of a special-care baby unit.

A breastfed pre-term or small-for-dates baby whose mother cuddles him (when he can leave the incubator) is greatly advantaged by the pleasure and stimulation of being near her, hearing her voice, heartbeat, breathing and tummy rumbles, sensing her delight and interest in him, smelling her natural body scent, and—when he's able—tasting the sweetness of her milk.

- Small-for-dates babies grow faster in the first year if breastfed. In particular, their head grows faster in the first three months, probably reflecting better brain growth.

Very-low-birthweight babies

Babies weighing up to 3 lb 5 oz (1500 g) need their mother's milk to be fortified (page 251). Some mothers find it difficult to produce enough milk, possibly because their short pregnancy hasn't allowed their breasts' glandular tissue enough time to mature. Others choose not breastfeed, in which case donated breast milk may be available from a breast-milk bank.

Be with your baby as much as you can. Touch and stroke him and talk to him. And when he can leave the incubator for short periods, cuddle him.

- A UK study found that very-low-birthweight babies who had plenty of cuddling next to their mother's naked skin cried less at six months old and were breastfed for longer (*Archives of Disease in Childhood*, 1988).

What about formula?

While pre-term formula is better than standard formula for pre-term babies younger than 34 weeks post-conception age, mother's milk is superior to both. However, some very-low-birthweight babies need human milk fortifier added to breast milk. And some slightly larger pre-terms also need made-up or powdered formula added to their breast milk.

Formula manufacturers continue to try to copy pre-term breast milk, which is why many add docosahexaenoic acid (DHA), for example. But they can't add such things as live cells, antibodies, growth factors, and lactoferrin. And they don't add good ("probiotic") bacteria. Breast milk is best for all babies, pre-term and full-term. If you can't provide enough milk, the hospital can give your baby a supplement of donated breast milk or pre-term formula.

Babies fed breast milk and pre-term formula grow faster than those given breast milk and donated milk, possibly because donated milk is usually drip milk, which is relatively low in calories, and also because pasteurization (heat treatment to destroy bacteria) of donated milk destroys the fat-releasing enzyme lipase.

If a baby receives no breast milk, he should ideally have ready-made liquid formula rather than made-up powdered formula. This is because ready-made liquid formula has been sterilized in the bottle by the manufacturer, so there's no risk of infection from it.

Intravenous (IV) feeding

The smallest (2 lb 3 oz/under 1000 g) and most unwell babies need liquid feed given via a drip into a vein. At first this contains sugar (glucose) and salts, later, perhaps, amino acids, vitamins, minerals, and fats as well.

Milk feeds

There's every chance you'll be able to provide enough milk, given good information and support from skilled nurses and doctors. If you want to increase your milk supply, do more frequent expressions, pumpings or feeds, and read chapter 10. Aim to relax and enjoy this time of mothering your baby in such a special way. And share tips with other mothers who are providing breast milk or actually breastfeeding a pre-term baby.

One alternative to your milk is donated breast milk. A possible snag is that it may not come from the mother of a baby similar in maturity to yours, so may not ideally match your baby's needs. Also, if it's collected as milk that drips from the donor's opposite breast while she's pumping, it'll be relatively low in calories, so your baby may need some milk forti-fier as well.

Another alternative is pre-term formula. Depending on his post-conception age and state of health, your pre-term baby will take your milk by

- Tube.

- Tube, cup, and breast.

- Cup, breast, and, perhaps, supplementer.

- Breast and, perhaps, supplementer

- Breast.

Fortifying/enriching breast milk

Although most pre-terms over 32 weeks post-conception age do well on expressed or pumped milk, the very smallest tend to grow slowly and have a higher risk of the bone-softening disease rickets, so breast milk may need to be fortified (enriched) with human-milk fortifier containing protein, vitamins (such as E), and minerals (such as calcium, copper, iron, phosphorus, and zinc). After about two weeks such a baby may benefit from an iron supplement too.

If your baby is receiving donated breast milk, it'll almost certainly need to be enriched with fortifier or combined with pre-term formula so he gets extra protein, calories, and minerals. This is because donated milk is generally mature milk, which differs in composition from pre-term breast milk. Donated milk is also likely to contain a high proportion of relative low-calorie, low-fat milk from early in a feed, as it's likely to have been collected while dripping from the donor's breast.

A tube-fed baby may need extra calories to replace those lost when milk fat sticks to the lining of the feeding tube.

Once a baby weighs just over 4 lb (2,000 g) or is discharged from the hospital, it's usually no longer necessary to add fortifier to breast milk.

Expressing or pumping

For the first few days it's better to collect your milk by expressing rather than pumping.

- One study found that pumping didn't help milk come in more quickly, and the researchers concluded that it should be strongly discouraged until the milk comes in (*Pediatrics*, 2001).

When your milk comes in, you can pump and express it.

Start collecting milk as soon after delivery as you can. It's just as important to start expressing or pumping soon after birth as it would have been to breastfeed soon after birth had your baby's size been normal. It also helps prevent engorgement. Collecting it won't take long in the first few days because colostrum is produced only in very small amounts. But this early milk is especially valuable for small babies, so treat it like liquid gold. Pumping may produce more milk than expression. But expressing may be associated with longer-term breastfeeding, possibly because mothers prefer it.

- In a US study, 68 mothers of 12- to 36-hour-old newborns (not pre-terms) either used a hospital-grade electric pump that pumped both breasts at the same time, or hand-expressed, for 15 minutes. Pumping produced an average of 1 mL (range 0–40 mL), expressing produced 0.5 mL (range 0–5 mL). Two months later, 96 percent of expressers were still breastfeeding, compared with 72 percent of pumpers (*Archives of Disease in Childhood*, 2011).

During the day, express or pump every two to three hours. Although your baby won't need large volumes yet, frequent expression or pumping helps builds up your milk supply. Aim for at least eight to ten sessions in 24 hours as six to seven are too few to stimulate optimal milk production and help make your let-down reliable. At night, it's best at first not to let more than four or five hours pass without expressing or pumping. However, some women can go six or seven hours without being woken by full breasts and still manage to fit in enough expressions in the day.

Day or night, express or pump any time if your breasts start feeling full. Don't let them become uncomfortable.

Clean your hands first with disinfectant solution or an alcohol wipe. Encourage milk to let down by keeping warm and gently massaging each breast or stroking it toward the nipple. When pumping, continue for 10 minutes each side. Expression takes longer, at least in the earlier days. Whether expressing or pumping, switch sides several times—every two to three minutes if necessary—to encourage milk to flow.

Store any milk your baby doesn't immediately need. Put the amount needed for a feed into a bag or other container, close it securely, and label it with your baby's name and the date. Repeat with as many other bags or containers as necessary.

If you have plenty of milk, you may be advised to discard the milk from early in a pumping or expressing session and instead collect the higher-calorie, higher-fat milk from later in the session.

Tube-feeding

Milk is given directly into the stomach via a fine feeding tube (a "naso-gastric" or "gavage" tube) to any baby who

- Weighs less than 3 lb 5 oz (1500 g).

- Is less than 32 weeks post-conception age.

- Isn't well enough to suck.

- Breathes faster than 75 breaths a minute.

- Can't yet coordinate sucking, swallowing, breathing, and gagging.

A nurse passes the feeding tube down the baby's nose, back of his throat, and gullet, into his stomach, where it usually stays between feeds. Most babies don't seem to mind the tube remaining in place between feeds. If your baby objects, a new one can be inserted for each feed. You may want to learn to do this yourself.

You or a nurse can then give tiny and frequent—perhaps hourly—feeds of your milk down the tube. Tube feeds are small. A 2 lb (900g) baby, for example, might need 2–3 teaspoons (10–15 mL) of milk an hour. The milk is either propelled down the tube with a syringe at frequent intervals (perhaps 1–3 times hourly, depending on size and need). Or it's pumped continuously.

Practice at the breast for tube-fed babies—When your baby can come out of the incubator, give him lots of opportunity to be at your breast even if he can't yet suck.

Ideally, choose somewhere quiet and comfortable. Hold him by your breast several times a day to get him used to its warmth, smell, and feel. It's also a good idea to hold him at your breast while he's receiving milk down the tube. Smooth a few drops of expressed milk over your nipple and bring him close enough to smell it. One day, when he's mature and interested enough, he'll lick the milk and, eventually, try practice-sucking. Be guided by your intuition and keep trying. Keep your milk supply going by frequent expression or pumping.

Practice at the breast boosts your milk supply. And babies allowed to practice-suck have higher oxygen levels, are more alert between feeds, gain weight better, develop earlier coordination of breathing, sucking, and swallowing (allowing them to cup-feed or breastfeed sooner), and go home earlier. One explanation is that practice-sucking during a tube-feed enhances digestion, perhaps by stimulating the vagus nerve—which then decreases the level of the hormone somatostatin so milk stays in the stomach longer. It also boosts insulin, which helps a baby to use glucose. And it increases gastrin, a hormone that releases stomach acid, boosts stomach movements, and encourages gut-lining cells to grow. Another explanation is that a baby who practice-sucks spends more time being calm, which frees energy for growth.

This time spent with your tiny baby practicing being at the breast helps you bond and is very worthwhile for both of you.

Tube-feeding, cup-feeding, and breastfeeding
(30–32 or 34 weeks post-conception age)

Tube-feeding continues to sustain the baby but as his feeding reflexes mature he can learn to feed from the cup and breast.

The swallowing reflex may develop as early as 11 weeks post-conception age and his rooting reflex from 28 weeks. The sucking reflex begins at 32 weeks but doesn't mature and strengthen fully until 32–34 or even 36 weeks. Pethidine (meperidine) in labor, or jaundice or other problems, can temporarily dampen effective sucking. Interestingly, studies show that babies coordinate sucking and swallowing earlier at the breast than at the bottle.

Your baby can drink from a cup or the breast when he

- Has a gag reflex. This stops milk going down the wrong way and develops from 26–27 weeks post-conception age.

- Can coordinate breathing, sucking, and swallowing without choking.

Some babies manage the cup or breast from 30–31 weeks and when they weigh 2 lb 14 oz (1300 g); others not until they are 32–34 weeks post-conception age and weigh over 3 lb 5 oz (1500 g).

Start teaching him to cup-feed with his feeding tube in place. He'll like it because he'll be able to taste the sweetness of your milk. Some people use a spoon or a dropper instead, but a cup is generally preferable. Don't use a bottle because this would teach him the technique of bottle-sucking, and so make it harder for him to learn the technique for breastfeeding

Put about 1–2 teaspoons (5–15 mL) of expressed milk into a sterilized baby cup. Hold your baby on your lap, half upright, preferably by your naked breast so he can smell your milk. Put a drop of milk on to his tongue with your finger, so he can taste it. Gently tilt the cup so it touches his lower lip and allows a little milk to enter his mouth, taking care not to swamp him. If he's very immature, he'll simply swallow the milk. As his sucking reflex appears and matures, he'll start sucking the milk from the cup. Within a few days or weeks he'll start lapping it like a kitten. Don't worry how much he takes; the nurses will work out whether he needs a supplement by tube. Make this time as peaceful and relaxed as possible, so he associates cup-feeds with pleasure and tranquillity.

Practice at the breast—Don't be surprised if he just licks your breast, or often sleeps for up to 20 minutes. Coordinating sucking and swallowing is challenging and tiring at first, but every day makes a difference.

Eventually he'll take three, four, or five sucks, and you'll hear him swallow or see the angle of his jaw moving toward his earlobe as he swallows. At this stage he'll be getting only a very little milk. This comprises milk that leaks from your nipple if your breast is full, or drips or flows during a let-down, as well as milk he can suck from the reservoirs. Eventually he'll be mature enough to learn to milk your breast too.

Time spent encouraging your baby gives you the opportunity to hold him and get to know him. The physical contact also helps him deal with the bright light, lack of movement, and other stresses of living in an incubator.

Give less by tube as he takes more from the cup and breast. Eventually, the tube can be permanently removed. This will be a red-letter day.

Cup- and breastfeeding (32–36 weeks post-conception age)

As your baby's sucking matures, he'll suck more strongly from your breasts and take more milk.

Encourage your milk to let down before he starts sucking. The nurses will advise on positioning so he gets as good a mouthful of breast as possible for his size and feeds most effectively. Switch him from side to side several times during a feed and let him feed as long as he wants. He'll need frequent breaks because he'll get tired. When he seems to have finished, express or pump your remaining milk and give it by cup another time.

It's important that between you and your baby you empty your breasts frequently, as stimulation from frequent feeding/expression/pumping will build up your milk supply. So, as he gets used to the breast, aim to fit in at least 8–12 breastfeeds a day, with no long gaps at night. A full-term baby would have this number and a pre-term baby, who takes smaller amounts, needs at least the same and ideally more to get enough milk.

A supplementer that supplies your expressed milk (or donated milk, or pre-term formula) while he's breastfeeding can be useful because it enables him to get more milk more quickly, which is useful if feeding tires him a lot. A disadvantage might be that he gets it so quickly that he doesn't give your breasts the stimulation they need to make plenty of milk. Overcome this by allowing him to comfort-suck as much as he wants, then expressing after each feed. Store the expressed milk to put in the supplementer for his next feed. Using a supplementer may mean you can give up cup-feeding sooner than you otherwise would have done.

As your baby takes more milk from the breast, you can give less from the cup until he can give it up completely.

Full breastfeeding (about 36 weeks post-conception age)

Only now is a pre-term likely to suck well enough to take adequate nourishment from the breast alone. A small-for-dates baby may manage this sooner.

Your baby may be sleepy, so you may have to wake him for feeds. Give him plenty of encouragement to keep at it during a feed. Pre-terms often don't "ask" for feeds until their post-conception age nears the equivalent of being full-term.

Going home ahead of your baby?

When breastfeeding a low-birthweight baby who needs hospital care, you'll find it much easier if you live in the hospital, ideally alongside your baby, until he comes home. You're then there whenever he needs a feed. He'll also benefit from the anti-infective properties of fresh breast milk. Some special-care baby units have beds for mothers.

If you go home but your baby stays in the hospital, you may want borrow an electric pump so it's easy to collect milk at home. Store this milk safely and take it to the hospital each time you visit, so the nurses can give it to him by cup when you aren't there. Use a cool bag with ice packs for transporting containers of milk.

Mothering your pre-term baby

Pre-terms are nursed in incubators to keep them warm and protect them from infection. But physical contact is very important for your baby and for the development of your mothering instinct. So if possible, hold him as often as you can. If he has to stay in his incubator, stroke him gently through the armholes. Some special-care baby units have beds for mothers.

Once your baby is out of the incubator, it may even be possible to sleep with him in the hospital. In a study at Pithiviers, France, pre-terms that slept in their mother's bed gained weight faster than other pre-terms.

Nurses don't have time to give their charges all the cuddling, stroking, holding, attention, and talking they ideally need. It's up to you to mother your baby as warmly and intimately as possible, even if this feels awkward at first. A lack of physical contact and mothering may be partly why pre-terms tend to cry twice as much as full-terms.

When you take him home, take all the time in the world to get to know one another and enjoy one another's company.

Kangaroo care

Pre-term babies can go home sooner if their mothers have spent a lot of time with them next to their body, safely tucked into their clothing between their breasts, like a young joey kangaroo in his mother's pouch. Researchers at the Hammersmith Hospital, London, found that babies weighing more than 3 lb 5 oz (1500 g) did better if cared for like young kangaroos! And according to South American researchers, most babies weighing 2 lb 10 oz (1,200 g) or more can be cared for this way. Your partner can carry the baby next to his naked chest in the same way if he likes.

Looking after yourself

As the breastfeeding mother of a pre-term you're a very special person. You also need a lot of help. So look after yourself and ask for all the support you need from family, friends, and hospital staff. This is especially important if you have other children or no partner. The more support you have, the longer you're likely to breastfeed.

In hospital, take every opportunity to relax, and make sure you're as comfortable as possible. To avoid boredom, take in a radio or a music player. If you have a smartphone or a tablet computer, you could ask the nurses if it's all right to use it in the hospital to watch films or TV, for example. Or use the hospital's radio or pay-TV. Ask relatives and friends to bring in favorite foods and drinks, or take you out for a meal. Your partner could give you a shoulder or back massage as you feed the baby and all three of you could have a cuddle together.

Confidence, support, and encouragement

Although pre-terms do so well on breast milk, nurses and doctors sometimes seem reluctant to encourage mothers to provide it. This may be because they perceive it as difficult and time-consuming for the mothers and themselves. Or perhaps they don't want to make women who don't breastfeed feel guilty (page 335). Or the special-care baby unit may simply have a bottle-feeding ethos.

Hold on to the fact that if you know what to do and have enough good advice, support, and encouragement, you're very likely to be able to breastfeed.

One study in the UK, for example, found that encouraging mothers to breastfeed their pre-term baby raised the proportion who left hospital exclusively breastfeeding from 1 percent to 58 percent! Another, in Mumbai, India, found that 95 percent of mothers of pre-terms breastfed successfully when encouraged.

Home with your baby

Two weeks after taking your pre-term home you may notice a turning point, suggests a study in the US. Most mothers now find that their baby stays awake at the breast longer and breastfeeds more effectively. This is obviously much more rewarding for the mother.

Amidst the novelty of having your baby at home, remember that you've been through a lot of stress, however excited and delighted you may be. And you may be tired out. So don't forget to look after yourself and ask for the help you need.

twelve

Some Special Situations

I f you're mothering and breastfeeding a newborn while managing a special situation, you need good information and support, not to mention plenty of tender loving care. You're doing a very important job!

You have twins—or more

Two babies stimulate the breasts twice as much as one, so you'll automatically make more milk. Many mothers breastfeed twins successfully for as long as they want, without giving formula feeds or complements. It may help to bear in mind that the average healthy woman can completely nourish a baby from one breast only.

However many babies you have, it's good if you can provide at least some milk for each one. Mothers of "multiples" say the more support and encouragement they have while breastfeeding, the better. Ask for as much as you need and be clear what you'd like done.

The Twins and Multiple Births Association (www.tamba.org.uk) provides information about breastfeeding, details of support groups, and telephone support, for mothers of twins or more.

Last, but not least, take as much care of yourself as you can. For example, you'll need plenty of good food, plenty of help and plenty of rest.

Feeding them together

At first it's easiest to feed each twin separately, but later, to save time, it's worth learning the knack of feeding both at once. This said there'll always be times when you'll enjoy the luxury of feeding them individually.

You can feed twins together in one of several positions. The easiest is probably to hold each one in the "football" hold. Or you could hold the first twin in the conventional position, while the second twin lies at the other breast, facing the same way as the first twin and parallel to him, with you supporting his head with your hand. Another idea is to have both babies in the conventional position, with one lying across the other.

Position each baby carefully and check they are well latched on (page 113) as this discourages sore nipples. Once you're used to feeding them both, you'll find it works well.

Should you feed the second baby every time you feed the first?

The answer is "yes" if you want to save time, or want to increase your milk supply, and "no" if you like the occasional chance to suckle one at a time.

Should you alternate the breast each twin feeds from?

The usual advice is "yes," so the twin that sucks more strongly stimulates each breast alternately.

In many mammalian litters, for example, a dog's, every newborn usually keeps to one particular nipple, and it's possible that human babies might prefer this too. Certainly in the first few weeks, if you always feed one baby from one breast and the other from the other, and if one sucks more strongly and so drinks more each time, your breasts will become lopsided.

Triplets

Many mothers have successfully breastfed triplets, though sometimes formula is necessary as well, especially early on.

Your baby has difficulty sucking, milking, or swallowing

We've discussed the most likely causes in chapter 11. But there are many other less common ones.

Possible mechanical reasons include a large tongue, a cleft lip or palate, abnormal gums or jaws, and severe tongue tie. Difficulty with swallowing can result from a cleft palate, a small lower jaw, or inflammation from the insertion of a tube down the windpipe for a breathing difficulty. A baby who finds swallowing difficult milks the breast poorly too. Less common reasons for difficulty with sucking, milking or swallowing include an underactive thyroid and certain neurological and neuromuscular problems.

Some of these conditions are relatively easy to treat, and the baby's sucking and milking improve afterward. Others improve spontaneously.

But a baby with an untreatable or less easily treatable condition may need a lot of help to breastfeed (page 240).

Your baby is ill or in the hospital

A sick baby needs the very best nutrition. He also needs the comfort of being at his mother's breast. Unless your baby is so ill or immature that he can't have milk, he'll do better with yours than any other. He'll also recover more quickly after any illness if he doesn't have the physical stress of digesting formula. If your baby has a respiratory illness with difficulty breathing, breastfeeding is easier than bottle-feeding. This is because a bottle-fed baby tends to breathe between swallows in a gasping fashion, and a respiratory illness can make the gasping more pronounced.

If your baby has to go into the hospital, it's best if you go too so you can give him comfort and breast milk. If you can spend only the daytime with him, leave expressed or pumped milk for the nurses to give from a cup at night.

If you can visit only infrequently, take in enough milk for several days. It calls for real patience to express or pump your breasts frequently—and more often than your baby would usually feed directly from the breast—day after day. But it can be done and will be easier if you hire or buy an electric breast pump.

Jaundice

In newborns there are three main causes of jaundice (yellow skin caused by high levels of the bile pigment bilirubin): normal "physiological" jaundice, breastmilk jaundice and starvation jaundice. There are also several other possible causes (below).

The diagnosis depends on when the jaundice began, on blood tests, and on the baby's weight gain. Treatment aims to prevent very high bilirubin as this can cause cause deafness, cerebral palsy or other signs of brain damage.

Physiological jaundice—This affects 40 percent of all babies, whether they are breast- or bottle-fed. It appears on days 2–4, nearly always disappears by the end of the first week, and there's no evidence of long-term problems. It results from the breakdown of red blood cells after birth, decreased liver metabolism of bilirubin, and increased absorption of bilirubin from the gut into the blood. All these are normal in newborns.

Jaundice is more likely in babies whose first breastfeed after birth is delayed beyond the first hour; in those fed on an infrequent and restricted basis; and in those who aren't well latched-on. Such babies get too little colostrum, and what they do get they don't get early enough. This early milk helps expel meconium, the first bowel motions that take with them a lot of bilirubin. When meconium excretion is delayed, more bilirubin is absorbed.

One expert says that having at least 10–12 breastfeeds a day discourages this type of jaundice. Studies show that giving water to a jaundiced baby isn't helpful and may interfere with his mother's milk supply. This is because he'll want fewer breastfeeds if his tummy is full of water.

Breast-milk jaundice—In 50 percent of breastfed babies, jaundice continues into week two and worsens in weeks two and three. It often lasts up to 8–12 weeks or even 16 weeks. One theory is that some component of breast milk enhances the absorption of bilirubin from the gut. Another is that breast milk's high lipase level releases fatty acids that inhibit the breakdown of bilirubin. Breast-milk jaundice is sometimes confused with starvation jaundice (see below). Eventually, even if breastfeeding continues, the jaundice goes and the high bilirubin falls.

Brain damage has never been attributed to breast-milk jaundice, and there's considerable evidence that this jaundice has no serious long-term effects.

However, phototherapy (see below) is often recommended to help prevent the bilirubin rising too high. If it rises to 2–3 mg/dL (35–50µmol/L) or more, then, depending on the age of the baby, many pediatricians opt for caution by suggesting, as well as or instead of phototherapy, one of two things.

Either carry on breastfeeding, but also give formula, as formula inhibits bilirubin absorption from the gut. Hydrolyzed protein formula ("elemental formula") is more effective at lowering bilirubin than standard formulas and less likely to cause cows'-milk allergy or intolerance. Ideally, give formula via a supplementer as you breastfeed. Alternatively give it by cup after a feed. Express after each breastfeed because your baby may feed for less time as he's also getting formula. Also, it increases the stimulation of your breast-milk supply. The hospital staff will measure the bilirubin frequently, perhaps even every 4–6 hours. This will fall more slowly than if you interrupt breastfeeding (below), but continuing to breastfeed will be more comfortable for you and will allow your baby to go on getting your milk.

Or stop breastfeeding for 24–48 hours. Keep your milk supply going by expressing or pumping more frequently than you would have fed the baby, and discard the milk. Meanwhile, feed your baby with donated milk. This works because although something in your milk must have made him jaundiced, another woman's milk won't have the same effect. When the baby's bilirubin has fallen significantly, you can resume breastfeeding. The bilirubin then usually rises slightly before falling slowly and steadily. If it rises significantly again, interrupt breastfeeding once more. If it doesn't fall significantly after a short break, extend the break by 6–12 hours. The hospital staff will measure the bilirubin every 4–6 hours. If it rises during the break from breastfeeding, the jaundice isn't caused by breast milk. Note that stopping breastfeeding may not work as well as phototherapy alone in babies less than five days old.

"Starvation" jaundice—This most often begins in the first week. Getting too little milk raises raises the blood's bilirubin by increasing its absorption from the gut. It also increases bilirubin absorption by delaying the excretion of meconium. Pre-term babies are at increased risk. So too are those babies who lose more than 10 percent of their birthweight. This happens, for example, to 10–18 percent of exclusively breastfed babies in the US.

It can be difficult to distinguish this jaundice from physiological jaundice or breast-milk jaundice. What's more, it may coexist with either.

To help prevent it, babies need their first breastfeed in the first hour after birth, then frequent and uncurtailed breastfeeds thereafter. They need to be well positioned and well latched-on. Ideally, all mothers should see a nurse trained in lactation assistance, or a lactation consultant, on the first day, then as often as necessary.

If starvation jaundice is suspected, and if your baby loses more then 10 percent of his birthweight, the treatment is more milk. So focus on improving your breastfeeding technique. You may also be advised to give him either your own milk (expressed after each feed and also between feeds), or donated milk or formula. You can give this extra milk after a breastfeed, via a cup. Or you can give it during a breastfeed, via a supplementer.

Phototherapy (light therapy)—is often recommended for moderately raised bilirubin from whatever cause. This usually entails the baby lying naked in a cot below a fluorescent blue or blue-green light, his eyes covered with a mask or colored perspex shade. You can take him from the light when you need to breastfeed. It's important not to let phototherapy interfere with how often you feed. An alternative is to wrap a fiberoptic blanket that emits blue light around him as he lies in a cot or as you cuddle or feed him. His eyes don't need to be covered.

The colored light changes the shape of the bilirubin molecules in the blood, which allows the body to eliminate them.

A pediatrician may approve phototherapy at home for a baby aged one or two weeks with breast-milk jaundice, a stable or only slightly rising bilirubin, and no other risk factors for brain damage. Or he or she may agree to you giving him "daylight phototherapy" at home. Do this by placing him naked in a cot or somewhere else safe, either by a window inside, or outside, in strong daylight. Ask how long, if at all, your baby can be exposed to actual sunlight. Avoid sunburn and don't let him get too cold or too hot. One advantage of being at home is that you can breastfeed much more easily.

Wherever and however phototherapy is done, your baby will need frequent blood tests to monitor his bilirubin.

Pre-term babies are more vulnerable to a raised bilirubin than are full-term babies, so any treatment must be started sooner.

Other causes of jaundice—include bruising, prematurity, infection, rhesus disease and bowel obstruction in the baby, and diabetes in the mother. Jaundice from any of these can coexist with any of the three main causes of jaundice (see above).

Affected babies are yellow at birth, or within 24 hours. Whatever treatment is necessary, they need early, frequent, and unrestricted breast-feeds for the reasons outlined above.

Your baby has diarrhea

Breastfed babies are very much less likely to get a bowel infection, but if they do, it's better and safer to carry on breastfeeding. Babies who stop are five times as likely to become dehydrated as those who continue. If your baby is severely ill he may need to drink an oral rehydration salts solution (recommended by a doctor) from a cup, as well as continuing to breastfeed. Even if he becomes so dehydrated from the diarrhea that he needs intravenous fluids, he can continue to breastfeed. Only extremely rarely must such a baby stop breastfeeding.

Your baby has low blood sugar (hypoglycemia)

Blood sugar (glucose) provides a baby's cells with energy, and your milk is a good source of sugar and of other nutrients from which he can make sugar. Low blood sugar is unusual in a healthy full-term normal-weight baby whose mother breastfeeds as soon as possible after the birth and then continues without restricting the number and length of feeds. This is because early and frequent feeds help to keep his blood sugar level within normal limits.

- A Danish study of 223 healthy breastfed full-term babies found that very few developed low blood sugar. The researchers said there is no reason for such babies to have routine blood sugar tests (*Archives of Disease in Childhood*: Fetal and Neonatal Edition, 2000).

Quite a few pre-term newborns develop low blood sugar as they adapt to intermittent feeds instead of the continuous supply of nutrients, including sugar, they received in the womb via the umbilical cord. Very immature pre-terms can have difficulty digesting any type of milk, especially formula. The milk therefore stays in their stomach for a long time, which delays the release of glucose and allows blood sugar to fall further than it otherwise would have done.

Babies with an increased risk of low blood sugar

These include those who

- Are pre-term.
- Are small-for-dates.
- Have an infection.
- Were short of oxygen during labor.
- Have become chilled.
- Had a delayed first breastfeed.
- Have infrequent breastfeeds.
- Have had sugar water—which causes a sudden rise in blood sugar followed by a sudden fall.

Or whose mother

- Had preeclampsia.

- Had an intravenous glucose drip in labor.

- Has diabetes.

- Has taken certain drugs.

Signs of low blood sugar

These include sweating, weakness, limpness, floppiness, disinterest in feeding, tiredness, a high-pitched or weak cry, blue lips, a rapid pulse, irritability, and frequent shuddering or shaking movements ("jitteriness")—particularly when disturbed. Some babies have seizures (convulsions or fits). At worst, a baby goes into a coma or his circulation fails. If the blood sugar repeatedly falls, or stays low for days, his brain could be damaged. Such a baby may also need other tests to find out whether an underlying condition (such as an infection) is responsible.

Definitions of low blood sugar vary. One is a level below 35 mg/dL (1.9 mmol/L) in his blood. But if there are no symptoms, some doctors are unconcerned if a full-term baby's level drops to 30 mg/dL (1.6 mmol/L), or a pre-term or small-for-dates baby's level falls to 20 mg/dL (1.1 mmol/L). In one study of newborn babies who had a level below 20 mg/dl but no symptoms other than jitteriness, and who continued breast-feeding, neurological tests some years later showed they had no problems.

What they need

All babies with an increased risk of low blood sugar, or signs of low blood sugar, need routine blood sugar tests.

All, including pre-terms that are mature and well enough to have milk, should ideally have undiluted breast milk (preferably from their mother), by tube, breast, or cup as soon as possible after birth.

All need breast milk frequently and on an unrestricted basis.

If you aren't producing enough, increase your milk supply (chapter 10). Meanwhile, your milk can be topped up if necessary with donated breast milk, or a suitable formula.

If you don't want to breastfeed, your baby can have formula.

Tongue tie

A baby's frenulum is the little central sheet of tissue between the root of his tongue and the floor of his mouth. In a few babies it is shorter (from top to bottom, with the baby upright), longer (from back to front) and thicker or tougher than usual. This can "tie" the tongue by tethering it to the floor of the mouth. So the tip of the tongue can reach neither the upper nor the lower gums. And because the tip of the tongue is restrained, the back of the tongue may roll forward over the lower gums. This can make its leading edge appear notched, puckered, or heart-shaped.

Such a baby may be unable to breastfeed effectively because he can't push his tongue far enough forward to take a good mouthful of nipple and areola between his upper gums and his tongue. Instead, he holds the breast in his mouth between his upper and lower gums. He may also make a clucking noise as he tries to milk the breast. And milk may dribble from the side of his mouth. His poor positioning at the breast means his milking action is poor. So his mother is more likely to get sore or cracked nipples, a poor milk supply, and blocked ducts.

The best way of dealing with minor tongue tie is to be particularly careful over your breastfeeding technique. The odds are that your baby will manage, and the more practiced he becomes at feeding, and the older he gets, the easier breastfeeding should be.

However, tongue tie that causes continuing breastfeeding problems responds very well to minor surgery to cut the frenulum.

- A study of babies with feeding difficulty and tongue-tie found that breastfeeding improved in 96 percent of those who had their frenulum surgically divided, compared with only 3 percent who had no surgery, but whose mothers had breastfeeding help. There were no complications after surgery (*Journal of Paediatrics and Child Health*, 2005).

Cleft lip or palate

The shock and disappointment of discovering that your baby has a cleft lip or cleft palate) may make you reluctant to breastfeed. Once you get over your initial reaction, it may help to bear in mind that you never see older children or adults walking around with a noticeable deformity of their lips. Plastic surgery is so good today that the defect can be almost perfectly repaired.

Cleft lip

A cleft lip needn't interfere with breastfeeding. Some milk may leak from your baby's mouth but you'll soon learn to make a seal by molding your breast around the cleft. You couldn't do this with a bottle! Your baby will be able to suck (unless the cleft is exceptionally severe) and milk your breast. Prevent engorgement, and try not to let your breasts become too full, as both these conditions make it more difficult to form a seal. If your breast is very full before a feed, soften it by expressing.

Many hospitals repair a cleft lip within two days of birth; others wait the traditional three months or so. Early surgery makes breastfeeding easier for the baby, and his mother more inclined to breastfeed.

Different surgeons advise waiting for different lengths of time before letting a baby breastfeed after a cleft-lip repair. Because of the danger of the wound splitting, some suggest waiting 3–4 weeks; others allow sucking at 10 days; and some allow it immediately after surgery. For the mother, the sooner her baby starts breastfeeding, the better, though obviously wound healing has first priority.

- 60 of 100 babies resumed breastfeeding immediately after surgery in one survey. There were no complications and breastfed babies gained weight faster than those fed from a cup (*Plastic and Reconstructive Surgery*, 1987).

While you wait to resume breastfeeding after surgery, keep your milk supply going by frequent and regular expression or pumping, and give your baby the milk from a cup. If the operation is postponed for several months, you'll need a lot of patience while breastfeeding, as babies with a cleft lip tend to take a long time over feeds.

If his lip is severely cleft and you find it impossible to breastfeed, give him your milk from a cup, a specially shaped spoon, or a bottle with an adapted teat ("nipple"). Ask your pediatrician about these.

Cleft palate

A baby with a cleft palate can't suck well because he draws in air from his nose when he tries. Make up for the loss of suction by holding your nipple and areola in his mouth while he feeds. He'll be able to suck and milk satisfactorily with practice. A supplementer may also be useful while he's learning.

Milk may enter his nose, but breast milk won't irritate the nasal lining, whereas formula might. Breastfeeding with you and your baby relatively upright will minimize the chances of milk entering his nose. Babies with a cleft palate are particularly prone to middle-ear infection, but this is less likely in breastfed babies than in bottle-feds.

An affected baby can have a plastic feeding plate (dental plate) until the cleft is repaired, often after a year old. This is made from impressions taken of his palate. It may be inserted as early as three days after birth (sometimes not until 10 days). It helps him feed satisfactorily and improves the shape of his dental arches. Some hospitals make plates routinely, others only for severe clefts.

Learning difficulty

There's every reason to breastfeed a brain-damaged baby. He'll gain the same benefits as any other and it will help your relationship develop. Many mothers feel their affected baby deserves every possible chance in life and know that breastfeeding gives the best start.

Like your baby, you'll need plenty of encouragement and support as you learn to breastfeed, so ask the hospital staff, family, and friends for as much as you need.

Down syndrome

One mother of such a baby commented, "I'm sure that breastfeeding and the closeness that came with it helped me to love and accept him just as he was."

These special babies are prone to infections, especially respiratory ones, so the protection offered by breast milk is particularly valuable.

Some feed slowly, weakly, or with little interest because of muscle weakness, a poor sucking reflex, or sleepiness. With patience you're highly likely to succeed with breastfeeding and you'll be sure you're doing the best for your baby. Just as with any baby, avoid using a bottle because learning to bottle-suck interferes with learning to breastfeed. Bottle-feeding would be just as time-consuming as breastfeeding anyway. If he is too tired to suck for long, express milk and give it from a cup. Encourage him to suck by giving him lots of skin contact, and by getting your milk to let down, and by putting a few drops into his mouth before you put him to the breast. Feed him before he has to cry, to avoid tiring him. If he's so sleepy that he doesn't wake very often, wake him for a feed every two hours or so if necessary by day, and every three hours at night.

Neurological or neuromuscular condition

Conditions such as cerebral palsy, infantile spinal muscular atrophy, congenital muscular dystrophy, neonatal myasthenia gravis and infections of the central nervous system can all prove challenging when it comes to feeding. For example, a baby with cerebral palsy may sometimes arch his back while feeding. Some babies are apathetic during feeds, or have difficulty sucking because of a poor sucking reflex, uncoordinated sucking, or muscle weakness.

See page 240 for information on how to encourage your baby to suck, milk, and swallow more effectively, and while feeding pay attention to the position of his whole body as well as his tongue, jaw, and lips. It's well worth persevering because most such babies can breastfeed with enough help and become much better at it as time goes by.

Your baby isn't thriving

The terms "failure to thrive" and "weight faltering" mean a baby isn't growing as he should. Something may be wrong if your baby continues to lose weight after ten days of life, hasn't regained his birth-weight by three weeks, gains very slowly after the first month, or gains increasingly slowly. There's particular reason for concern if he's also unwell.

There are many reasons why your breastfed baby may not grow as he should. For example, he may

- Not drink enough—probably because of poor positioning at the breast, infrequent short feeds, or poor sucking or swallowing.

- Be losing nutrients—because of malabsorption, diarrhea or vomiting.

- Have an infection—for example, in his urine.

- Have high energy needs that aren't being adequately met—for example, if he's small for dates or has a congenital heart disease.

And you may

- Not be producing enough milk—because of poor technique, an unhealthy diet, illness, or exhaustion.

- Not be letting down your milk well—perhaps because he's poorly positioned, or you're tired out, or because you're a heavy smoker or drinker or take certain drugs.

- The pediatrician will take a careful medical, social, and dietary history, examine your baby thoroughly, watch a feed and arrange for any necessary tests.

Your baby needs an anesthetic

If a baby needs an anesthetic before surgery, breastfeeding can safely continue until up to three hours before the operation. If he wants a feed after that, he can have water until up to two hours before.

Your baby has a rare illness with implications for breastfeeding

One such condition is galactosemia, caused by an enzyme deficiency. It can be fatal in a baby not on a diet free from lactose ("milk sugar"). There's no alternative but to stop breastfeeding and give special lactose-free formula.

Phenylketonuria, another "inborn error of metabolism," causes a high level of phenylalanine in the blood. This can cause brain damage and learning difficulties. Breast milk contains less of this amino acid than does formula. So an affected baby can be breastfed. If his blood's level of phenyl-alanine becomes dangerously high, he can have a combination of breast milk and special low-phenylalanine formula, or, if necessary, this formula alone.

Your baby's immunizations

Soon after immunization your baby may go off breastfeeding and be more fussy than usual for about 24 hours. If your breasts become very full, express a little milk every so often.

The five-in-one vaccine (diphtheria, pertussis/whooping cough, teta-nus, polio, and HiB—*Haemophilus influenzae* B) isn't affected by breast-feeding, and a breastfed baby can have it at the usual recommended times. The same applies to rubella, mumps, measles, yellow fever, cholera, and typhoid vaccines.

Rhesus antibodies

Some mothers with rhesus antibodies in their blood and a rhesus-pos-itive baby worry that breastfeeding may pass the antibodies to the baby. A woman with rhesus antibodies in her blood has them in her milk too.

But they won't affect her baby because they're inactivated by his gut. So it is perfectly safe to breastfeed. Indeed, it's the best way to feed such babies, according to several studies. It's also safe to breastfeed after an injection of anti-D immunoglobulin.

You are unwell

If you're too unwell to have your baby by your bed, you'll need someone to look after you both and give you the baby when he needs a feed.

If you're in the hospital, you may be able to take him with you, depending on what's wrong and on the hospital's facilities. If not, see if someone can bring him to you for feeds. This entails a lot of work and commitment, and means you'll need to be in a hospital close to home. Another way of continuing to breastfeed in the hospital is to express or pump your milk and send it home. It should be stored in a refrigerator, taken home in a insulated bag by a friend or relative, and refrigerated until needed. It can then be given to your baby from a cup.

A few illnesses rule out breastfeeding. Others do so temporarily because of the drugs needed. If you have a long-standing illness such as severe asthma or kidney disease, you may feel too tired and run down to breastfeed. But some mothers find breastfeeding makes them rest and tires them less than bottle-feeding would.

Diabetes

Type 1 diabetes affects affects from 1–30 people in 100,000, depending on the country, and can run in families. Breastfeeding for at least 9–12 months reduces the risk of a baby with a family history of type 1 diabetes getting it himself one day

- In a Danish study of 102 mothers with type 1 diabetes, 86 percent were breastfeeding at 5 days, and 68 percent at 4 months— 54 percent of them fully (*Diabetes Care*, 2006).

A mother with type 1 or type 2 diabetes or pregnancy diabetes, whose baby goes into a special care unit after delivery, should be particularly sure to breastfeed or express or pump frequently. This helps establish her milk supply early, which will help balance her dietary needs and insulin dose.

Most women need less insulin in the 4–6 weeks after childbirth than before their pregnancy. If a woman uses too much, her blood sugar (glucose) falls. This releases adrenaline, which in turn decreases the blood flow into her breasts and can inhibit her let-down.

Traces of insulin and adrenaline in milk are largely inactivated by a baby's digestive enzymes. Any minute amounts of insulin that enter his blood simply mean he temporarily produces a little less of his own.

Infections are more common in women with diabetes, and any antibiotics taken must be safe for their baby. They should particularly watch out for thrush.

Any breastfed baby sometimes wants more or less milk. A change in the amount a mother with diabetes needs to produce can make her blood sugar dip or rise, in which case she must adjust her diet, exercise, and insulin.

Some breastfeeding women find their blood sugar is more stable than it was before.

- Of 809 women who'd had pregnancy diabetes, the 404 who breastfed had better glucose metabolism, according to a study in California.

The researchers thought this might reduce or delay their risk of developing type 2 diabetes in later life (*Obstetrics and Gynecology*, 1993).

Infection

Breastfeeding by a mother with certain infections can act as a natural vaccine by supplying her baby with white cells (B lymphocytes) that produce antibodies against that infection. But this doesn't happen with all infections. And with certain infections breastfeeding isn't safe.

If you're advised to interrupt breastfeeding, keep your supply going in the meantime by frequent expression or pumping, and discard the milk. Once your baby is allowed breast milk again, you'll then have plenty.

Chickenpox—If your chickenpox begins within five days before or two days after childbirth, being with your newborn risks giving him a severe form of this infection. So you need to be separated from him until all your spots are crusted over. You also need an injection of varicella-zoster immunoglobulin (VZIG) as soon as possible. Your baby must be monitored until 21 days old. Although it's unclear whether chickenpox viruses are present in breast milk and, if so, whether they could infect the baby, experts nevertheless advise giving such a baby expressed breast milk. If he gets chickenpox he should be treated with the antiviral drug acyclovir.

If your chickenpox begins more than five days before delivery or after the third day afterward, you'll produce and transfer antibodies to your baby via your placenta or your milk. In this case, he risks getting only the mild form of chickenpox, so there's no need for separation or a VZIG injection. You can breastfeed, though it's sensible to reduce the risk of infection by washing your hands before you touch him, wearing a mask and covering as yet uncrusted spots.

Herpes cold sores or other herpes infections—infection with Herpes simplex type-1 viruses can cause "cold sores" (usually on the lips but sometimes in the mouth or on the breasts). Herpes simplex type-2 viruses generally cause sores in the genital area. A herpes infection can be very serious for newborns, so no one with a cold sore should kiss a baby.

Women with sores on the breast should stop feeding until the sores have healed.

If there are no sores on the breast, experts recommend strict hygiene, treatment of the infection, and continued breastfeeding. It's extremely unusual for breast milk to contain herpes viruses.

A few experts, however, advise a woman with a first herpes attack, especially of the genital area, not to breastfeed. This is because of the risk of infecting a newborn with viruses that are potentially very dangerous to him, as his immune system is vulnerable and breast milk hasn't yet had a chance to develop much anti-herpes activity. Such experts also say there's more chance of developing a sore on the breast during a first attack.

A woman advised not to breastfeed can keep her milk supply going by frequent expression or pumping but should discard the milk. Once the infection has cleared and she's no longer shedding viruses, she'll then still have a good milk supply and can start to breastfeed again. The antiviral drug acyclovir has considerably brightened the treatment outlook.

Hepatitis—Women who are carriers of hepatitis B viruses can breast-feed, as there's no evidence that this increases their baby's risk of the infection, especially if they receive hepatitis B vaccine and hepatitis B immune globulin soon after birth.

Tuberculosis (TB)—If you've had lung TB but have been infection-free for two years, you can safely breastfeed.

If you had active lung TB in pregnancy, and your treatment (with triple therapy) was begun at least a week before your baby was born, you needn't be separated from him and can safely breastfeed, provided he is also treated with isoniazid.

If you're bacteria-negative, you can breastfeed even if you've only just begun treatment, provided he too is treated with isoniazid (in a smaller dose than if you were bacteria-positive). It's important that he doesn't have too much isoniazid because he'll also get some in your milk, and an overdose can cause a type of nerve damage called peripheral neuritis. Some experts suggest monitoring a baby's liver function to make sure this doesn't happen. The commonly used drug para-aminosalicylic acid isn't recommended for the mother of a breastfed baby, as no one is sure how much gets into milk, so she might be given streptomycin or kanamycin instead. If other drugs are used, special precautions may be advisable.

If a breastfeeding mother contracts active, bacteria-positive TB, separation from her baby may be recommended for safety while treatment begins and until a laboratory culture of her sputum and stomach fluid are bacteria-negative. If her milk isn't infected, it's reasonable for her baby to have expressed or pumped milk from a cup. Treatment usually renders a woman noninfectious in a very short time.

It could be argued that if a mother and baby have been together before the mother's TB was diagnosed, there's no point separating them. But because the complications of TB are more hazardous in newborn babies, it's worth taking every precaution to prevent them catching it.

In some developing countries, and among certain peoples such as some American Indians, it's virtually always safer to leave a mother with active TB and her baby together, because breastfeeding is so much safer than bottle-feeding when there's insufficient money for formula, a lack of clean water, fuel and other bottle-sterilizing necessities, and a high risk of infections in general. In such circumstances the risk of drug toxicity is relatively unimportant. These breastfed babies should be carefully treated with isoniazid, however, and vaccinated with a special type of BCG vaccine (isoniazid-resistant). The mother's TB needs treatment at the same time.

Gonorrhea—If this is diagnosed at delivery, your baby shouldn't have your milk, or be with you, until 24 hours after treatment has begun.

HIV—Breastfeeding by a mother with HIV gives her baby up to a one-in-five chance of getting HIV if neither she nor he has antiretroviral drug treatment. The reasons why not all such babies become infected is probably because

- Breast milk's anti-infective factors help protect the baby. For example, white cells called B cells in the milk of infected mothers can generate antibodies that may inhibit HIV.

- Breast milk helps protect a baby's gut from damage by allergenic-foreign proteins, discouraging the passage of HIV through the gut lining into blood or lymph vessels.

- The hormone erythropoietin may strengthen the lining of the milk glands and ducts, and the breasts' blood vessels, making viruses less likely to enter milk.

An HIV-positive woman should base her decision on how to feed her baby by setting the risks and benefits of breastfeeding against the risks of formula-feeding in her particular circumstances.

In many industrialized countries, including the UK, the US, Canada, Australia, and France, experts advise HIV-(type 1)-positive women not to breastfeed, because they consider the risk of their babies acquiring HIV infection greater than the risk of not being breastfed.

An HIV-positive pregnant woman in a developed country is best treated with several antiretroviral drugs in pregnancy and afterward, and having a cesarean section (C-section). The overall risk of her baby being infected is then "only" 1–2 percent. However, it's better for her to for-mula-feed if she isn't prepared to take this risk.

However, in areas of those developing countries in which many babies die because of diarrhea, other infectious diseases, and malnutrition, HIV-1-positive women almost certainly should breastfeed. Not being breastfed here means a child has nearly six times the risk of dying from these conditions. Early exclusive breastfeeding reduces the risk of a mother transmitting HIV-1 to her baby. A South African researcher said in 2002, "The overwhelming majority of babies born to HIV-infected women, and all babies born to uninfected women, benefit from exclusive breastfeeding for about six months."

- Of 1,276 exclusively breastfed babies of HIV-infected mothers, 14 percent became infected with HIV-1 by 6 weeks, and 19 percent by 6 months. Those on solids or formula as well were more likely to become infected. Of the exclusively breastfed babies, 6 percent died in the first 3 months, compared with 15 percent in the others (*Lancet*, 2007).

In resource-poor settings in certain developing countries, 20 percent of the babies of HIV-positive mothers are born with HIV. Some acquire it in the womb, others during delivery. But, if a mother receives one dose of an antiretroviral drug (for example, nevirapine) in labor, and her baby has one dose immediately after birth, the proportion of infected babies falls to 12 percent. The infection is more likely to progress to AIDS (acquired immune deficiency syndrome) if such a baby is not breastfed, partly because breast milk contains several anti-HIV factors.

So it seems wise for an HIV-positive breastfeeding woman living in such circumstances to breastfeed exclusively.

It is also wise for her to

- Have antiretroviral drug treatment. Her baby needs this too.

- Make sure her partner uses a condom for sex, since if he's HIV-positive too, sex without a condom could increase her body's viral load.

- Look after her general health, for example, by eating a healthy diet, so the infection is less likely to progress.

- Have skilled support with breastfeeding so she avoids sore nipples and mastitis as far as possible.

- Avoid feeding from a cracked nipple, or a breast with an abscess.

When her baby is a year old, she should stop breastfeeding if he isn't yet infected. This is because the ongoing benefits of breastfeeding after a year may not outweigh the potential risk of becoming infected.

Heat-treating expressed breast milk to 62.5°C (144.5°F) for half an hour, or boiling the milk, reduces its HIV load, but it's challenging for a mother always to have to express, and giving expressed milk means she has to sterilize a cup or spoon—which requires water and fuel, or water and a chemical sterilizer, all of which may be in short supply.

The infection is more likely to be present in the milk of a woman who becomes infected during the time she breastfeeds than if she became HIV-positive before or during pregnancy.

Because so few babies catch HIV (type 2) from their mothers, there are no specific recommendations yet.

Syphilis—Infection of the skin on the breasts means a baby shouldn't breastfeed, but may, depending on medical advice, be able to have expressed or pumped milk.

Leprosy—Breastfeeding is valuable enough to outweigh any danger from contact. However, a mother may be advised not to hold her baby at other times. Both mother and baby can have drug treatment.

Cytomegalovirus infection—can be transmitted by breast milk. Infection in a healthy newborn is unlikely to cause symptoms. But infection in a low-birthweight baby can cause potentially life-threatening illness.

The viruses are usually passed on from infected people by contact with body fluids such as urine, saliva, or breast milk. They can also be sexually transmitted and spread via transplanted organs and blood transfusions. In healthy people it usually causes no symptoms.

Infection by breast milk doesn't usually cause disease in a baby. But it can do so in a very-low-birth-weight baby. So if you have such a baby and know you know you have this infection, your pediatrician may recommend either freezing your breast milk at 30°F (-20°C) to reduce the number of viruses, or pasteurizing it to eliminate the viruses.

HTLV infection—human T-lymphotropic virus (type 1 or type 2) infection can result, for example, from years of sex with an infected person; an infected blood transfusion; or a drug injection with a needle used by an infected person. Up to 1 in 20 infected people develop T-cell leukemia; spinal infection with progressive muscular weakness; or inflammation of the eyes, joints, lungs, muscles, or skin.

If you know you have this virus, you shouldn't breastfeed as you could give it to your baby,

Osteoporosis

Women with osteoporosis can breastfeed. They may, like other women, experience a temporary loss of bone-mineral density during pregnancy and breastfeeding.

When breastfeeding, sit comfortably and in a well-supported position. If possible, ask someone to pass your baby to you so you avoid lifting.

Research suggests that breastfeeding reduces the long-term risk of developing osteoporosis, and it's possible, though unproven, that it may also be beneficial long-term for women who already have the condition.

High prolactin

Treatment with bromocriptine dries up milk, but women with high prolactin are traditionally advised not to breastfeed anyway. This is because breastfeeding raises prolactin further. Also, the risk of a breast abscess seems higher, and, in a sizable proportion of women, high prolactin results from a pituitary tumor called a prolactinoma, and it's feared that raising prolactin more could enlarge this, which could cause visual disturbances, including blindness. However,

- A Swedish study of 38 women with a prolactinoma concluded it's safe to stop bromocriptine in pregnancy and while breastfeeding, provided a woman has had at least a year's treatment before pregnancy, and has monthly prolactin tests and visual-field measurements so she can start it again at the first suspicion a tumor is growing. Eight in ten women breastfed successfully for up to two years (*Acta Endocrinologica*—now *European Journal of Endocrinology*, 1986).

Preeclampsia

Severe preeclampsia can precede several breastfeeding challenges. For example, the baby may have a low birthweight and be in an incubator. The newly delivered mother may still be at risk of a seizure (convulsion or fit) and need blood-pressure-lowering drugs, sedation and bed rest in a darkened room. The good news is most mothers recover within 24–48 hours of delivery.

If a woman can't put her baby to the breast, or early feeds are unsuccessful and stressful, she can express or pump temporarily instead. Some doctors consider this too stressful and therefore too risky for a woman who may have a fit, but expert nursing can make it as easy and stress-free as possible. Anyway, the stress of having engorged unemptied breasts is considerable. And a mother who wants to breastfeed but is told not to may feel more anxious, unless heavily sedated.

If an affected mother is treated with the sedative phenobarbitone it's vital to check that her baby (especially if ill or pre-term) doesn't become sedated by drinking her milk, as a sedative hampers a baby's ability to feed. If your doctor is reluctant for your baby to drink your milk because of its high drug levels, you or the nurses can keep your milk supply going by expressing or pumping until your medication level is reduced.

If you're too ill to breastfeed, or for you or the nurses to pump or express your breasts, you can get your milk supply back when you're well again.

Cesarean section (C-section)

Many babies today are born by cesarean section—more than half in some US hospitals. There's no reason why you shouldn't breastfeed, but you'll need to be determined. One helpful thing before the operation is to ask the doctor to insert your intravenous (IV) drip into your forearm, rather than into the back of your hand. This will make it easier for you to hold your baby afterward.

The main challenge to breastfeeding is that your tummy will be tender, which makes it uncomfortable to feed with your baby on your lap. You'll need to find a position in which his weight isn't on your tummy and your abdominal muscles aren't strained by holding him to your breast. Enlist a nurse's help to position him. One option is to lie on your side in bed. When you want to change breasts, you can then lean over more toward him, or call the nurse to help you turn over and to move the baby. Other options, if your scar is horizontal, are to sit with your baby in the football hold, or to sit with him lying on a pillow at your side, his legs across your thighs, and his head supported by another pillow or by your arm on a pillow. Sit straight, without slumping, so you don't strain your abdominal muscles.

Unrestricted breastfeeds are particularly important for stimulating a good milk supply. One reason is that women who've had a cesarean generally produce less milk than do other mothers for the first few days. Another is that any IV fluids you've had might encourage fluid retention in your breasts and so make them more tense. This could make it more difficult for your baby to latch-on. Breastfeed frequently, day and night, make each feed as long as your baby wants, and express a little milk before each feed if your breasts are tense.

- A study in South Australia found that by day 6, only 1 in 5 breast-fed cesarean babies had regained their birthweight, compared with 2 in 5 breastfeds born normally. But by then all were getting similar amounts of milk. So the slow start didn't last long (*Archives of Disease in Childhood: Fetal and Neonatal Edition*, 2003).

Nowadays many women who have a cesarean are given an epidural. This is an injection of local anesthetic, or an opioid medication, or both, into a space within the spine to block pain. This means breastfeeding can start without delay. If you've had a general anesthetic you may not be able to breastfeed immediately, but ask for your baby to be brought to you as soon as you're awake and well enough.

If your baby is in an incubator after delivery and you can't be with him for feeds, express or pump your colostrum or milk. The nurses can then give this milk by tube or cup.

Breastfeeding aids recovery after a cesarean as it produces oxytocin, which helps shrink the womb to its former size.

A cesarean often leaves a mother very tired, so it's important to get rest. This doesn't mean that nights must be unbroken, with your baby given a bottle by the nurses. But between feeds the day shouldn't be crammed full of activity on the ward or at home. Allow ample time to sleep or catnap.

Painkillers may be necessary, especially in the first day or two, because the healing scar hurts, especially when moving or coughing. Ibuprofen and paracetamol (acetaminophen) are considered safe for a breastfeeder.

A cesarean, especially if unplanned, can undermine a mother's confidence in herself as a woman, but breastfeeding should help change her mind.

By the end of the first week you should feel very much better, though it will take many months before you're back to normal.

Breast surgery

Some women have had a breast lump removed before they ever get pregnant; a few need a lump biopsied (sampled via a needle) or removed while breastfeeding. Others have had plastic surgery to make their breasts larger or smaller. Whether surgery interferes with the success of any subsequent breastfeeding depends mainly on its type and extent.

Biopsy or removal of a lump before breastfeeding

If you are to have a lump biopsied or removed, and there's any chance you might one day want to breastfeed, have a thorough discussion with your surgeon first. As little breast tissue as possible should be removed, and the incision should sever as few milk ducts as possible.

If you've had a biopsy, you won't know whether you can breastfeed until you try. If—even with the best advice and support—you can't feed from that breast, let its milk dry up by not feeding from it, and by expressing only the least amount needed to stop it hurting. You're highly likely to be able to make all the milk your baby needs from the other breast.

Biopsy or removal of a lump during breastfeeding

Make sure your surgeon knows you are breastfeeding and wish to continue. Breastfeed your baby as near the start of the operation as possible, and ask the nurses to bring him to you as soon as possible afterward. They will help you breastfeed from the other breast. Feed from the operated side as soon as you can. You may find it helps to press very gently over the dressing while you feed.

Breast-reduction surgery

Whether you can breastfeed fully after "reduction mammoplasty" depends on how much glandular tissue was removed, how many milk ducts were cut, whether severed ducts have managed to join up so milk can get to the nipple, and whether those milk glands with intact ducts can produce enough milk.

If you contemplate this operation before having children, and think you might ever want to breastfeed, be sure your surgeon knows so he can leave as many milk ducts intact as possible.

In one operation, the nipple and areola are cut away completely before being transplanted higher up. In another, they are left attached to some breast tissue so some ducts remain intact.

The longer the gap between surgery and pregnancy, the more successful breastfeeding is likely to be. The only way you'll know whether you can breastfeed successfully is to try. Even if you manage to give your baby only a little milk each day, it's worth it for both of you. If you have to give formula as well, you can give it while breastfeeding, by using a supplementer.

- An Australian survey of 30 women who'd had a baby after breast reduction found that of the 93 percent who wished to breastfeed, 73 percent were doing so on leaving hospital, and 27 percent three months later—though only one was exclusively breastfeeding (*British Journal of Plastic Surgery*, 1994).

Breast-enlargement surgery

Many women with breast implants breastfeed successfully. But this surgery can cause problems with breastfeeding. For example, it increases the risk of not being able to produce enough milk.

- A US study found that 64 percent of breastfeeding women with implants had insufficient milk, compared with fewer than 7 percent of those without implants (*Obstetrics and Gynecology*, 1996). Most complications can be minimized with good surgical technique and post-operative management, but they can't always be avoided. Most women don't consider in advance whether surgery might affect their future ability to breastfeed exclusively. But it's important to be well informed before taking this big step.

The effects depend on the

- Type of incision. An incision around the areola is more likely than one beneath the breast to endanger your milk supply.

- Positioning of the implants. For example, there may be long-term breast pain and other effects of pressure from the implant on the breast.

- Complications of surgery. First, severing either the lateral and medial branches of the fourth intercostal nerve, or the nerve endings of the nipple-areolar complex, reduces sensation in the nipple and areola, which in turn reduces milk production. Second, a post-operative hematoma (internal bruise) encourages gradual contracture of the capsule around the implant, which requires further surgery. Third, infection may also need more surgery.

Silicone implants—have become much less popular following publicity over many women in whom they had ruptured.

The scare dating from 1994 about whether breastfed babies of mothers with these implants might develop a stiff gullet because of drinking milk contaminated by leaking silicone has died down, partly because of a Canadian study.

- In this study, the silicone level in the milk of 15 women with implants was very similar (55 ng/mL) to that in the milk of mothers without implants (51 ng/mL). Astonishingly, silicone levels were 80 times as high in 26 brands of cows'-milk formula (4,402 ng/mL) and 12 times as high in store-bought cows' milk, as they were in mothers with implants (*Journal of Plastic and Reconstructive Surgery*, 1998).

X-rays

Rest assured that if you have an X-ray, your milk will be safe for your baby.

If you need a mammogram, note that a breastfeeder's breasts are denser than those of a non-lactating woman, which can make it harder to read a mammogram. Their density is less after a feed. So take your baby to the X-ray unit early and feed him before your mammogram.

Medications or other drugs

Virtually every drug passes into breast milk, some in higher concentrations than others. This said, most are present in such very low doses or have such low known risks that breastfeeding is considered safe. On average, less than 1–4 percent of the mother's dose of a drug goes via her milk to her baby. The older the baby, the less milk he takes and therefore the smaller the drug dose he gets in proportion to his weight. As he grows he's also better able to metabolize and eliminate most drugs.

Drugs that enter breast milk do so most easily in the first three days after birth. The good thing is that the amount of colostrum produced is very small, so the potential dose to a baby is also small.

A very few drugs are potentially harmful because they

- Have side effects which affect adults as well.

- Have a different action in a baby.

- Are concentrated in milk.

- Aren't broken down by a young baby.

- Cause a sensitivity or allergy which could be dangerous with repeated doses.

Knowledge of how such drugs affect breastfed babies is far from complete. It's clearly unacceptable to give a healthy woman a drug to see what happens to her baby. The number of breastfeeding women taking any but the most common of drugs is very small. And it's difficult to measure drugs in breast milk.

If a drug is considered unsafe for a breastfed baby, there's often an alternative. If a particular drug is essential for a woman but risky for her baby, she'll have to stop giving him breast milk while she takes it. But this happens only very rarely.

Babies with a low birthweight, jaundice, a kidney problem, allergy in the family, or deficiency of an enzyme called glucose-6 phosphate dehydrogenase (G6PD) may be particularly susceptible to adverse effects from certain drugs.

A few drugs enter milk in doses of more than 1–4 percent of the mother's dose. They include anti-convulsants, antidepressants and anti-mania drugs. But there's rarely any concern until the dose in milk is higher than 10 percent of the mother's dose. Such drugs include metronidazole, atenolol, lithium and potassium iodide.

If you need prescribed medication, remind your doctor you're breast-feeding so he can check the drug's safety if necessary. If you're concerned about a drug not listed below, your doctor may know, or can check a drugs-and-breastfeeding database. Or you can look it up on the Internet (see below) and discuss your findings with him if necessary.

Many over-the-counter medications are safe in normal doses, but ask a pharmacist if you are unsure.

Useful websites

These enable you or your doctor to retrieve reliable information fast. Note that while trade names of medications sometimes vary from one country to another, their generic (chemical) names are the same.

UK—The West Midlands and Trent Drug Information Service's Quick Reference Guide for Drugs in Breast Milk is at ukmicentral.nhs.uk.

US—The US National Institutes of Heath's Drugs and Lactation Database (LactMed) is at toxnet.nlm.nih.gov/cgi-bin/sis/htmlgen?LACT.

Canada—The MotherRisk Program at the Hospital for Sick Children, Toronto offers information at Motherisk.org/women/breastfeeding.jsp.

Global—The World Health Organization's Drugs in Pregnancy and Lactation is at whqlibdoc.who.int/hq/2002/55732.pdf.

Here is a list of drugs known to be unsafe or best avoided by a breast-feeding woman, including some possible adverse effects in her baby.

Anti-infective drugs

Antibiotics—can cause diarrhea; other adverse effects are uncommon.

Chloramphenicol—causes sleepiness and vomiting, and theoretically could harm the bone marrow, leading to aplastic anemia and a low white cell count. Avoid.

Ciprofloxacin—High concentrations in milk might affect a baby's joints, for example. Avoid.

Clindamycin—Its concentration in milk can be several times that in the mother's blood. There's a risk of bloody diarrhea from bowel inflammation. Avoid.

Co-trimoxazole—could cause jaundice and a deficiency of folate (an important B vitamin). Avoid for two weeks after birth. If your baby is under 24 weeks old, his doctor should monitor him.

Dapsone—can cause hemolytic anemia and jaundice. Your baby's doctor should monitor him.

Metronidazole—can cause poor appetite, vomiting and diarrhea and a theoretical risk of cancer. High doses aren't advised. Avoid if possible. If needed for trichomonas infection, store enough milk for a day, take one 2 g dose, then discard your milk for 24 hours and meanwhile give your baby the stored milk.

Nalidixic acid—One baby whose mother was also on amylobarbitone developed hemolytic anemia. It has also caused raised intracranial pressure. Take only if absolutely necessary. Report any abnormal signs in your baby to his doctor.

Nitrofurantoin—Its level in milk is insignificant. But it isn't advised for mothers of pre-terms or those with a G6PD deficiency.

Novobiocin—Can cause jaundice. Avoid.

Penicillins—appear in trace amounts in milk so could cause allergic sensitization in a susceptible baby. They also encourage thrush. Otherwise they are safe in their usual dosage. Report any abnormal signs in your baby to his doctor.

Sulphonamides—can cause jaundice and a rash. Hemolytic anemia has been reported in a G6PD-deficient baby. If your baby is under a month old, his doctor should monitor him. Some experts recommend avoiding them.

Tetracyclines—could theoretically cause mottling of a baby's developing teeth, though absorption from a baby's gut is poor. Avoid.

Anticancer drugs

Breastfeeding must usually be abandoned, though methotrexate and busulphan seem to present little hazard.

Anticoagulants

Bleeding has occurred after surgery or trauma in babies of mothers on anticlotting medication, but is more likely in a baby deficient in vitamin K. Warfarin and heparin are suitable. Be cautious when using other anticoagulants. The baby will benefit from a vitamin-K supplement.

Antithyroid drugs

These can cause a potentially fatal blood disorder, so your baby's doctor will monitor his development and blood count. Iodides (also in some cough medicines) can suppress a baby's thyroid, so his doctor will monitor his thyroid-hormone levels. They can also sensitize a baby's thyroid to certain other drugs, including lithium, chlorpromazine, and methylxanthines. Carbimazole can be used in doses of up to 30 mg a day. Propylthiouracil is less concentrated in milk than is carbimazole.

Central-nervous-system drugs

If your baby becomes abnormally drowsy while you are on one of these medications, he might not feed as well, and his doctor should monitor his weight gain.

Alcohol—in amounts large enough to make you tipsy, alcohol can inhibit your let-down and make your baby sleepy. Very large amounts taken regularly could damage his brain.

Amantadine—can cause vomiting, urinary retention, and rashes. Avoid.

Antidepressants—may make a baby sleepy. Limited evidence suggests selective serotonin-reuptake inhibitors (SSRIs) and tricyclics don't cause toxic side effects or adverse long-term developmental effects in a baby. The best SSRIs to take are probably paroxetine or sertraline, but not fluoxetine as it takes a long time to break down. Tricyclics are excreted in milk but not metabolized by a young baby, so could accumulate in his body. But no side effects have been reported, and they seem safe provided the dose isn't too high, and the baby thrives. Imipramine is probably preferable to amitriptyline for short-term use. Doxepin encourages sedation and breathing problems in a baby.

Antipsychotics—are present in small amounts in milk. Many are unsuitable when breastfeeding.

Barbiturates—can make a baby drowsy and lethargic, encouraging poor feeding and weight loss. They may react with other drugs. One case of cyanosis (blueness) caused by a condition called methemoglobinemia occurred in a baby whose mother was also taking phenytoin. Avoid if possible.

Bromide—usually produces drowsiness and may cause a rash.

Cannabis—can accumulate in a baby's body. There have been reports of delayed motor development at one year in babies of marijuana-smoking mothers. Avoid.

Carbamazepine—is not advised in high doses or along with other antiepileptics, as it can accumulate in a baby's body.

Chloral hydrate—can cause drowsiness.

Chlorpromazine—could cause drowsiness, so it may be better avoided.

Cocaine—can concentrate in milk and accumulate in the baby. Avoid.

Diazepam—There's one report of lethargy and weight loss. It can accumulate in a baby's body and increase physiological jaundice. Use high doses only with caution.

Dichloralphenazone—causes slight drowsiness.

Ecstasy and MDMA—Few safety studies exist. Avoid.

Ethosuximide—Significant levels can accumulate in a breastfed baby. Poor sucking and over-excitability have been reported.

Heroin—can cause addiction in an unborn baby if taken by the mother during pregnancy. Breastfeeding and very gradual weaning is one way of withdrawing the drug from a baby. But the American Academy of Pediatrics recommends that heroin-addicted mothers should not breastfeed.

Lithium—might cause lethargy, floppiness, or blueness.

Morphine—Significant amounts can be excreted in the milk. Avoid.

Phenytoin—Many mothers on this medication have breastfed safely. But it has been associated with vomiting, tremors, and rashes, as well as an idiosyncratic reaction of blueness due to a condition called methemoglobinemia.

Primidone—The high levels in milk can make a baby sleepy.

Sulpiride—can be associated with adverse affects in a baby. Avoid.

Hormones

The pill—The combined (estrogen plus progestogen) pill can suppress the volume of milk a woman makes and reduce her duration of lactation. Two studies have shown a decrease in protein, fat, and minerals in milk. Small amounts of the pill's synthetic steroids also appear in the milk. Isolated reports exist of breast enlargement in male babies, proliferation of the vaginal epithelium in females, and changes in bones, though all occurred with oral contraception containing higher doses of hormones than are currently used. Many experts recommend the progestogen-only pill for breastfeeding women.

Progestogen contraceptive implants/progesterone vaginal contraceptive ring—Studies suggest these have no adverse effects.

Syntometrine—a combination of oxytocin and ergometrine that is often given after the second stage of labor (see page 120). Ergometrine is a smooth-muscle stimulant that makes the womb contract, makes blood vessels contract, and is related to lysergic acid diethylamide (LSD). The dose given to a mother is ten times too small to cause mind-altering effects like those of LSD but can cause a variety of adverse effects. Certain researchers recommend that women who want to breastfeed should not have it (page 120).

Miscellaneous

Allopurinol and oxipurinol—enter breast milk in high concentration, so a baby risks the same side effects as his mother.

5-aminosalicylic acid (mesalazine)—is considered safe but can cause diarrhea.

Antidiabetes (hypoglycemic) drugs—Your baby's doctor should monitor his blood sugar level.

Aspirin—carries a very small risk of rashes, gastrointestinal side effects or, if a baby has a blood-clotting disorder, jaundice and bleeding into the brain. There's also a small risk of potentially fatal brain and liver damage called Reye's syndrome. Safe in usual dosage but report any abnormal signs in your baby to his doctor.

Atropine—is said to diminish milk flow and cause constipation and retention of urine in the baby, though there's no good evidence.

Beta blockers—Atenolol can slow a baby's heartbeat. Propanolol is preferable, but while only small amounts appear in milk, it could theoretically accumulate in the baby. Your baby's doctor should monitor his heart rate blood sugar level.

Digoxin—Even if a mother takes a high dose, the amounts in her milk are small. Your baby's doctor should monitor his heart rate.

Dihydrotachysterol—This may encourage bone-mineral loss. Possibly better avoided.

Diuretics (thiazide type)—can decrease the milk supply. Your baby's doctor should monitor his weight.

Ergometrine—lowers prolactin so might suppress lactation. In some obstetric units ergometrine is given after delivery only if the womb fails to expel the placenta naturally or there's bleeding from the womb. See also page 120.

Ergot alkaloids—cause diarrhea, vomiting, a weak pulse, and unstable blood pressure in 9 in 10 breastfed babies. They can also lower prolactin and therefore suppress lactation. Avoid.

Fluoride—can cause mottling of developing teeth. Use with caution (page 23).

Ginseng—There's one report of the breastfed son of a woman on large amounts of Siberian ginseng developing pubic hair, a hairy forehead and swollen nipples. He returned to normal when breastfeeding stopped. Avoid.

Gold salts—can cause rashes and a low white cell count. Avoid.

Indomethacin—There's one report of convulsions. It's probably better avoided.

Laxatives—may cause diarrhea. Your baby's doctor should monitor his weight.

Nicotine—may reduce the milk supply and interfere with the letdown. Smokers are more likely than nonsmokers to give up breastfeeding early. There's one report of restlessness and circulatory disturbance in a baby. It can also cause abdominal pain, nausea, vomiting, and diarrhea. Avoid.

Phenylbutazone—there's the possibility of a potentially serious blood disorder. Avoid if possible; if not, your baby's doctor should monitor him.

Pseudoephedrine—in cold remedies. It might inhibit milk production. Avoid.

Reserpine—There's one report of significant nasal stuffiness, slowing of the heart, and an increase in mucus production in the breathing passages. Avoid if possible; if not, your baby's doctor should monitor him.

Sulphasalazine—There's one report of bloody diarrhea. Avoid if possible; if not, your baby's doctor should monitor him.

Vitamin B6 (pyridoxine)—One study showed a decrease in milk supply with doses over 100 mg a day. Avoid.

Radioactive tests and treatments
Experts differ in their advice, but this is a safe summary:

67Gallium citrate, 75Se-methionine, Sodium 32P phosphate and Chromic 32P phosphate—Significant amounts enter milk. Different experts advise interrupting breastfeeding and discarding milk for between 72 hours and two weeks. Ask if your hospital's nuclear-medicine department will measure your milk's radioactivity so you can return to breastfeeding as soon as possible.

Iodine isotopes—Radio-iodine thyroid studies shouldn't be done in breastfeeding women. Hyperthyroidism and thyroiditis can be diagnosed using pertechnetate- (technetium 99m-) imaging together with clinical criteria and plasma-hormone levels.

99Tcm-pertechnetate (technetium 99m)—Express and discard your milk for 12 hours.

99Tcm-MAA—Express and discard your milk for 6 hours.

99Tcm-DTPA, 99Tcm-EDTA, 99Tcm-MDP, 99Tcm-erythrocytes, 51Cr-EDTA and 111In-leukocytes—There's no need to stop breastfeeding but some experts seek to reassure mothers alarmed by radioactivity by suggesting they express and discard the milk produced in the 4 hours after a test.

If you're advised to have a radioactive-isotope investigation or treatment, ask if there's an alternative—either one that doesn't use an isotope or one that enters milk only in small amounts.

If the interruption to breastfeeding is to be short, store expressed or pumped milk in the refrigerator or freezer to be given to your baby during that time.

Environmental contaminants

Breast milk can contain environmental contaminants to which a mother has been exposed via food or air. But the good news is that their levels in breast milk are mostly decreasing. Experts believe breast milk may help detoxify some of them. And the many advantages of breastfeeding are thought to greatly outweigh any possibility of harm except for an extremely small minority of exposed babies. The greatest risk is during pregnancy, not breastfeeding.

Formula can contain environmental contaminants too.

Organochlorine pesticides

Some of these, including chlordane, DDT, dieldrin, hexachlorobenzene and heptachlor, are restricted in some countries and banned in others. They can persist in the ground and in the body for years.

Chlordane—The "acceptable daily intake" of this insecticide is easily exceeded in contaminated areas. Its effects on breastfed babies are unknown.

DDT—Although present in breast milk in contaminated areas, and in the milk of mothers who smoke or have ever smoked (as DDT is used on some tobacco crops), no ill effects have been observed in babies.

Dieldrin—Some people in contaminated areas consume up to 22 times the acceptable daily intake of this insecticide. Dutch research (1992) showed that the more often a woman ate meat and dairy produce, the higher her milk's level of dieldrin.

Heptachlor—The acceptable daily intake (ADI) of this insecticide from breast milk is exceeded in exposed babies, according to one study. Some intakes are up to 7 times the acceptable daily intake. Long-term exposure in animals can damage nerves, kidneys and immunity.

Hexachlorobenzene—Many infant deaths occurred in Turkey after mothers ate wheat treated with this now globally banned fungicide. It is one of the most persistent organophosphates, and the acceptable daily intake (ADI) from breast milk is easily exceeded in contaminated areas. Some babies' intake from the milk of exposed mothers contains up to 48 times the ADI.

Dioxins and furans

These are released by burning PVC plastic and wood treated with preservatives and are among the most toxic poisons. They enter breast milk in areas of industrial contamination and it has been suggested that severe contamination of milk could lead to a bleeding disorder (late hemorrhagic disease of the newborn) caused by vitamin K deficiency in young breastfeds.

PCBs (polychlorinated biphenyls)

Their industrial use is banned in some countries and restricted to closed electrical systems in the European Union. The disposal of PCB-containing articles (such as transformers, capacitors and painted items) is a problem. However, PCBs aren't thought to harm breastfed babies, and their levels in breast milk have only rarely (after unusual exposure) been found to exceed safe limits.

Flame retardants

These are used to treat carpets and soft furnishings and can find their way into breast milk. High exposure from any source to the older flame retardants, most now phased out in many countries, can affect thyroid hormones and, when older, performance in intelligence and developmental tests; any effects of the newer ones are as yet unknown.

Breastfeeding an adopted baby

Many women have fully breastfed their adopted baby. Once a pregnancy has prepared your breasts for lactation, they'll always retain the ability to produce milk. If they've produced milk for any length of time, they'll be even more able to do so years later. This is why grandmothers in many parts of the world can breastfeed their grandchildren.

All women can stimulate their milk production and build up their milk supply over time by breastfeeding, expressing, or pumping frequently. You can do this even if you've never had a baby—in which case it's called "induced lactation"—though you'll have to persevere and supplement your milk with other food. And you'll need a cooperative baby.

A woman who breastfeeds her own baby has had months of pregnancy for her breasts to prepare for breastfeeding. So you must expect to take a long time to prepare your breasts too. Start building up your milk supply at least six weeks before you expect to take delivery of your adopted baby.

When he arrives, you'll probably need to give formula as well. However, some mothers have fed an adopted baby with breast milk from his birth mother, a breast-milk bank, or a breastfeeding friend until their own milk became plentiful enough.

A supplementer is very useful for relactating mothers. The original one was developed by a man to help his wife breastfeed their adopted baby.

How long will it take to build up your milk supply? It has been done within two weeks by mothers who weaned their own baby as long as six years before. It usually takes much longer. The pleasure it gives can far outweigh the difficulty involved.

Feeding someone else's baby

Historically, wet nurses have sometimes fed other women's babies. A wet nurse is either a woman who is still feeding her own baby and can therefore build up her milk supply to feed someone else's as well (rather as if she had twins or was "tandem nursing"—page 304), or one who has just finished feeding her own baby.

It was relatively popular among the wealthier, land-owning classes in Britain in the nineteenth century because it enabled a rich man's wife to return to her normal menstrual cycles sooner and, as a result, to have another child more quickly.

In France in the eighteenth and nineteenth centuries, wet nursing was accepted in Paris, for example, as a means of enabling mothers of young babies to return to paid work. This sort of wet nursing was a paid occupation, so it behooved the wet nurse to make sure the baby was well nourished and well cared for. Indeed, her own baby was sometimes put second.

In some cultures throughout history, a baby's father has been involved in, or has actually managed, the choice of wet nurse. This stemmed partly from the notion that a wet nurse's milk, breastfeeding, and mothering conveyed aspects of her health, character, and moral standing to the child. The baby's father also sometimes dictated how long his baby was to be breastfed, and when and what other foods were to be introduced. These behaviors were ways of exerting his power over his wife and asserting his position in the family.

In developing countries today grandmothers sometimes feed their daughter's baby.

The younger a baby, the more likely he is to accept a feed from someone else. But no one should feed someone else's baby unless she has his mother's permission and has had the same tests she would need to have if she were donating milk to a bank. Infection of the nipple with herpes viruses or thrush can be transferred to a breastfeeding baby, for example, and HIV (human immunodeficiency virus) infection can be transferred via infected breast milk.

thirteen

Feeding an Older Baby

Weaning" comes from the Old English word for "accustoming." It's generally used to mean stopping breastfeeding. But it can also mean accustoming a baby to other foods while still breastfeeding.

When, how, and why you start giving other foods and when, how, and why you stop breastfeeding are up to you and your baby. However, a wealth of experience gained from other mothers, plus years of scientific research, provides useful guidelines.

Most important, don't cut down on breastfeeds when you start giving solids. Your milk is still very valuable to your baby, and breastfeeding is valuable to you both.

Introducing other foods

The day you give your baby something other than your milk is a big milestone. Some babies take to it enthusiastically; others are less eager.

When should you start solids?

Weaning foods are traditionally called "solids," however runny they might be. The World Health Organization (WHO) recommends exclusive breastfeeding for six months, which means no other drinks or solids until then. So too do the UK Department of Health and the American Academy of Pediatrics.

Around six months seems a natural time to start offering solids, because many babies allowed to decide for themselves don't start picking up pieces of food or taking an intense interest in their mother's food until about then. It's also when many get their first tooth.

Before the WHO recommendations, quite a few mothers gave solids before four months. But mothers seem to be taking the recommendations on board, if only to some extent.

For example, in the UK the percentage of babies given solids early fell between 2000 and 2005:

Babies receiving solids at different ages

	2000 (%)	2005 (%)
3 months	24	10
4 months	85	52
6 months	98	98

(*Infant Feeding* 2000; *Infant Feeding* 2005)

Why not earlier?

Mainstream thinking is that starting solids before six months might

- Trigger allergies in susceptible babies.

- Encourage the early appearance of gluten sensitivity, which can show up with celiac disease or other symptoms.

- Hazard a mother's milk supply.

However, a few experts are investigating whether the risk of allergy and, perhaps, nonallergic food sensitivity might be reduced if very small amounts of potential triggers were to be introduced from three months (page 22).

When's the latest?

A few babies are satisfied and well nourished on breast milk alone for up to eight or nine months or even longer.

How to start solids

Many mothers start by spoon-feeding or, the first few times, by offering a little taste of appropriate and suitably prepared food from their (washed) finger. Others wait until their baby picks up food for himself. If your baby likes it, give a little more.

When giving your baby anything other than root vegetables for the first time, don't give it again for four days, so you can see whether he develops any symptoms (such as diarrhea, a runny nose, or a rash) that could mean he's sensitive to it. It also gives him the chance to get used to each new taste.

After the first two or three weeks of starting solids, you can give two or more foods in the same meal. However, some babies (like some adults) prefer foods to be kept separate.

Be sensitive to his appetite and let him guide how much you give.

Spoon-feeding—Give your baby the breast, then offer food in a spoon with a fairly flat bowl. Put the spoon into his mouth, then gently withdraw it against his upper gum and lip so some of the food stays in his mouth. He may try to suck in some. End by giving another drink of milk from your breast. Choose a food that's soft enough to swallow easily. Babies start chewing at around six months, and as they become more used to solids you can give them gradually lumpier foods. However, the average baby doesn't become efficient at chewing for another month or so.

Finger foods—Some inquisitive six-month-olds like to investigate by grasping food from their mother's hand or plate. This is fine if it's suitable and not too hot. Good "finger foods" to pick up and suck on, chew, or bite include raw fruit, such as a large piece of peeled apple, a rusk of oven-baked salt-free, whole-wheat bread, and anything hard that won't break into pieces and choke him. He'll probably like the taste and will eat some by gradually dissolving it in his mouth.

Many babies love the new sensations from eating solids. They smack their lips and look for more. Others are surprised, but a screwed-up face or a look of amazement won't necessarily mean your baby doesn't like the food, just that it's unfamiliar. Wait for a moment so he doesn't feel pressured and then try again. A lot of what goes into his mouth will probably come out again, but simply scoop this up gently from his chin with the spoon.

What should you give?

From 4 months at the earliest—ideally not before 6
Offer

- Vegetables—avocado, broccoli, carrots or other root vegetables, cauliflower, zucchini, squash.

- Grains without gluten—rice, corn (such as polenta), millet, and other starchy carbohydrate foods, such as tapioca, sago.

- Fruit—apple, apricot, banana, pear.

From 5 months at the earliest—ideally not before 6

- Chicken, turkey.

From 6 months
Add

- Dairy food—full-fat cows' milk, cheese, yogurt.
- Other meats.
- Peas.
- Gluten-containing grain (wheat, barley, rye, oats) foods—for example, bread, baked-bread rusks, breakfast cereal, flour-based sauce.

From 8 months
Add

- Beans, tofu, lentils (avoid these in your baby's last meal of the day if gassiness at night stops your baby sleeping).

From 9 months
Add

- Eggs—cooked well so the yolks are more digestible; raw or lightly cooked eggs are unsuitable for children under age one because of the risk of salmonella infection.
- Fish.
- Almonds or hazelnuts—very finely ground, to a child without a history of food allergy.

From 1 year
Add

- Nuts—offer a child without a history of food allergy ground-up nuts, but don't give whole or chopped nuts to a child under 5 years, as there's a small risk of inhalation.

You can purée a food if your baby can't yet chew. Do this by mashing, pushing it through a sieve or mouli, or whizzing it in an electric blender.

Meat is one of the most difficult foods to chew, so finely chop it, or blend or mince it, until your baby is around ten months, when it may be all right simply cut up small.

To make a savory purée more liquid and thus easier to eat, add a little of one of the following:

- Expressed breast milk (its familiar sweet flavor makes new foods more attractive).

- Water in which you've cooked vegetables.

- Water.

- Vegetable or chicken stock (previously frozen in an ice-cube tray then used cube by cube).

To make a sweet purée easier to eat, add a little of one of the following:

- Expressed breast milk.

- Water in which you've cooked fruit.

- Water.

A healthy diet

At first your baby will still get nearly all his nourishment from your milk. So you needn't worry about balancing his diet until he's eating more solids, and breast milk plays a less important role.

Go easy on added sugar, and avoid it for children under age one where possible. Sugar encourages tooth decay and provides only "empty" calories, which means it doesn't contribute worthwhile or irreplaceable nutrients. The intrinsic sugars in fruit, vegetables and milk often taste pleasantly sweet anyway. Occasional foods containing added sugar won't hurt older babies. But it's wise not to give sweetened snacks or drinks between meals or at bedtime, unless you clean your baby's teeth and gums afterward.

Salt added by you or by manufacturers is best avoided as it can be dangerous for a baby if given in excess.

Don't give your baby breakfast cereals containing added bran, as this can prevent iron, calcium and zinc being properly absorbed. It's also very filling, which could spoil his appetite.

Many experts, though not all, recommend that children under age one should not have honey, as there's an extremely small risk of food poisoning from bacteria producing botulinum toxin.

Homemade or commercially made?

Many mothers like to give homemade food most of the time, often giving their baby what they themselves are going to eat, perhaps mashed or sieved first. This is cheaper than commercial baby food, and accustoms your baby to family food. If you cook especially for him, it's convenient to freeze portions in ice-cube trays, so you have something for when the family meal isn't suitable.

But up to 95 percent of mothers in westernized countries give their babies some commercially prepared foods, perhaps mainly when it's particularly convenient.

Drinks

While your baby is under 6 months old, it's ideally best to breast-feed exclusively. However, some successful breastfeeders occasionally give small amounts of other drinks, such as water or even formula. This is unlikely to do much, if any, harm to your baby or you, provided that breastfeeding is well established, provided he isn't very young, and provided you give the fluid by cup, not bottle.

When your baby is over 6 months, breast milk should ideally remain his main drink for some time. You can gradually introduce other drinks, but remember that giving a lot of fluid other than breast milk could diminish your milk supply.

Water

Your baby will do very well if you give him only water. However, note that some experts believe it's better for a baby under a year not to drink water that's been artificially fluoridated because of the risk of this encouraging mottling of developing teeth.

Sugary drinks can harm teeth

Give drinks that contain fruit juice, squash or syrup only infrequently, if at all. Ideally always clean your baby's teeth and gums afterward, because these drinks contain natural or added sugars, and acids, which encourage tooth decay. This can begin before a tooth comes through the gum. These drinks are especially hazardous if given between meals, at bedtime, or by bottle. A baby's newly erupted teeth are more susceptible to tooth decay than when he is older.

Fruit juice—Try the occasional drink of pure orange juice diluted with water or on its own. This is best given at mealtimes, as its vitamin C encourages the absorption of iron from other foods.

Fruit drinks containing artificial sweeteners are best avoided.

Fruit squashes or diluted syrups—Squashes and syrups diluted with water are popular but contain a lot of sugar. While some contain vitamin C, not all do, and many contain no natural fruit juice at all.

Herbal baby drinks—Dentists report that fruit-containing herbal baby drinks are among the worst culprits for damaging teeth.

Cows' milk—In developing countries, babies are traditionally weaned on to a diet that doesn't include cows' milk. But they tend to get the benefit of breast milk for far longer than infants in developed countries.

In many developed countries in which the traditional diet includes cows' milk and other dairy foods, women are used to incorporating milk into their family's diet. Indeed, most expect to give their babies cows' milk and if they don't they might find it difficult, without extra information or help, to ensure their baby gets a balanced diet, with enough fat and calcium particularly.

Whether you give cows' milk depends partly on your baby's age. If you stop breastfeeding before six months, you should substitute your breast milk with cows'-milk formula. You can carry on giving formula until your baby is a year old. "Follow-on" milk is completely unnecessary. And undiluted cows' milk is arguably better avoided for the children under age one as it's saltier than formula.

After a year old, full-fat cows' milk is a good source of calcium and fat. Growing babies need more fat in their diet than do older children and adults. Giving an older baby some milk each day in addition to family food readily fills this need. But semi-skimmed milk is unsuitable for children under two years old, and skimmed milk is unsuitable for children under five years old.

How long to continue breastfeeding

The World Health Organization recommends breastfeeding exclusively for six months, then continuing to breastfeed along with giving other foods and drinks for up to two years, or beyond. This recommendation is based on an enormous amount of research into babies' and mothers' health. More than 70 countries now recommend breastfeeding for a year or more.

Breastfeeding—along with other foods—after 6 months

There are three major advantages to this:

1. A breastfed baby receives some protection against infection for eight months in developed countries and much longer in developing countries.

2. You and your baby probably enjoy the intimacy of feed times.

3. You may reduce your risk, in later life, of getting breast cancer, ovarian cancer, rheumatoid arthritis, osteoporosis, high blood pressure, high cholesterol, diabetes, metabolic syndrome, a heart attack, or a stroke.

How long will your milk supply last?

It'll last as long as you want if breast milk is your baby's major fluid intake. However, as soon as you give him meaningful amounts of other drinks, with only one or two breastfeeds a day, your supply will begin to dry up. Having said this, some women continue with only one feed a day for many months.

It isn't unusual for women who breastfeed into the second year to produce over about a pint (half a liter) of milk a day. Wet nurses used to feed one baby after another for years, and many mothers the world over feed their children, or even their grandchildren, for several years. The Western idea that milk automatically dries up after a few months is totally wrong.

Breastfeeding an older child

You can breastfeed your baby until he's one, two, three, or even older. Your milk supply will slowly dwindle as he feeds less often and gets increasingly more of his nourishment from other food and drink. Breastfeeding an older child is more important for comfort and pleasure than for nutritional reasons. A breastfeeding mother and child have a very special relationship and many mothers and their children like this to continue. It's perfectly normal in the scheme of things for a child this age to want to go on breastfeeding, though it's unusual to see it in developed countries.

An older child who's learning to explore his world may run back to you for the occasional quick feed then return to doing what he was doing. Touching base in this way reassures him that all is well and restores his energy and enthusiasm for other action.

He may feed to get off to sleep or during the night for comfort. Or there may be no obvious pattern to his feeds. He may want one when he feels like cuddling and being close, perhaps when he's tired, stressed or otherwise upset, or unwell. A working mother and her child may see the morning and evening breastfeeds as precious times when they can be together and share its unparalleled intimacy.

You may notice a patch in the first year, perhaps when he's four to six months old, when you wonder whether you want to continue breastfeeding. You may be feeling livelier and wanting to do more in the outside world. But if you do fit a lot more in, you could easily find your time for breastfeeding squeezed, which could compromise your milk supply. If you feel that breastfeeding has gone on long enough, it's much better to stop rather than to resent feeding him. If you've had enough, give up gradually.

Some women whose older child breastfeeds whenever and wherever he wants look somewhat overwhelmed or drained, especially if he does it often, or in company. As you carry on breastfeeding an older child, it's perfectly reasonable to help him learn that he can't necessarily feed at any time he likes. He's old enough now to learn to give and take. So teach him, gently but firmly, that sometimes it's "no" to a breastfeed. Be creative, for example, by thinking ahead of ways to distract him, or other ways of meeting his needs—for example, for a drink, for food, for comfort, or to relieve boredom.

If you continue breastfeeding as your baby passes his first birthday, your main challenge will probably be coping with criticism from friends and relatives. Many will be surprised you're going on. This can be off-putting, but if you and your baby want to continue, it's up to you. It's scarcely surprising that a society that sometimes finds it hard to deal with the sight of a young baby being breastfed, finds it even more difficult to cope with seeing an older one at the breast. If your child tugs at your clothing, or asks for a feed when you're out visiting, feed him in another room if you prefer.

How long you continue is your choice. However long it is, you'll know you've done your best for him, and it'll probably have given you a lot of pleasure too.

Breastfeeding during a period

This won't harm you or your baby. Some women find their breasts are more tender than usual during a period. Changes in milk volume may occur because of altered blood flow in the breasts. Some babies have slight diarrhea for a couple of days; others seem to dislike the taste of the milk.

Some babies are more fractious for the few days before their mother's period. This could be because they sense she has premenstrual tension.

Breastfeeding in pregnancy

You can breastfeed throughout your next pregnancy if you want, though some women find their breasts are more tender than usual.

Your milk supply may decrease, probably because pregnancy hormones affect milk production, but a month or so before your next baby is due it will automatically increase again.

Breastfeeding an older child and a baby

Carry on feeding your toddler when your new baby arrives if you want, but let your newborn have first call on your milk. Breastfeeding two children of different ages is called tandem nursing.

Researchers aren't yet sure whether mature milk made by pregnant breastfeeding women becomes enriched when their next baby is born by the extra antibodies; protein; zinc and other minerals; vitamins A, E, B6, and B12; and live cells normally found in colostrum. However, it seems highly unlikely that a newborn baby would be at any disadvantage.

Stopping breastfeeding

Some women decide themselves when to stop; others pick up on cues from their baby and make a joint decision; and others let their baby decide. Whoever decides, many women experience mixed feelings of loss, and pleasure at moving on. Or you may simply feel that breastfeeding has gone on long enough—in which case it's much better to stop rather than to resent feeding him.

Baby-led weaning from the breast

"Baby-led" means your baby decides when he wants to stop. Some babies lose interest in the breast relatively soon, others want to go on much longer, and some don't want to give up at all.

Sudden baby-led weaning

Sometimes a happily and fully breastfed baby will suddenly refuse to feed. There may be an obvious reason such as a cold, teething, or an unpleasant experience (such as a loud noise) while at the breast. At other times there's no apparent cause.

Sometimes a fully breastfed baby will suddenly refuse to feed.

It's upsetting for your baby as he has to get used to another source of milk and comfort. And if his "nursing strike," as it's known in the US, has no obvious cause, it's upsetting for you too as he turns down not only your milk but also, by implication, you.

If a cold is making it so difficult for your baby to breathe through his nose that he gives up on breastfeeding, try

- Putting decongestant nosedrops containing phenylephrine (from a pharmacy/drugstore) into his nostrils 5 minutes or so before a feed. Use them according to the packet's instructions.

- Washing out some of the nasal mucus with saline nosedrops. Make these by stirring ¼ teaspoon of salt into a cup of warm water. Before a feed, tilt his head back a little then put 2–3 drops into one nostril with a rubber-bulbed dropper (from a pharmacy). Wait for 10 seconds or so. Then hold his head gently but firmly against you so it can't move, squeeze the bulb, carefully insert the end of the dropper just ¼ in (½ cm) into one nostril and release the squeeze to try to suck out some of the mucus. Repeat with the other nostril. Make fresh saline each day and wash the dropper well after each use.

- Using steam to help liquefy the mucus. One way of doing this is to have a saucepan of simmering water on the stove, shut the kitchen door and window, and sit with your baby nearby. Put a few drops of eucalyptus essential oil into the water for extra decongestant effect.

- Letting him sleep with his head slightly raised rather than with him flat on his back. Raise his head safely by putting something under the head-end of the mattress rather than directly under his head.

If for whatever reason he won't breastfeed, give him expressed or pumped milk from a cup for the time being, but always calmly offer the breast before and after each cup feed. He may be having a temporary feeding strike, or he may be ready to quit.

The easiest way

If you want—or have—to stop breastfeeding, it's easier to do so gradually. If you stop quickly, you'll probably have a fractious baby and painful, engorged breasts. There's no place for drying-up pills.

1. Give up first the feed at which you have least milk. Most women find this is in the later afternoon or early evening. Give him something else to drink. If you have to wean early, remember that young babies benefit from sucking, so a bottle may be better than a cup.

2. After a week or so, give up another feed. Carry on cutting out one more feed every week or so until you're feeding only once a day. You may find it's most comfortable to give up the earliest morning feed last, as you'll probably have most milk then. But many mothers prefer to give up the final feed of the day last, as their babies enjoy this the most and sleep well afterward.

Weaning from the breast is best done unhurried and unworried. Don't wean in an emergency if you can avoid it. Your baby will find it hard to understand why he's suddenly denied the breast, and might be upset for some time.

If he asks for a feed by nuzzling against your breast several days after you've stopped feeding him, and you let him suck, he'll soon realize there's little, if any, milk there—though he may want to try anyway.

If you find yourself wishing you hadn't stopped so soon, or for some reason your baby needs to continue, you can always stimulate a new supply of milk and start again.

fourteen

Breastfeeding and Sex

Juxtaposing the words "breastfeeding" and "sex" still raises eyebrows, even though it's hardly possible to open a newspaper or magazine, surf the net, or watch a TV program without being confronted by a sexual message of some sort.

Mother, lover . . . or both?

Surprisingly many women harbor the belief that a woman should shut off her sexual side once she becomes a mother. Some come to the end of their first pregnancy feeling somewhat ambivalent about breastfeeding from the sexual point of view. Until now they've seen their breasts mainly as sexual objects that gave pleasure to themselves and their man. Now another function is asserting itself, and confusion reigns. Some men, too, have difficulty seeing their partner as "Mother" and "Lover" and some, often unwittingly, to be fair, force her to make a choice. As a result, breastfeeding can suffer.

The pleasures of breastfeeding

Part of this confusion is that breastfeeding can be highly pleasurable for a woman, and for some even sexually arousing. In fact, some women find feeding their baby one of the more sensual experiences they've had. But breastfeeding, like intercourse, must have been enjoyable throughout history, or the human race would have died out.

But a few women feel uncomfortable, even guilty or ashamed, about any perceived link between sexuality and breastfeeding. Such women say they are particularly concerned if they feel aroused when breastfeeding a boy, or notice he occasionally has an erection while feeding. How, a woman's unconscious may wonder, could she possibly cause such a response in her own son? Incest is a major taboo, and this sort of incident puts some women off breastfeeding.

309

Men's and women's views of sex and breastfeeding

Men largely think of sex in terms of their desire for penetrative inter-course, with them and, perhaps, their partners, having an orgasm. But most women think differently. Sex to them is closely bound up with other factors, such as their wish to find a lifetime partner who will look after them and father their children, the need for contraception, and the pos-sibility of having a baby. In other words, women tend to view intercourse differently because it's they who carry and nurture babies. It's also part of a much larger "sexual" and emotional picture than it is for the average man.

While to most men breastfeeding is simply a way of feeding a baby, to many women it's an extension of their commitment to getting pregnant with a particular man—a commitment that in some mystical, let alone practical sense, they ideally want to last a lifetime.

In traditional cultures many millions of women are pregnant or lac-tating for most of their reproductive lives, and breastfeeding is still by far the most important form of contraception. The average western woman, though, doesn't want to be ruled by her cycles, and doesn't have babies every two or three years. On the contrary, she spends much of her repro-ductive life avoiding pregnancy. Such a woman increasingly wants very few babies, and prefers to look flat-bellied, slim, and even somewhat mas-culine in body style. However, most women want to experience the whole range of female sexuality, including pregnancy, birth and breastfeeding. Not surprisingly, these diverse desires are sometimes difficult for her to reconcile, let alone for society as a whole. Men too have problems with these conflicting concepts.

What breasts represent

Breasts are the erotic focus for millions of men in many countries. But in the many cultures around the world that don't eroticize breasts as we do, women tend to breastfeed for much longer.

Could it be that over the last century "breast-erotic" societies have become so deprived of the experience of being comforted and nourished at the breast—and so habituated to seeing images of the eroticized and "unmotherly" breast—that men seek to replace their unmet infantile needs and primitive drives in other ways, albeit later in life? Such ways could, perhaps, include compulsive behaviors such as promiscuous sex, and various methods of oral gratification, including overeating, smoking, and drinking.

Or could society's eroticization of the breast make women less likely to want to breastfeed and men less likely to support them? With both men and women putting such an emphasis on breasts as sex objects, it's hardly surprising that erotic overtones can militate against breastfeeding. Studies have shown that some women won't even consider breastfeeding because they believe it will ruin their figure and render them sexually unattractive.

Breastfeeding and sex

Both sexual arousal and lactation make a woman's breasts larger and more sensitive, and many women feel protective or motherly both after intercourse and when breastfeeding. This is because the level in a woman's blood of the powerful sex hormone oxytocin increases during both intercourse and lactation.

More than half of all women get a lot of pleasure from their breasts when making love; some, indeed, claim they can have an orgasm from breast-play alone. And breast stimulation during breastfeeding makes some women at least partially sexually aroused. All this is hardly surprising, given that the nipples and genitals are interconnected by nervous pathways in the brain.

The degree of sexual arousal caused by breastfeeding is variable. Some women notice nothing; some report feeling "nice"; others have increased vaginal moisture; and a few feel they could actually climax. Some women feel euphoric or contented after a feed in a similar way to after an orgasm. Some such women find these experiences make them feel emotionally and sexually closer to their man. Indeed, studies show that breastfeeders return to having sex earlier after childbirth than other women. However, whether lactating women in general tend to feel sexier than bottle-feeders in general isn't at all clear. Some feel more sexy, others less so. And any one woman may feel different from one baby to another, or while breastfeeding any one baby.

- One interesting study suggests that women who spend time with breastfeeding mothers experience greater sexual desire. This is thought to be partly because they produce pheromones (hormone-like substances in sweat and other skin secretions) whose scent affects nearby women at an unconscious level. It's possible that they act as a signaling system to inform a woman's body that it's safe for her to reproduce (*New Scientist*, 2002).

Off sex after childbirth?

Recently delivered women are traditionally advised to wait for several weeks before having actual intercourse. When they get the all-clear from their doctor, some women find their sex drive is dampened, while some simply don't feel sexy. There are several possible reasons:

Fatigue

Probably the biggest reason for not feeling sexy is exhaustion. Many mothers of young babies who are waking at night, whether breastfeeding or not, are too tired even to think about sex! Fathers may be tired too. If your baby wakes often, consider having him by your bed so you can easily feed him without having to wake properly. Or you could have him actually in your bed. You can make love while your baby sleeps near you.

Stretched or stitched vagina

The second most likely reason is that a woman's vagina is still recovering from being stretched or stitched during childbirth. Time and patience will prevail, but it may help to insert a finger (yours or your partner's) into your vagina the first few times you feel like making love. Then, over several days or weeks, insert two, then three fingers, then his penis, using a lubricant if necessary.

Tender breasts

Your breasts may sometimes be so full and tense that they're tender to the touch. A way around this is to express some milk. Or you could encourage your partner to suck your nipples as you start making love; there's no need to worry about him taking milk from the baby—there'll be plenty there. Relieving the tension in your breasts will eliminate any tenderness and may also help you get aroused.

Leaking milk

You may feel embarrassed about leaking as you get aroused or have an orgasm, or you might be concerned about milk wetting your bedclothes. Some men, too, are put off by leaking. You can reduce the chance of leaking by taking off a little milk before you make love, as above. Some women feed their baby before lovemaking, for this reason.

Too much responsibility

A few women, first-timers especially, find having total responsibility for a baby and all the other pressures of motherhood too much and feel so anxious and overwhelmed that they lose interest in sex.

Not ovulating

Another possible reason for feeling less sexy in the early months after childbirth is that exclusive unrestricted breastfeeding suppresses ovulation, and for many women their peak of sexual interest is around the time they ovulate.

Shocked by childbirth

Some women are so shocked by giving birth that they consciously or unconsciously avoid sex because they don't want any chance of another pregnancy.

No need for the previous intimacy you had with your partner

It is common for some women to find their relationship with their baby and their sensations from breastfeeding so powerful and fulfilling that they no longer need the sensual and erotic experiences they used to have with their partner. This may make him feel excluded, though whether he's upset by this depends on his background and personality. A woman's intense interest in her newborn is normal; it's also relatively temporary. Prevent or deal with any challenges this presents to your relationship by being open and frank with each other.

Shows up your lack of intimacy with your partner

Some women say the intimacy and delight they share with their baby, and their feeling of being needed by him, and special to him, stand in stark contrast to the poverty of emotional intimacy and pleasure they share with their partner. A few such women stay with their man only because they get rewards from their relationship with their baby.

However, relying for your emotional sustenance on your relationship with a baby is at best short-sighted, at worst even abusive. Young children rely on parents to meet their needs, but parents shouldn't rely on their children to meet their own—this is the wrong way round.

If you have an unsatisfactory relationship with your partner, consider seeing a counselor or therapist for help in making your relationship more rewarding to you both.

Want to avoid intimacy with your partner

A few women unconsciously use their commitment to breastfeeding and mothering as a way of avoiding sexual or emotional intimacy with their partner. Certain women, unconsciously, or even consciously, will have wanted this all along.

Need a "comfort blanket"

The first year of their child's life is one of the most common times for a man to have an affair or the couple to break up. A woman betrayed in this way may focus intensely on breastfeeding or mothering as a way of diverting her attention, consoling herself, boosting her self-esteem, and obtaining some degree of emotional intimacy.

Focusing on your partner

Experience and studies show that if a woman's partner encourages her in breastfeeding, she is more likely to do it successfully. Some men, though, resent their baby intruding into their sexual and emotional life, and want their previous life back as soon as possible. Their spoken or unspoken messages make their partner less likely to breastfeed for as long as she wants.

If this happens to you, find verbal and nonverbal ways of letting your man know he's still central to your life and that you love him. Obviously you'd like him to be a tower of strength as you adjust to being the parent of a newborn baby. But this particular challenge is happening to both of you at the same time, and at an unconscious level may well be making this grown man feel like a needy, frightened, or angry little boy. Psychologists call new parenthood the "third childhood," because its challenges can evoke emotional issues unresolved since infancy (our "first childhood") or adolescence (our "second childhood").

A loving couple can usually work on this by addressing the situation honestly and explaining how they feel about parenthood, breastfeeding, and sex—or the lack of it. But both of you may temporarily need support and encouragement from someone wise and trusted.

A problem can occur if a man who's psychologically thrown by the experience of new fatherhood, and his partner's concentration on her baby, continues to feel rejected and abandoned.

Some of these feelings will stem from his experience of being mothered in babyhood. Part of an infant's emotional development is to see important experiences or things as either all good or all bad. For example, the breast that isn't there when a baby boy is desperately hungry becomes a "bad" or even "punishing" breast belonging to a "bad" mother.

As he grows, provided he is exposed to "good-enough" mothering, he's likely to resolve this "splitting" of important experiences, things or people into good and bad, and comes to see the breast—and, indeed, his mother—as good and bad, not either/or.

But if he doesn't resolve this splitting, then any important future stressor, including new parenthood, can bring up his original infantile tendency to see things as all good or all bad. Although this operates at an unconscious level, it can have far-reaching effects on his attitudes and behavior.

Your man has a responsibility in all this, and it will help if he tries to become more aware his feelings and practices sharing them with you—or with a trusted friend—rather than acting them out in unhelpful and inappropriate ways, such as by storming off, criticizing your lack of interest in him, or even having an affair in an effort to find the love he fears he's lost.

When discussing any of this, make a pact to express your feelings using "I" language, rather than "you" language. For example, say, "I feel such and such . . . ," rather than, "You make me feel such and such . . ." This is more honest, less confrontational, and less threatening.

Focusing on you

Some women think their lactating breasts, with their initially increased size, look rather sexy and enjoy showing them off to their man. Others are shy about them. Others find that large, full, possibly tender, and leaky breasts make them feel anything but sexy and attractive. If your lactating breasts make you feel more womanly and "female," your perception of breastfeeding will be different, and its chances of success better, than if you dislike the way they look and the way you feel about them.

Breastfeeding is most likely to be successful if a woman likes her breasts, enjoys them being touched, and sees them as a vital part of her \ femininity. One US study found that women with sexual hang-ups were much less likely to breastfeed successfully. Other studies looking at women's reasons for not breastfeeding as they intended reveal that in a substantial minority this was because they found it "distasteful" or "immodest." Such women see their breasts as "private," and the notion of having to expose them other than for washing or medical examination completely unacceptable.

Indeed, a few women are actually revolted by the thought of a baby sucking their breasts. They say it's too animalistic, too primitive, not what they want at all. The roots of such feelings are often very deep. Just as the experience of new fatherhood can make a man think at an unconscious level of the breast, breastfeeding, and his partner as the symbolic mother, as bad, so too may this happen to a woman.

Whether you feel like a mom or a sexual playmate in bed, you may be happy for your partner to play with your breasts as he did before. He may also want to suck your nipples and taste your milk, which is fine if it's okay with you.

Once you start making love again you'll probably notice a few changes. Some women say their nipples don't erect and their breasts don't swell like they used to. This is most likely when their breasts are full of milk. The solution is to take off a little. And try changing the positions in which you make love if your larger breasts get in the way.

The foundations for successful breastfeeding are influenced by a woman's early experiences with men. If she's learned to value and enjoy her breasts in her sexual relationships, she'll be more receptive to breastfeeding.

Once you have your baby, involve your partner in your enjoyment of breastfeeding, if he wants. And aim to keep up some aspects of your "lover" image, so you don't give your partner messages that you've gone off him in favor of mothering. It may take time before you begin to feel sexy again, though, so be gentle and patient with yourself.

Honest communication between new parents is at the heart of a successful relationship. It also encourages enjoyable and effective parenting, and successful breastfeeding.

Many couples make breastfeeding a time of personal growth, and succeed in nourishing not only their baby but also their emotional and sexual relationship.

fifteen

Breastfeeding and Work

You don't need to stop breastfeeding just because you're going back to work. Millions of women around the world successfully combine the two. And this is just as well because women are an important part of the workforce, and most young women see themselves as economic units. For most, raising young children has to fit in with working full or part time.

Some mothers with young babies work because they must, some so they don't slip off the career ladder, others because they'd rather work than stay at home. Most, though, say they would prefer to stay at home with their young children. Many feel anxious about leaving their children. And almost all would prefer not to work full time after having a baby.

It's difficult to know how many mothers of young children work, because so many of those who do so work part time or at home, and their activity is unrecorded by government agencies.

- A survey of nearly 19,000 women in the UK showed that 3 in 4 middle-income mothers worked when their babies were under a year.

But only one in five lower-income mothers did (*Journal of Epidemiology and Community Health*, 2011).

- Of 228,000 mothers of new babies in the US, only 26 percent of those who worked full-time were still breastfeeding at 6 months, compared with 35 percent of the whole sample. Those mothers who didn't work were more than twice as likely to be still breastfeeding at six months as were mothers who worked full time (*Women's Health Issues*, 2006).

- In a large UK survey (*Infant Feeding*, 2005), mothers who returned to work before their baby was 6 months old were more likely to have stopped breastfeeding by 6 months than mothers who returned when their baby was older, or who weren't working at all.

If you're pregnant and planning to return to work when your baby is very young, and if you're wondering if it's worth bothering to breastfeed for a short period before you go back, the answer is a definite "Yes." No matter how short a time you do it you and your baby will benefit.

Breastfeeding women either stop before they return to work, or somehow find ways of continuing when they go back after maternity leave. With planning and determination, even exclusive breastfeeding is compatible with full-time work outside the home.

Support at home

It's particularly vital if you're a breastfeeding working woman to get all the support you need to help you look after your baby and yourself, maintain a home, and enjoy your relationship with your partner, family, and friends. Your partner may be the obvious person to help at home, but he may be too busy with his work or insufficiently motivated or knowledgeable. Of course, you may not have a live-in partner—or, indeed, a partner at all. But whoever helps, you must be clear and specific about what you need done. Management skills are very important for working breastfeeding mothers! Assess the situation regularly so you can use your resources more effectively.

Some partners and helpers are worried that they know too little about breastfeeding to be of any real help. This is understandable but wrong. It'll be you who'll make the decisions about what you'll do and how you'll do it—your helper only needs to know how to help you achieve your goals. Reading this book will be a great start, as you'll then be aiming for the same things.

HOW YOUR PARTNER CAN HELP

Here are some practical suggestions. He could

1. Discuss your joint "management strategy" so you work out between you what needs doing and how you can best share it. It'll certainly help to work as a team.

2. Do some chores, such as making a shopping list, shopping (or inputting the Internet shopping list), unpacking the shopping and putting it away, deciding what to eat, cooking, serving food, clearing the table, dishwashing, cleaning, bed-making, laundering, putting clothes away, refueling the car, paying bills, remembering birthdays, organizing celebrations, mending things, and, perhaps, gardening. Helping to keep the "nest" in order is vital if your partner goes back to work.

3. Change diapers, help with bath time, play with the baby, bathe him or have a bath with him, soothe him by walking around with him, get him off to sleep by carrying him in a sling or rocking him. If you have other children, get him to help as much as he can with them.

4. Give you a massage or a cuddle.

5. Be encouraging and affirming (page 191).

6. Be your ally and your friend.

Support at work

But however good your domestic arrangements, you'll need a helpful, understanding employer if you're going to succeed at being a breastfeeding working mother.

- Researchers in Chile found that 53 percent of working mothers who were given support with breastfeeding continued with exclusive breastfeeding until 6 months, compared with only 6 percent of those not given special support (*Journal of Tropical Pediatrics*, 1999).

Talk with your employer early in your pregnancy about your plans to breastfeed. Facilities and support at work are very important if women are to breastfeed exclusively for six months and perhaps even for longer. This is now well recognized in many countries and most have laws that ensure employers make breastfeeding easy. This said, individuals in your particular workplace may not to be up to speed on these regulations and you may have to take them gently through your expectations and see what can be achieved.

At this stage it makes sense to think about arranging flexible working hours and, if you want to breastfeed in "company time," you'll need to let your employers know in writing. Attitudes have changed dramatically all over the world on this subject and campaigners and legislators have so improved matters that in most countries a working breastfeeding woman no longer finds herself banished to a bathroom or dressing room to feed or express milk.

Most employers now have a policy that includes: break allowances for the mother who wants to feed or to express milk; a clean, decent place where she can express or feed; a fridge for storing expressed milk; and work hours that make breastfeeding possible.

The International Labour Organization recommends that breastfeeding mothers should have two breaks of at least half an hour each in the working day. Many countries recognize these breaks. They mean a breastfeeding woman can express or breastfeed once during a morning nursing break, once in the lunch break, and once in an afternoon one.

In the US, a new amendment to the Fair Labor Standards Act was made law in 2010. This requires employers to provide a breastfeeding mother, for a year after her baby's birth,

- Reasonable break time to express milk during the working day.

- A private place that isn't a bathroom in which to do this.

It's important to remember that there are also benefits to your employer in all this—he's not doing you a favor. Research shows that employers who make breastfeeding easy have reduced absences caused by child sickness; increased staff morale; a higher rate of return to work; lower recruitment and training costs; and a really good incentive to offer future female employees. This is certainly not a one-way street.

Combining work and breastfeeding

If you work, the easiest solution is to work at home if possible. Your employer may facilitate this now that so much can be done remotely in our linked-up, Internet-based world. Most women try to continue with their existing employment if at all possible, but if this can't be arranged there are hundreds of home-based jobs, from making things, word-processing and writing, to telephone selling. There are numerous working-from-home websites that can help.

The next easiest option is to work part-time and locally. Working locally cuts down on commuting which means you can easily and quickly get home to your baby in an emergency. If you are really close by he may need feeding only once while you're away. If you leave him with a babysitter, you can leave expressed breast milk in the refrigerator to be given from a cup. As it'll always be so fresh, it'll never need freezing.

Working part time a long way from home or full time anywhere means being away from your baby for a lot longer. You can express or pump enough milk to leave for him while you're away, but this requires considerable effort, time, and determination. While it's good because he'll have only breast milk while you're at work, and you'll keep your milk supply going, it also means both you and he will miss out on the pleasure of actual breastfeeding. As a result, he won't be able to be at the breast when he wants to be particularly close to you for reassurance or comfort.

A few women manage to leave enough milk for their baby while they're at work just by expressing or pumping after the early-morning feed, when their breasts are fuller than at other times of day. But most need to express or pump after each feed at home. While breastfeeding, expressing, or pumping, they may also collect "drip milk" from the other breast. One way of doing this is to put a breast shell inside their bra cup to collect the drip milk, though make sure that any holes in it are at the top so it doesn't leak.

However, in order to leave enough milk for your baby to have while you're away, you may also have to express or pump at work and take the milk home at the end of the day for him to have the next day.

Well before you go back to work, practice expressing or start using a pump so you become confident. This will be one less thing to worry about once you're combining work and breastfeeding. As part of this preparation phase it makes sense to do some trial runs of collecting milk and being apart from your baby.

Don't forget that when you're back at work you'll need some backup tops and breast pads. It could be embarrassing to discover this the hard way in that vital meeting! You might also want to keep a duplicate set of a insulated bag, ice pack, and milk-collection containers in case you ever forget to bring them to work in the morning.

Expressing milk

Aim to express at least every three hours while you and your baby are apart—and more often if necessary. Express after feeds at home too. You'll probably get only a very small volume when you express after a feed, but several small volumes added together soon mount up. You'll quickly discover what's best.

Make sure your babysitter knows how to warm and swirl your milk, and unless you're sure you've left enough, tell her what to give if he's still hungry after having the milk you've left. Boiled, cooled water will fill his tummy for a while. But if he ever does need water, take steps to increase your milk supply so you'll be able to leave more in future. Formula should be the very last resort.

Reasons for expressing at work include the following:

1. So you can add it later to the milk you express at home, and thereby leave enough for the next day.

2. So your breasts don't become too full. If they do, you risk discomfort, a blocked duct, breast infection, and a gradual reduction in your milk supply. You can always throw away any excess milk your baby doesn't need.

3. So you can keep up your milk supply. Expressing encourages your breasts to produce more. But it doesn't stimulate them as well as your baby does, so you may have to express more often than you would feed, or use a pump too.

Expressing at work will take longer than feeding your baby at home and calls for privacy and somewhere comfortable to sit. Express your milk into a clean plastic container and then cover it and keep it cold. If you can't refrigerate it, put it into a wide-necked vacuum flask containing some ice put in before you left home in the morning. The flask will also protect the milk on your journey home. Alternatively, use a small cooler bag containing an ice pack frozen at home. Put the ice pack into the refrigerator at work so it's ready to go back into the cooler before you take your milk home.

If you don't want to express at work, you can breastfeed before you go in to work in the morning and as soon as you get back, as well as in the evening and at night.

When deciding whether to go back to work, bear in mind that getting up at night and working full time can be very tiring. Also, some babies so like being with their mother that they get in the habit of waking very frequently at night, as if to make up for lost time during the day. For your sake, make nighttime feeds as boring as possible! This might involve having the light dimmed or off, and keeping quiet and nonstimulating.

Of course, when you're with your baby during the day you can breast-feed as often and for as long as you both want. Combined with continued regular expression at work, this should keep your milk supply going.

Get him used to the bottle?

Many women ask whether they should accustom their baby to a bottle before returning to work. In the first few months, before breastfeeding is properly established, it's better not to. When your baby is hungry he'll almost certainly take your expressed breast milk from a cup given by the babysitter (though he may understandably refuse a cup if you offer it). If he isn't interested at first, the babysitter should persevere and all will eventually be well. In the early months a cup is better than a bottle because some babies given a bottle soon learn to prefer it to the breast then make a fuss when breastfed. Giving expressed breast milk from a spoon is another option.

If your baby is older than four months, drinking your milk from a bottle shouldn't interfere with him breastfeeding when you're there.

Looking after yourself

If you're a working breastfeeding mother, the odds are you'll be tired, especially if you have older children as well. So it's particularly essential to look after yourself. I look at this in some detail on page 173.

Enjoying your baby

Without a doubt leaving your baby to go back to work can be a real wrench—and even actually stressful, especially if you're returning within weeks rather than months or years. Even if you are looking forward to getting back to friends and intellectual stimulation, being parted from your young baby will be hard—for both of you. This is normal, if painful.

Spend time with baby and your intended caregiver together well before you start leaving him. This gives him an opportunity to get used to her while you're still there.

When you pick him up at the end of the day, spend time showing him that the caregiver and you are extensions of one another. Ask her about his day. Remember that in preindustrial societies several women would care for a baby over any given day. And such childrearing has been shown to be highly successful.

Some working mothers encourage their babies to stay awake in the evenings so they can spend more time with them. It has to be said that some babies have similar ideas! Night feeds can be precious times when you and your baby take a delight in each other's company but you'll need to balance this with your need for sleep as a working woman. Carrying him around in a sling when you are with him in the day can help provide maximum connection. It's also important to remember that unless you're running a major corporation you'll be with your baby far more than you'll be without him over any seven-day period.

Whatever you do, bear in mind you'll probably have only one or two babies in a lifetime and they'll only be really tiny and dependent on you for a short time. All life involves making compromises and with thought, planning, help, and determination, you should be able to enjoy both your job and your baby.

sixteen

Mainly for Fathers

The role of fathers has altered a lot over the four decades since the first edition of this book and looks set to change even more. In the 1970s, most people expected a young child's parents to be married and living together, with the man the main breadwinner and the child's biological father.

While this is still the case for many young children today it has become less so, and things are on the move. A man living with a woman may not be her child's biological father. In the US, more than one in three children lives apart from the biological father. In the UK, nearly one in five firstborn babies begin life without their biological father living with them. Similar trends are happening in some other westernized countries too. Even when the man in the home is the biological parent, his lifestyle is likely to be considerably different from that of a father of similar age 30 years ago.

Fathering today tends to fall into one of two types. In the first, the man works to support his family. Many such men find the workplace insecure and stressful. In the second, the father is either out of work or employed on a temporary basis, so feels financially insecure. He may even feel panicky over whether his family has security of tenure in their home.

So both groups can find themselves either overstretched or otherwise stressed and with less time or energy for their family than they'd like.

It's a paradox that social-welfare systems aren't always beneficial to family life. Some of the more recent changes, such as the option for paternal leave or shared parental leave after a child is born, can benefit breastfeeding. However, a stressed man may not welcome a request from his partner for him to take time off work after the birth. He may also fear that his colleagues and employers will interpret his absence as a lack of commitment to his job.

In addition, if his partner previously contributed significantly to the family income, or was the major breadwinner, he may prefer to see her back at work as quickly as possible to take the pressure off him. If he imagines that her work and breastfeeding won't mix, he may encourage her to formula-feed.

Some men don't much care about breastfeeding because they don't know about its many advantages. Once they learn, though, they usually see how important their contribution to supporting it can be.

Why you're so important to breastfeeding

The father of a breastfed baby is a very important person and can play several helpful roles.

For example, a few hospitals even today still give breastfed babies water or formula unnecessarily, especially at night. If this isn't what your partner wants (which it almost certainly isn't if she's aiming to breastfeed successfully) you can prevent it happening. Remind the staff that you and your partner want your baby to be totally breastfed. Don't be put off by someone saying it doesn't matter if he has the occasional bottle. It may very well matter if breastfeeding is to have the best chance of success.

Stay with your partner during and after the birth if she wants you there. This is one of the most important events in her life and she may need your company and support. She may also feel emotionally and physically keyed up, or exhausted, and anything you can do to help, support, love and encourage her could help get breastfeeding off to a good start.

In the US some women are asked immediately after childbirth whether they want to breastfeed, and if the answer is "no," they're given an injection to dry up their milk. This happens in certain other countries too. However, if a woman hasn't made her final decision, she'll probably be in no fit state to decide in the few minutes after giving birth. Some women who decide at this time to bottle-feed wish later that they'd had more time to think. In the UK dry-up drugs are given only rarely, but if your partner is offered them, ask if she really needs them, or whether, if she's going to bottle-feed, she could instead let her milk dry up of its own accord. If she's had dry-up drugs, then changes her mind, she should be reassured that she'll be able to get her milk back, although this takes time and determination.

Some women feel low in the first week after childbirth. It's then that they may need most help with breastfeeding. One experienced breast-feeding counselor says she thinks that successful lactation depends on a woman's helpers, not her ability to produce milk. You could be your partner's most valuable helper.

However useful you are in the hospital, you can help even more when your partner gets home. Take a couple of weeks off work if you can, so you can be there for her, especially if you have other children. You'll be particularly important as a provider, protector, and general helper over the next few weeks, and you'll play an even more valuable part in family life than usual. Many women hope, or expect, the home to run as it did before they had the baby, and many men feel much the same. But if your partner is to breastfeed successfully, and you can't take time off work, you'll almost certainly need help in the home from family or friends or, if you can afford it, paid assistance.

Fathers who've been taught how to manage common challenges with breastfeeding can be a very real help in enabling a woman to continue breastfeeding for as long as she wants.

- Researchers in Naples, Italy, worked with 280 expectant fathers, giving some of them training in breastfeeding management, the others just an ordinary fathers' prenatal class. Twenty-five percent of the partners of those who'd had special training breastfed at birth, compared with only 15 percent of the others. What's more, 19 percent were still partially breastfeeding at 1 year, compared with 11 percent of the others; 5 percent thought at some time they had insufficient milk, compared with 27 percent of the others; and 4 percent were still breastfeeding at 6 months despite experiencing difficulty, compared with 24 percent of the others (*Pediatrics*, 2005).

Your partner will need emotional backup too, because breastfeeding is a deeply emotional business. So listen empathically whenever possible. This involves three steps:

THREE STEPS TO EMPATHIC LISTENING

1. Put your own concerns aside so you can focus on her.
2. Try to understand how she's feeling so you can identify her main emotions.
3. Let her know what you sense is going on for her emotionally, using "feelings" words such as "anxious," "angry," "afraid," "disappointed" and "jealous." It doesn't matter if you're wrong.

Most of us like to know that someone understands where we're at. Good listening can also help fend off postpartum depression, as this is particularly likely in women who feel emotionally alone in their new role. Research has shown that mammals of many species (including humans) produce less milk, or even stop producing it, if disturbed or stressed while breastfeeding. Serenity fosters successful breastfeeding, and having you to listen to how she's feeling will allow her to let off steam and enjoy her baby. Having her feelings heard makes her realize you care, and that she isn't alone.

Many women feel very emotional after having a baby, partly because of the physical, hormonal, and emotional upheaval of childbirth and becoming a mother, and partly because of the changes in lifestyle. This could be challenging for you to understand.

It's wise to be especially sensitive, and careful what you say. A casual or thoughtless remark could destroy her confidence and make her feel inadequate.

If you have other children, you'll need to look after them or organize others to do it so your partner can get the rest she needs. You can also be a buffer between her and the outside world. Relatives and friends may be keen to see her and the new baby, but make sure they come in small doses. Many's the time a recently delivered mother has become so exhausted by visitors that she hasn't the energy to get breastfeeding off to a good start.

Encouragement is another thing you can provide. Studies show that if a woman's partner doesn't want her to breastfeed, she rarely manages to do so. Even if he's simply neutral, the chances of successful feeding are greatly reduced. One American breastfeeding counselor who guaranteed success wouldn't accept a woman as a client unless her man approved of breastfeeding. It's better if your attitude is positive from the beginning, as your partner may find breastfeeding particularly challenging in the first few days while she's learning how to do it. She'll need loving encouragement and support and will especially value it coming from you.

Some common concerns

Two things that concern men most about breastfeeding (or at least the things they most often talk about, which isn't necessarily the same) are whether their partner will (a) go off sex and (b) lose her figure. There's more about sex and breastfeeding in chapter 14 but let's look at the figure question here.

Virtually every man thinks of his partner's breasts first and foremost as sex objects. Of course breasts are for feeding babies too. But during a couple's life together, which could be up to 40 to 60 years or more, their erotic role is important for a much longer time. So it's foolish to ignore any fears a man may have about his partner having droopy breasts after breastfeeding.

But let's consider what actually happens. All breasts enlarge during pregnancy. If she breastfeeds, they stay bigger for longer. This can be a bonus for the man who likes large breasts! Indeed, some such men are greatly turned on by their breastfeeding partner's larger breasts and more erectile nipples. Wearing a well-fitting bra night and day in later pregnancy, and while breastfeeding, supports heavier-than-usual breasts and prevents their skin becoming overstretched, which maintains their original shape. Many women find their breasts are softer after they stop breastfeeding. This is because the milk glands and ducts shrink quite abruptly after stopping. But as the weeks and months pass, a woman's body fat is redistributed, and her breasts' contours gradually fill out again. Research suggests that any change in breast size and shape results from pregnancy, not breastfeeding.

But whatever happens, does it really matter? The fashion for perfect breasts isn't just crazy—it's also wholly unrealistic.

You and your baby

Many fathers say they like the idea of their partner breastfeeding partly because it's such an intrinsically feminine thing to do. But it can leave them feeling there's little they can do for their baby. Indeed, some men like the idea of bottle-feeding because they can then give their baby the occasional feed. And at a time in history when increasing numbers of young men feel useless, helpless, or even hopeless, feeding their baby is something they feel they can do to contribute.

This certainly isn't a good reason for persuading your partner not to breastfeed, because there are innumerable things you can do with your breastfed baby, including cuddling, playing, and bathing—all of which are much more fun than bottle-feeding!

Some new fathers feel shut out of the excitement of the first few days. Your partner is closely involved with her newborn, and you may feel she and the baby are hogging the limelight and excluding you. However, although you aren't center stage, this can be a wonderful time for you and potentially for your self-development too. You can be proud of bringing a new life into the world. You also have the opportunity to practice being selfless and learning how to back up your partner while she finds her feet looking after and breastfeeding your child. For many fathers of a newborn baby this "mothering" role is a completely new experience. Many enjoy it a lot.

While this all comes easily to some men, others find it a challenge. You may have been used to being looked after by your partner, just as your mother looked after you before that, and can't easily change roles.

Talking all this through may help you accept and enjoy your new role. Discussing it with men who've been here can be particularly useful.

Caring for your breastfeeding partner can add a new dimension to your relationship—one in which you mature from being a big boy to a real man who gives as much, or more, than you receive. This could lead to positive growth and change.

Benefits of breastfeeding to you

Having a breastfed baby and a breastfeeding partner can provide you with benefits you might not have considered:

- You won't have to get up at night to take your turn preparing and giving bottle-feeds.

- You can't run out of milk powder at awkward times. And it's one thing less to buy!

- There's much less equipment to carry when going out, traveling, or going on vacation.

- You'll get pleasure from seeing your partner enjoying the feelings of femininity, fulfillment, and intimacy so many women experience with breastfeeding, and also from knowing you're contributing by being there to support her.

Looking after yourself

With all the fuss, commotion, and excitement over your new baby, it's all too easy to forget yourself and your needs. But you'll enjoy this time more and have more to offer if your energy, health and well-being are being cared for. This checklist might help:

- Are you getting enough sleep? If you're waking a lot when your partner breastfeeds at night, you may find yourself dropping off during the day. Perhaps you could learn to catnap during your lunch break at work, sleep in another room for part of the night, or take a short nap in the early evening or when you've helped get any other children to bed.

- Are you getting a healthy diet? You need to keep up your stamina if you're to support your partner.

- Are you keeping up your interests and hobbies? While you may need to put them on hold, in the early weeks in particular, there's no need to give up all your interests and become a second mother to the baby. Balance is everything.

- What about exercise? Time is often short at this stage of life, but if you work those muscles and get your circulation going you'll enjoy higher levels of "feel-good" cannabinoids and keep yourself fit for your new role.

- Is there anyone around for you? Your partner may be too absorbed while she's getting used to the new baby and, if it's her first child, to motherhood. Yet you may need someone to help you adjust to your new role. Many men benefit from talking about the feelings, changes, and responsibilities that accompany their new lifestyle. Few men find it easy to "let it all hang out." But a shared joke, and the relief of being honest about the highs and low of your new lifestyle, can be a godsend. Getting out with friends can also help keep everything in perspective.

Pass on the message

As the dad of a breastfed baby, and partner of a breastfeeding woman, you're in a position to do some very valuable work. This could involve letting some of the men and boys in your local community know about the benefits of breastfeeding and the value of being a supportive father. So if circumstances permit, consider asking a local prenatal teacher if she'd like you, your partner, and the baby to attend a class to talk about your role, your feelings, and the pleasure of breastfeeding. And if you have an "in" to a local school, you could do the same with whoever teaches biology or personal and social development.

Most boys today never see a baby being breastfed, and never get the chance to talk about being a father. If their own father has left the family, they may never be exposed to a positive role model for fathering either. So your contribution, however small it may seem to you, could have an enormous and lasting significance. You may feel you'd be vulnerable to criticism if you went public as a "breastfeeding dad," but experience suggests you'd be very warmly received by fathers-to-be at prenatal classes and by boys at school.

seventeen

A Word for Helpers

Various people, including a woman's partner, relatives, friends, neighbors, breastfeeding counselors, lactation consultants, doctors, and nurses, may offer advice encouragement or other help with breastfeeding.

Note that the support of a breastfeeding mother by a woman who has herself breastfed successfully has been found to be a significant factor in helping such a mother to breastfeed for as long as she wants.

"Mothering the mother" is very important. Indeed, it's considered vital in many cultures. This is perhaps especially so if she is breastfeeding her first baby, when she has everything to learn, may be anxious about doing things right and needs all the help she can get to encourage her in her new adventure. If she has other children she'll also need help of a more practical kind as the new addition puts further pressure on her time and energy.

If you're helping someone to breastfeed, these tips will guide you in being really useful

7 tips for helping effectively

1. Be encouraging—as just a few words can give a breastfeeding woman confidence when she most needs it. I vividly remember being in a postnatal ward at King's College Hospital, London, giving my first baby one of her earliest feeds with a midwife, Staff Nurse Benjamin, watching. Smiling, she said, "Mrs Stanway, you're a wonderful mother." Her warmth and encouragement have stayed with me ever since. If a woman has a breastfeeding problem, simply identifying something she's doing that she can be pleased about—then telling her—can help her find a way through simply by generating feelings of self-esteem and instilling the belief that she can succeed. This is especiallyimportant for a beginner. There's always something to encourage—even simply the readiness to seek help.

2. Be positive about breastfeeding—though never ever pressure or bully a woman to breastfeed. And however strongly you feel, try not to be evangelistic. Studies show that a health professional's enthusiasm encourages women to start and to continue. The attitude of a mother's partner or mother or other supportive helper, can make all the difference too.

3. Develop empathic-listening skills (page 327)—so you can recognize from a woman's words and body language how she feels about breastfeeding and any challenges or special situations she's facing. Then check out with her how you think she's feeling, so she feels understood.

4. Listen to yourself—so you're aware of your emotions too. Then put them aside so they don't interfere with listening to and being there for the breastfeeding woman you're helping. Note that a mother's (page 95) and a father's (page 329) feelings about breastfeeding can apply to a helper too. If you have uncomfortable feelings about breastfeeding, they may stem from difficult situations in your past or current life. For example, they may concern the mothering you had, or the love you have or don't have today. And if you've had children, they may stem from your experiences of feeding them. Such emotions could include fear, helplessness, jealousy, envy, feeling unloved, anger, yearning, and neediness. If none of these sound familiar, either they don't apply to you, or you might be unwittingly suppressing them. It might be helpful to discuss your feelings with someone you value if they're getting in the way of your being an effective helper.

5. Observe your own behavior—We're unaware of suppressed emotions because our unconscious mind has built defenses to stop them hurting us. But observing the deeply significant, symbolic and primal act of breastfeeding can sometimes break down these defenses enough to let painful suppressed emotions surface. You might then feel so uncomfortable that you find yourself unwittingly encouraging formula-feeding. You're now no longer an effective breastfeeding helper. This could be your unwitting way of preventing the pain. It might even be because at an unconscious level you want to punish your own mother for having been a "bad" mother—and this breastfeeding mother now somehow represents your mother.

Wha tever the reason, you might unconsciously want to separate a breastfeeding mother from her baby by putting a bottle between them. But you're getting your stuff mixed up with hers. If you think you need to come to terms with painful emotions or explore unwanted behaviors, you may want to discuss your feelings with a trusted friend or even a counselor.

6. If you're explaining the benefits of breastfeeding,

- Put aside any fear that doing so will engender guilt in a woman who decides not to breastfeed, or can't. Such a fear is unrealistic. Your job is to aid her decision-making. Her decision will be well informed only if she has good-quality information. If, after weighing the pros and cons as she sees them, she decides not to breastfeed, your job is then to give her the opportunity to discuss her reasons and her feelings about what's she's decided. Doing this respects her and honors her decision. She's then much less likely to suppress uncomfortable feelings which could seep out as guilt. She needs to know you'll support her in her decision, whichever way it goes.

- Be open to learning as new research continues to elucidate the benefits of breastfeeding.

- If you don't know the answer to a question or problem, say you'll find out.

7. Give yourself the credit you deserve for being a breastfeeding helper.

Resources

Recommended reading list

The Womanly Art of Breastfeeding, La Leche League International.
The Politics of Breastfeeding, Gabrielle Palmer.

La Leche League (page 357) and the NCT Shop (page 358) sell a wide variety of leaflets on breastfeeding.

Breast pumps

A useful selection, including several of the electric and hand pumps listed below, is available from johnlewis.com.

Electric pumps

Ameda Egnell Ltd. (ameda.com)

Egnell Elite Breast Pump—This works by suction and by stimulating the nipple and areola. It is quiet, efficient, and has variable suction with a resting phase, and two sizes of funnel (for different shaped breasts). Its two cups mean you can pump both breasts at once; the extra stimulation this provides encourages let-downs and halves pumping time. In the UK you can rent the pump you used while you were in the hospital, or have one delivered to your home the next working day. It's also available for rent in the UK from many National Childbirth Trust branches.

Ameda Lactaline Personal-Dual Breast Pump—lets you pump both breasts at once.

Medela (medela.com)

Symphony—has "2-phase expression technology," which mimics a baby's sucking and milking rhythm. It pumps both breasts at the same time. You can buy or rent it, perhaps from a hospital that acts as an agent.

Lactina—can pump both breasts at the same time. Has single-phase expression. You can rent it from the company or from a hospital that acts as an agent.

Freestyle—has two-phase expression technology. One of the smallest pumps to pump both breasts at the same time.

Swing—has two-phase expression technology.

Mini Electric Pump—outlet- or battery-powered; useful when traveling.

Hand pumps

Avent (philips.co.uk)
Manual Comfort Pump—has an easy-to-use piston-action with a squeeze handle.

Ameda (ameda.com)
Ameda One-Handed Pump.

Ameda Lact-h Hand-Operated Pump.

Medela (medela.com)
Harmony—mimics a baby's sucking and nursing rhythm.

Freezer bags
Freezer storage bags for expressed breast milk are available from the NCT Shop (nctshop.co.uk).

Feeding cups
Feeding cups for pre-term and older breast-fed babies are available from the NCT Shop (nctshop.co.uk).

Nursing bras
The NCT Shop (nctshop.co.uk) has an excellent range of drop-cup and zip-cup nursing bras in a variety of sizes up to 46J.

Blooming Marvellous (bloomingmarvellous.co.uk) has a good range of attractive nursing bras with matching knickers.

Breast pads

Waterproof-backed
These are readily available from pharmacies.

Washable
Ameda Breast Pads—Machine-washable 100% cotton pads from Ameda (ameda.com) and the NCT Shop (nctshop.co.uk).

Lansinoh Washable Nursing Pads (lansinoh.com).

Cone-shaped
Lansinoh Contoured, Non-slip Breast Pads (lansinoh.com)

Boots cone-shaped pads—from Boots in the UK.

Philips (philips.co.uk)—also has a range of breast pads.

Medela (medela.com)—sells hydrogel pads.

Nipple cream
Lansinoh cream (lansinoh.com)—pesticide-free lanolin cream for sore nipples.

Breast shells
Various types are available from pharmacies and from medela.com and philips.co.uk.

Breast shields
These are available from medela.com.

Avent Niplettes
These are available from pharmacies, possibly by special order, or as "Niplettes" from philips.co.uk.

Supplementers

Lact-Aid Nursing Trainer System (lact-aid.com)
The advantages of this are that you control milk flow simply by altering the height of the bag; it's less bulky and quieter than the Medela SNS, it's discreet to use, and only the permanent parts need cleaning.

The disadvantages are that it's harder to assemble, you need to buy disposable bags and you need to move the tube from one breast to the other.

Medela Supplemental Nursing System (medela.com)

The big advantage of this is that it has two tubes, one for each breast.

The disadvantages are that it works by gravity, so milk flows from an unclamped tube even when a baby isn't actively suckling, which encourages ineffective feeding. Also, you need to clamp and unclamp the tubes to adjust the flow, or use thinner or thicker tubing. And you have to clean all its parts.

Spare tubing in three widths is available from expressyourselfmums.co.uk (search for "SNS").

Open-sided cribs and cots

A variety of cribs and cots suitable for putting against your bed are available on the Internet, including at nctshop.co.uk, johnlewis.com, and amazon.com.

Useful features include a side that drops completely and multiple height options that allowing the mattress to be level with your bed.

Valley cushion

Valley Cushions (valleycushions.co.uk)

This "ring-doughnut" cushion prevents pressure on a painful perineum while sitting down in the early days after childbirth.

Fertility prediction

OvuTest Fertile Focus Personal Saliva Fertility Prediction Microscope (craigmedical.com)—If relying on breastfeeding and the sympto-thermal method for contraception, this microscope-like gadget the size of a lipstick can help by revealing the fern-like pattern in your dried saliva that is present only during fertile days (from three or four days before ovulation to two to three days after).

First Response Ovulation Prediction Kit (firstresponse.com)—This can be a useful additional guide for breastfeeding women who are also using the sympto-thermal method of contraception. Available from pharmacies, it can be useful when periods have returned, for predicting when ovulation is likely to occur. This is because, when used toward the middle of the cycle, it indicates whether you are likely to ovulate by measuring hormone levels in urine. If ovulation is on its way, you can use additional contraception in your fertile time during the five days before ovulation and the three days after.

If your periods haven't yet returned, it's too expensive to use each day but can be useful as an additional guide if you've observed changes in bodily signs (e.g., vaginal mucus) which indicate that ovulation is near.

Fertility Awareness Kit—This contains an explanatory video, thermometer and charts. Details from plannedparenthood.org.

Organizations

US

La Leche League International (llli.org)—this organization has offered breastfeeding women high quality information, encouragement and support for many decades.

International Lactation Consultants Association (ilca.org)—the professional association for International Board Certified Lactation Consultants and other health care professionals who care for breastfeeding families. It publishes the quarterly Journal of Lactation.

UK

La Leche League of Great Britain (laleche.org.uk)
LLL has many leaders and groups. It provides a wide range of information, including books and many leaflets, plus details of products including baby slings.

Also, for the blind or visually handicapped, there are many publications in Braille, on cassette-tape or reel-to-reel. Ask for LLLI's special publications list.

For a price list, send a stamped self-addressed business-size envelope. For information in languages other than English, ask for the translation list (No. 508).

National Childbirth Trust (nct.org.uk)
The NCT Breastfeeding Promotion Group has many counselors and a range of information sources including books and leaflets. Its Experience Register lists women who have breast-fed in special situations and are willing to discuss these with other parents.

The NCT Shop, nctshop.co.uk, offers a range of books, nursing bras, underwear, night-wear, and various baby-care products.

Association of Breastfeeding Mothers (abm.me.uk)

This organization has local groups and counselors who offer information and support.

Australia

Australian Breastfeeding Association (breastfeeding.asn.au)

Index

E

F

Dr. Penny Stanway

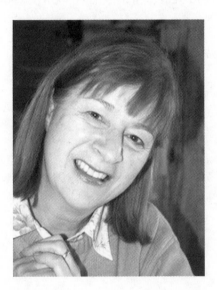

Penny Stanway worked both in general practice and as a senior medical officer in child health before becoming a health writer. Besides *The Breastfeeding Bible*, she has written more than 20 other health books, many on child health and nutrition, including *Good Food for Kids* and *Feeding Your Baby*, and most recently, a series of books on individual foods, including *The Miracle of Lemons*, *The Miracle of Cider Vinegar*, and *The Miracle of Garlic*.

She wrote *The Breastfeeding Bible* 35 years ago for two reasons. First, so pregnant women could easily access the up-to-date, accurate and unbiased information needed to make an informed decision on whether to breastfeed or formula-feed; and second, so breastfeeding women could benefit from the knowledge offered by decades of scientific research and from the practical experience of many hundreds of thousands of other women.

Since then she has updated and reedited this bestseller many times to ensure it remains the "breastfeeding bible" relied on by many women around the world. This edition is the sixth.

She is on the professional advisory board of La Leche League International and has taught mothers how to breastfeed and professionals how to help them do so successfully in many countries.

Penny's three children, now adults, were each breast-fed. Her elder daughter now has three children of her own—all of whom were breast-fed.